UPDATES ON BRUCELLOSIS

Edited by **Manal Mohammad Baddour**

Updates on Brucellosis
http://dx.doi.org/10.5772/59890
Edited by Manal Mohammad Baddour

Contributors

Pablo Yagupsky, Farhad Abbasi, Ricardo Alberto Gomez Flores, Ali Akbar Heydari, Suk Kim, Max Maurin, Ozlem Sahin, Mitra Ranjbar, Calvin Gomo, Julián Solís García Del Pozo, Javier Solera, Ana Cláudia Coelho, Juan Garcia-Díez, Adosinda Coelho, Marta Pérez-Sancho, Teresa García-Seco, Lucas Dominguez, Julio Alvarez, Ana Maria Cervan

Published by InTech

Janeza Trdine 9, 51000 Rijeka, Croatia

Publishing Process Manager Iva Lipovic

Technical Editor InTech DTP team

Cover InTech Design team

First published November, 2015

Printed in Croatia

Additional hard copies can be obtained from orders@intechopen.com

Updates on Brucellosis, Edited by Manal Mohammad Baddour

p. cm.

ISBN 978-953-51-2211-1

Meet the editor

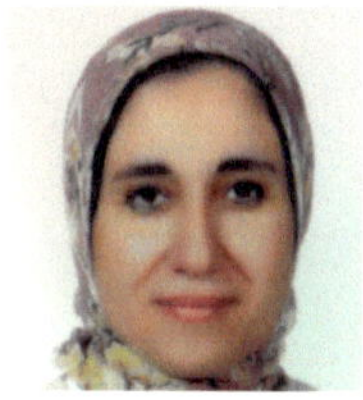

Manal Mohammad Baddour is a Professor of Medical Microbiology and Immunology, Faculty of Medicine, Alexandria University, Egypt. She serves as a Clinical Microbiologist and Microbiology Consultant in the Alexandria University Hospital as well as in several private sector hospitals. She has been the Principal Investigator or Coinvestigator of 18 research projects of various academic granting agencies. She has supervised 4 PhD and 13 master degree theses, and reviewed manuscripts for 18 international journals. Dr. Baddour has served as Editor and Associate Editor on the board of several international journals. She has published 32 microbiology articles mostly in renowned journals and has authored two internationally published books with an h-index of 9. She participates in many conferences and workshops related to microbiology and infection control.

Contents

Preface

Brucella spp., discovered by David Bruce in 1887, are Gram-negative, facultative intracellular coccobacilli that can multiply within phagocytes and have complex nutritional requirements. They can infect terrestrial and aquatic mammals. Currently, the genus includes 11 "species," each potentially containing several biovars of variable virulence: *B. melitensis* predominantly found in sheep and goats, *B. abortus* in cattle, *B. suis* in pigs and boars, *B. ovis* in sheep, *B. canis* in dogs, *B. neotomae* in desert wood rats *(Neotoma lepida)*, *B. microti* in the common vole *(Microtus arvalis)*, *B. ceti* in cetacean, *B. pinnipedialis* in pinnipediae, *B. papionis* in baboons, and *B. inopinata* isolated from human samples but of unknown animal reservoir.

Although named as species, recent DNA relatedness studies have shown there is only one species in the genus, *B. melitensis,* with multiple biovars.

Although each species of *Brucella* has a preferred host, all can infect a wide range of animals, including humans.

The common routes of infection in humans are the intestinal tract (ingestion of infected milk), mucous membranes (droplets), and skin (contact with infected tissues of animals).

B. melitensis, B. abortus, and *B. suis* strains cause abortion and infertility in their natural hosts – goats and sheep, cattle, and swine, respectively. Humans can also acquire a severe, debilitating febrile illness known as brucellosis, as a result of contact with infected animals or their products. *B. ovis* is a natural pathogen of sheep, where it primarily causes epididymitis and infertility in rams.

B. canis infection causes abortion and infertility in dogs. Although *B. ovis* and *B. canis* are important in animals, human infection with *B. canis* is rare, and human infection with *B. ovis* has not been reported so far. *B. neotomae,* a *Brucella* strain that infects only desert wood rats, is not known to be associated with clinical disease in any host species.

Human brucellosis, also termed Maltese fever, Bang's disease, undulant fever, or Mediterranean fever, remains a prevalent zoonosis worldwide, but higher incidences are currently observed in the Middle East, Russia, West Asia, Africa, and Latin America. However, imported cases are still observed in brucellosis-free countries because of frequent travels in endemic areas.

Brucella infection is one of the big imitators in infectious diseases and can mimic many other infectious and noninfectious diseases. Additionally, the course of the infection varies considerably from totally asymptomatic to a severe illness that is potentially fatal. Complications, chronic infections, and relapses are prone to occur particularly in patients with low immunity.

The infective dose is relatively low as 10 to 100 organisms are sufficient to cause the disease.

Contrary to other intracellular pathogens, *Brucella* species do not produce exotoxins, antiphagocytic capsules or thick cell walls, resistance forms, or fimbriae and do not show antigenic variation. The key aspect of the virulence of *Brucella* is thought to be due to their ability to avoid the killing mechanisms within macrophages. Granulomatous nodules that may develop into abscesses form in the lymphatic tissue, liver, spleen, bone marrow, and other parts of the reticuloendothelial system. The main histologic reaction in brucellosis consists of proliferation of mononuclear cells, exudation of fibrin, coagulation necrosis, and fibrosis.

Brucellae are hazardous in the laboratory. Most *Brucella* species are highly infectious in humans and are considered by the CDC to be biological agents needing Biosafety level III precautions. They are moderately sensitive to heat and acidity. They are killed in milk by pasteurization.

Diagnosis may be difficult and in many cases relies on serology because this fastidious organism can be difficult to cultivate even on selective media using prolonged incubation.

Sustaining a high index of suspicion is important particularly in high-risk individuals living in endemic areas, as early diagnosis and prompt therapy improve the outcome and prevent complications.

Since the global eradication of brucellosis will not be feasible in the near future, owing to socioeconomic and political factors, and since the evolution of an adequate human vaccine currently seems a utopia, there exists a need for optimal antibiotic treatment schedules based on well-designed clinical trials.

In animals, brucellosis can be considered as one of the most economically important zoonosis worldwide, resulting in clinical disease, abortion, neonatal losses, increased calving intervals, reduced fertility, decreased milk production, increased culling rates because of metritis, and the emergency slaughtering of infected animals, and also an impediment to free animal movement and trade.

Manal Mohammad Baddour
Professor of Microbiology and Immunology
Faculty of Medicine
Alexandria University
Egypt

Chapter 1

Risk Factors for *Brucella* spp. in Domestic and Wild Animals

Ana Cláudia Coelho, Juan García Díez and Adosinda Maria Coelho

Additional information is available at the end of the chapter

http://dx.doi.org/10.5772/61325

Abstract

Brucella spp. is the aetiological agent of brucellosis, a serious contagious disease that results in reproductive failure and that has profound public health significance because of its zoonotic characteristics. This disease also is responsible for a high economic impact associated with the application of prevention, surveillance and test-and-slaughter programmes in animals by national authorities. *Brucella* spp. infects a large variety of animals and their prevalence is variable worldwide, mainly associated with the presence or absence of control programmes and also with the vaccination of animals against brucellosis. To achieve the control and eradication of brucellosis, the identification of the risk factors of brucellosis that maintain the infection in animals and/or the environment is fundamental. Although several risks have been identified, the most important have been associated with the biology of the bacteria, animal management (age, sex, species or breed), herd management (herd/flock size, number of species, contact with wild animals or type of animal production), farm management (facilities, cleaning and disinfection or veterinary support) and farmers' knowledge about the disease. Thus, to benefit from proper risk identification of brucellosis, it is essential to put a cost-effective and efficient brucellosis control programme into place.

Keywords: Brucellosis, risk factors, animals, prevalence

1. Introduction

Brucellosis is a serious contagious disease that results in reproductive failure and has profound public health significance because of its zoonotic characteristics [1]. In animals, brucellosis can be considered as one of the most economically important zoonosis worldwide, resulting in clinical disease, abortion, neonatal losses, increased calving intervals, reduced fertility, decreased milk production, increased culling rates because of metritis and the emergency

INTECH
open science | open minds

slaughtering of infected animals and also an impediment to free animal movement and trade [2-4]. However, a high economic impact is associated with the human disease and also by the application of prevention, surveillance and test-and-slaughter programmes in animals by national authorities [4,5].

Brucella spp. infects a large variety of animals as described in Table 1. Classically, the genus *Brucella* includes six recognized species based on antigenic/biochemical characteristics and primary host species [6]. *Brucella abortus* (cattle), *Brucella melitensis* (sheep and goats), *Brucella suis* (swine, cattle, rodents, wild ungulates), *Brucella ovis* (sheep), *Brucella canis* (dogs) and *Brucella neotomae* (rodents). More recently, other species have been recognized such as *B. ceti* (cetaceans), *Brucella pinnipedialis* (seals), *Brucella microti* (voles) and *Brucella inopinata*. The last was isolated from a breast implant in a human with clinical signs of brucellosis [7].

Animals	*Brucella spp.* Hosts	Reference
Domestic/Farm animals	Alpacas, Cattle, Dogs, Goats, Horses, Llamas, Pigs, Sheep	[8,9,10-14]
Wild animals	Bears, Bison, Buffalo, Camelids, Caribou, Deer, Elk, Ferrets, Foxes, Rabbits, Rodents, Wolves	[15,16,17-22]
Birds	Partridges, Quails	[23,24]
Marine mammals	Dolphins, Dugongs, Manatees, Otters, Sea porpoise	[15,23-29]

Table 1. Hosts of *Brucella* spp. among the literature

The epidemiology of brucellosis is variable worldwide. In developed countries, brucellosis has been eradicated or presents low individual prevalence due to control programmes and vaccination of animals [30,31]. Currently, the brucellosis status of a country is based on the epidemiology in domestic animals. However, to consider a country free of brucellosis, it may also include epidemiological data regarding brucellosis in both wild animals and in marine animals [15,25].

According to the data available at the World Organisation for Animal Health (OIE) (2009), brucellosis (including *B. abortus* and *B. melitensis*) was not reported in several countries such as the USA, Australia and several European countries. Among the latter, Mediterranean countries such as Spain, Portugal, Italy and Greece are not brucellosis free today [32-35]. On the other hand, the picture of the prevalence of brucellosis has changed in South America, Africa, Middle East and Asia, where brucellosis is endemic because control programmes are insufficient or they basically do not have a great impact in animal and human health [5,26]. Since official data about prevalence of brucellosis in these countries is scarce, reports carried out in these areas show a large variability in the prevalence (Table 2).

The aim of brucellosis control is both to decrease the impact on human health and avoid economic consequences through reducing exposure to *Brucella* spp. and increase resistance to the infection among animal populations. To achieve this objective, several measures such as test-and-slaughter programmes and/or biosecurity measures (hygiene, control of animal movements, vaccination or reproductive management, etc.) should be performed [30].

However, to achieve success against brucellosis, the elaboration of control and eradication programmes must first identify all the potential risks that maintain the infection in animals and/or the environment.

Species	Country	Individual prevalence	Lab method	Reference
Cattle	Brazil	2.9%	RBT+2ME	[43]
	Libya	42%	RBT	[44]
	Bangladesh	2.66%	RBT + I-ELISA	[45]
	Nigeria	24.0%	RBT+ELISA	[46]
	India	5,00%	RBT + ELISA	[47]
	Uganda	14%	RBT	[48]
	Uganda	5%	ELISA	[49]
Sheep	Libya	24%	RBT	[44]
	Bangladesh	2.31%	RBT + I-ELISA	[45]
	Nigeria	14.5%	RBT + SAT	[49]
	Kyrgyzstan	8.9%	RBT	[50]
Goat	Libya	31%	RBT	[44]
	Bangladesh	3.15%	RBT + I-ELISA	[45]
	Uganda	17%	RBT	[48]
	Nigeria	16.1%	RBT+SAT	[49]
	Kyrgyzstan	2.5%	RBT	[50]
Horses	Iran	2.5%	RBT	[51]
	Nigeria	14.7%	RBT	[52]
	Pakistan	20.7%	RBT	[53]
Dog	Iran	4.90%	IA	[54]
	Argentina	14.7%	RBT	[55]
	Nigeria	5.46%	RBT	[56]
	Nigeria	28.6%	RBT	[57]
	Iran	10.62%	IA	[58]
Swine	Croatia	1%	RBT	[11]
Coyote	USA	18%	Card test	[59]
Camels	Egypt	5.7%	RBT	[18]
Wild boars	Switzerland	1.5%	RBT	[60]
	USA	23.4%	CT+STT+RT+CFT	[61]
Marine mammals	USA	0.03%	C-ELISA	[62]
	USA	38%	RBT+CFT+ELISA	[63]

IA: Immunochromatography assay; RT: rivanol test; C-ELISA: competitive ELISA; CT: card test; STT: standard tube test; LAB method: laboratory method for brucellosis diagnostic; ELISA: Enzyme-Linked Immunosorbent Assay; RBT: Rose Bengal Test; 2ME: 2-mercaptoetanol test; CFT: Complement Fixation Test; I-ELISA: indirect ELISA; SAT: serum agglutination test

Table 2. Seroprevalence of brucellosis among the different species

Identification of risk factors of brucellosis has been reported in epidemiological studies [36-41]. Although several risks have been identified, the most important are related to farm management, animal management and knowledge about the disease [42]. Thus, to benefit from proper risk identification of brucellosis, it is essential to put a cost-effective and efficient brucellosis control programme into place.

2. Risk factors of brucellosis in animals

The risk factors can be categorized into those associated with characteristics of animal populations, management and the parasite biology.

2.1. Risk factors associated with the biology of *Brucella* spp.

Brucella abortus is the aetiological agent of bovine brucellosis and responsible for an economically important cause of abortions in cattle [31]. *B. abortus* also affects other species such as bison, buffalo or elks representing an important risk for the maintenance of the agent in the animal population with special importance in areas where wildlife and cattle rearing occur together [15]. Moreover, infections in wildlife can hinder eradication efforts in cattle. *B. abortus* is still a human pathogen and outbreaks associated from infected cattle and also from ingesting contaminated dairy products represent an important risk of infection [4].

Brucella melitensis can affect most domestic animals, but dairy sheep and goats are especially susceptible. Sheep have different receptivity according to breed, while in goats this association has not been reported [64]. *B. melitensis* is the main etiological agent of brucellosis in small ruminants, although sheep can be also infected by *B. ovis*. Sporadic cases of brucellosis have been described in sheep and goats as *B. abortus* and *B. suis* [65,66]. The dogs that guard the herds and flocks can also be infected [67].

Dogs, cats and other wild carnivores such as foxes or wolves present an important role in the epidemiology of brucellosis, because they act as mechanical disseminators due to the transportation of infected foetuses or placentas from abortions in infected herds and flocks. Since pigs are susceptible to infection by *B. melitensis*, pig farms present some epidemiological importance where both species are reared [68]. In addition, wild ruminants with potential contact with infected sheep and/or goats could be infected with *B. melitensis*, maintaining the infection in natural environment [15].

Porcine brucellosis is caused by *Brucella suis* biovars 1, 2 or 3. The disease caused by biovars 1 and 3 is similar, while that caused by biovar 2 differs from 1 and 3 in its host range, its limited geographical distribution and its pathology [66]. In domestic pigs, risk factors associated with infection are ingestion of aborted foetuses, foetal membranes, abortion products and uterine discharges, or contaminated foodstuffs. Transmission during copulation is very common [66, 69,70]. Artificial insemination with contaminated semen or conjunctival mucosal should also be considered a risk [66,71].

The infection of a pig herd by brucellosis could be associated with the purchase/entrance of infected animals, contact with wildlife reservoirs, use of contaminated semen or feed [72] or the use of a lend boar. Other risk factors could be attributed to transmission of the disease by mechanical vectors due to contamination of vehicles, holding equipment or utensils and also to the introduction of infected offal (e.g. placenta and afterbirths) [70]. Serological screening and purchase from brucellosis-free herds should reduce this risk [70].

The likelihood of the introduction of the infection from potentially infected wild boar, free-range pigs or hares and its establishment in outdoor and backyard pig populations depends on housing management such as the type of housing (outdoor vs indoor), low levels of biosecurity, direct or indirect contact with infected wild boar, free-ranging pigs or hares, feeding practices (*i.e.* home prepared food vs commercial food), purchasing animals or semen without testing, no testing of live pigs, husbandry systems, lack of detection of unapparent infections, contamination of semen collection centres and equipment, contamination of transport vehicles, transport of pigs from different holdings or mixing of pigs [70].

2.2. Risk factors associated with the host

2.2.1. Age

Age has been referred to as one of the intrinsic factors associated with brucellosis. Higher seroprevalence of brucellosis has been observed in older animals, both in cattle and small ruminants with a prevalence odds ratio (POR) of about 2.0 in cattle over 5 years old and a POR of about 1.7 in small ruminants over 2 years old [43,73-77]. Similar results have been observed in wild boars and camels [78,79]. Brucellosis has traditionally been considered a disease of adult animals since susceptibility increases after sexual maturity and pregnancy [80]. However, variations in the age of sexual maturity among breeds could present differences between age and brucellosis positivity [81]. *Brucella spp.* presented a tropism to the reproductive tract due to the production of erythritol, a 4-carbon sugar produced in the foetal tissues of ruminants that stimulates the growth of *Brucella* [82]. Thus, it may also explain the higher prevalence in adult animals than in young [83]. On the other hand, a higher prevalence of brucellosis in adults has also been associated with longer contact with infected animals or with the environment. This potential risk may be significant in those herds without culling of positive animals [84]. It must be kept in mind though that this low prevalence might be faulty because young animals can be infected without clinical symptoms presenting serologic response for only one week [83,84].

2.2.2. Sex

The influence of sex in the prevalence of brucellosis has been studied in cattle, small ruminants and wild animals [74,77,79,80,84]. Female ruminants presented a higher odds of brucellosis infection, the same has been observed in female dogs compared to male dogs [85]. Although this is difficult to explain, it could be associated with the intrinsic biology of the microorganisms and its tropism to the foetal tissues as previously described. Since brucellosis infection in males presented clinical signs such as epididymitis and orchitis, the prevalence in males could be lower than females because they may be culled faster [86]. On the other hand, the absence of clinical signs such as abortion or metritis in non-pregnant infected females or the absence of farmers' observation/identification of abortions in extensive herds may also explain the higher prevalence in females. In addition, in non-pregnant females, brucellosis becomes chronic. This fact has important epidemiological implications since, after an initial immune response, animals may be asymptomatic carriers, the antibodies disappear from circulation and are difficult to detect with traditional serological techniques [87]. Since brucellosis in pigs may affect both males and females equally, sex susceptibility has not been fully demonstrated [72]. Regarding wild boars, the behavior of females living in matriarchal groups could explain the higher prevalence [79].

2.2.3. Species and breed

The prevalence of brucellosis is variable among species and region as described in Table 2. However, prevalence in farm animals seems to be lower in small ruminants than large ruminants [44,84] and lower in sheep than in goats [45,88,89]. Transmission of brucellosis occurs in ruminants through the excretion of contaminated materials from the female genital tract, which constitutes the main form of transmission to other animals and humans. In most of the circumstances, the main route of spread is the placenta, foetal fluids and vaginal discharges expelled after delivery or abortion. At that time, large numbers of *Brucella* are released [90]. The vaginal excretion of *Brucella* spp. in goats is greater and more prolonged than sheep, lasting for 2-3 months. In sheep, it is generally lower and normally ceases within 3 weeks after birth or abortion. It is also common that excretion occurs through milk or semen [91]. The excretion of *Brucella* in milk is generally intermittent and usually only appears 6 to 12 days after the abortion. In goats, the excretion is more abundant and more prolonged, so there is an increased risk of infection via the consumption of milk from this species [92,93].

The phenomenon of latent brucellosis in sheep was observed in lambs born from infected mothers that breast-feed with milk contaminated with *Brucella.* These lambs are seronegative to adulthood, while in females, the latency of brucellosis is maintained until the first pregnancy, a period in which the disease process develops [94].

Infected females thus present a high number of abortions with special importance in primiparous females [87].

In game animals, seroprevalence in wild boars seems to be higher than wild ruminants [8,95-98]. To the best of our knowledge, there is no evidence of higher susceptibility to brucellosis within specific species. In the case of horses, they have usually been considered more resistant to brucellosis than ruminants [51], but the variation of prevalence reported in endemic areas of brucellosis [99,100] seems to be discussible. The information available about differences of brucellosis infection by species is scarce. In sheep, pregnant dams do not present *Brucella* spp. in vaginal discharges, contrary to that observed in goats [101], where excretion may extend over two or three months [102]. Thus, the higher prevalence in specific species could be achievable through the intrinsic characteristics of the etiological agent [103].

Regarding the breed, a higher prevalence of brucellosis has been reported [104] in cross-breed cattle than local breeds, although other reports indicated no statistical differences among cattle breeds [46,105]. In small ruminants, Maltese and South American sheep breeds seem to present a greater resistance to brucellosis compared to the sheep breeds of Southwest Asia and the Mediterranean, such as the Awassi breed [13,106,107]. Although Husky and Chihuahua dog breeds appeared to be more prone to *Brucella* infection than other breeds, their infection seems most likely influenced by other factors such as the local dog population or owners than by dog breed [107]. In swine, some breeds such as Duroc and Jersey Red crosses may be less susceptible to experimental challenge with *B. suis*, suggesting some genetic resistance [108]. Previous studies showed that stray dogs demonstrated a greater than three-fold rate of infection versus non-stray dogs [109].

Keypoint: Risk factors associated with *Brucella* spp. and the host

Brucella abortus is the aetiological agent of bovine brucellosis in cattle although also infects other species such as bison, buffalo or elks. It represents an important risk to the maintenance of the agent in the animal population with special importance in areas where wildlife and cattle commingled. *B. melitensis* is the main etiological agent of brucellosis in small ruminants, although sheep can be also infected by *B. ovis*. Sporadic cases of brucellosis have been described in sheep and goats as *B. abortus* and *B. suis*. Porcine brucellosis is caused by *Brucella suis* biovars 1, 2 or 3. The disease caused by biovars 1 and 3 is similar, while that caused by biovar 2 differs from 1 and 3 in its host range, its limited geographical distribution and its pathology.

Several risk factors of brucellosis have been associated with the host such as age, sex, species or breed. Regarding age, higher seroprevalence of brucellosis is observed in older animals since susceptibility increases after sexual maturity and pregnancy. It could be associated with the tropism of *Brucella* spp. to erythritol, a 4-carbon sugar produced in the foetal tissues of ruminants that stimulates the growth of *Brucella*. This fact may explain the higher prevalence in adult animals than in young ones. With regard to sex, the odds of infection by brucellosis in ruminants are higher in female than male probably associated with the tropism to the foetal tissues as previously described. Species and breed have also been described as risk factors. In farm animals, the prevalence seems to be lower in small ruminants than large ruminants and lower in sheep than in goats. In this last case, the vaginal excretion of *Brucella* spp. in goats is greater and more prolonged than sheep, lasting for 2-3 months whereas excretion in sheep is generally lower and normally ceases within 3 weeks after birth or abortion. Regarding the breed, there is not consensus among the studies. Thus, some of them reported higher prevalence of brucellosis in cross-breed cattle than local breeds. In small ruminant, Maltese and South American sheep breeds seem to present a greater resistance to brucellosis compared to the sheep breeds of Southwest Asia and the Mediterranean, such as the Awassi breed.

2.3. Risk factors associated with herds

2.3.1. Herd/flock size

An important risk factor for brucellosis seropositivity is herd size, being higher in large herds and/or flocks. An increased odds ratio for seropositivity has been largely reported in cattle

[82,84,104,110] as well as in small ruminants [77,86,111]. In contrast, no statistical differences among goat flocks were observed in the literature [112,113].

The higher prevalence of brucellosis in large herds and/or flocks has been associated with several factors, such as a higher number of animals tested in larger herds means the probability of detecting at least one seropositive animal is greater [77] or the higher number of animals increases the likelihood of transmission of the disease by contact among them [114]. The low prevalence of brucellosis in small-sized herds could also be associated with the herd and/or farm management [86]. Thus, small-sized flocks usually graze at pastures near or contiguous to the farm, avoiding contact with other flocks or utilization of common paths and/or roads. Because premises for small herds or flocks are smaller, cleaning, disinfection and manure removal procedures are easier and less time consuming to the farmer. Disinfection is also facilitated by the low resistance of *Brucella* spp. to most disinfectant agents [115] and by the low cost of this operation. Farmers of small-sized herds may easily control the partum period and usually keep dams away from the flock during parturition. This measure is very important in case of abortions, to avoid pasture contamination. In these small sized herds, replacement is usually made by reposition and economic trade is not frequent. Thus, the absence of an elevated rate of animal movement decreases the likelihood of infection.

The health status of a flock may influence the predisposition to brucellosis infection. Thus, in small-sized herds, farmers can easily identify sick animals and veterinary and preventive treatments are usually carried out at low financial cost. Regarding the official control of brucellosis by the official veterinary authority, small-sized flocks are easily controlled and in the case of a positive finding, most farmers agree to cull the whole flock to maintain the brucellosis-free status and also to avoid a zoonotic infection [116,117]. In addition, the vaccination coverage of young animals with RB-51 or Rev-1 is more easily achievable in these herds.

On the other hand, the higher prevalence of brucellosis observed in large flocks may be also associated with the utilization of communal pasture areas, utilization of common paths and/or roads and due to contact with others flocks [114]. Cleaning and disinfection procedures of premises and manure removal in large-sized flocks is more difficult than in medium or small flocks because it requires the availability of mechanical equipment and consequently a higher financial cost. An increased prevalence of brucellosis associated with decreased of proper manure removal, cleaning and disinfection procedures has been described [118]. The control of reproductive management is difficult in large flocks, where parturitions on grazing areas are frequent and abortions are a source of pasture contamination. In addition, animal movement in large herds is frequent, both for replacement and/or trade, thereby increasing the risk of infection by brucellosis. Due to the higher cost of veterinary treatments and/or application of preventive programmes, animals in large flocks may be more susceptible to brucellosis infection. Moreover, associated with high numbers of animals unvaccinated and/or non-blood sampled animals may occur and remained unprotected and susceptible in case of infection. In addition, these animals act as a source of brucellosis contamination to the rest of the herds [74,118] and in the case of positive animals, farmers hesitate to slaughter the entire flock.

In dogs, the risk of transmission increases in kennel environments due to the high interaction among the animals and reduced space, which infected dogs share with other healthy ones to play, defecate or urinate [119]. Kennels with a history of abortion are 13 times more likely to be seropositive than kennels without this record [120].

Transmission studies have demonstrated that the exposure of healthy dogs to abortion products is an easy way for *B. canis* transmission [119]. The aborting bitch presents a high risk for the spread of infection to healthy dogs. *B. canis* is also found in the milk of infected lactating bitches, which might lead to the potential infection of nursing pups [121]. The high POR of seropositivity in kennels with a history of abortions could be associated with the presence of *Brucella* over long periods of time, caused by the absence of good reproductive practices and exposure to body fluids in the environment [120].

2.3.2. *Number of species*

Farming several species in the same herd has been described as a risk factor [78,80,84], although there is no evidence of higher susceptibility of brucellosis in specific species. Thus, an increase in prevalence where several species intermingle is difficult to explain but could be associated with higher chances of being *Brucella* seropositive because of multiple sources of infection.

It has been suggested that brucellosis is transmitted only rarely from sheep and goats to cattle, or among cattle [88]. However, the higher risk for cattle on farms which also had sheep or goats suggests that some of the cattle infections may have originated from small ruminants since *B. melitensis* biovar 3 was isolated from cow's milk.

Because *B. melitensis* is considered the most virulent of *Brucella,* it may explain the increased POR in cattle rearing with small ruminants [103]. In addition, the susceptibility of all ruminants to infection by *B. abortus* may explain the higher prevalence of brucellosis in cattle herds in contact with buffaloes or wild ruminants [37,122]. Horses seem to be resistant to brucellosis, although the risk of infection increases when they intermingle with cattle [46].

In regions where *B. melitensis* has been confirmed in sheep and goats, cattle can become infected with this bacterium [74]. It has not yet been determined whether *B. melitensis* can be kept alone in a population of cattle in the absence of small ruminants. *B. melitensis* causes abortion in cattle similarly to *B. abortus.*

As previously described, horses present a certain resistance against brucellosis, however, seropositivity has been associated with horses in areas without brucellosis control programmes for large and small ruminants. In addition, *B. suis* infection in horses has been reported in those commingling with swine [123].

The presence of swine could be a risk for brucellosis transmission to cattle [123] and is a public health concern. However, recent studies showed that cattle intermingling with pigs in the same area do not seem to be infected by *Brucella* spp. and do not contribute to its maintenance [125]. In contrast, the risk of cattle infection by *B. suis* from wild boar has been recently described [126].

The practice of mixing cattle, either through grazing or sharing watering points, is a significant risk factor for brucellosis [104,127,128]. Community pastures should be treated as livestock unit and control measures must be applied to all animals [129].

Other researchers [84] found that the disease is easily transmitted in areas where extensive production systems predominate, based on grazing and the high mobility of herds, the mixture of species in the same herd and where sharing pastures, roads and water sources occurs. Mobility increases the likelihood of contact with other potentially infected herds or wild animals that are reservoirs of disease.

The presence of dogs has been described as a risk for brucellosis infection in farm animals [125] and represents a potential epidemiological threat in endemic and/or brucellosis areas without brucellosis control programmes. However, dogs are a potential risk in the diffusion of brucellosis, acting as mechanical disseminators by feeding on aborted foetuses, dragging them along and spreading the bacteria [107].

Canine brucellosis is usually caused by *B. canis*, although infection by *B. abortus*, *B. suis* and *B. melitensis* have been reported [129]. Previous studies showed that dogs have been identified as a link in the brucellosis transmission chain. *B. abortus* and *B. melitensis* can be transmitted from cattle to farm dogs playing the role as vector. *Brucella* can produce disease in dogs via ingestion of infected reproductive tissues [9]. Infected dogs with *B. abortus* can spread organisms into the environment through urine, vaginal secretions, aborted foetuses or faeces. If a pregnant dog is infected with *B. abortus*, it may abort, and the tissues and vaginal discharges have a great potential for transmitting *Brucella* to susceptible cattle [9,129]. Dogs can also be infected with *B. suis* via ingesting aborted swine foetuses [71]. Thus, the elimination of infected cattle may not necessarily eradicate the disease [9].

2.4. Risk factors associated with farm management and environment

Several risk factors of brucellosis associated with farm management and environment have been referred to in the literature as presented in Table 3.

Regarding the main seroprevalence, dairy animals have a much greater chance of not only contracting brucellosis but also of spreading it faster than beef animals. The reason is not a genetic or physiological factor but due to husbandry. Animals that live in concentrated smaller areas come into close contact when they are grazing and when they are milked [129]. The zoonotic transmission of brucellosis by improper milking procedures was observed [128] associated with skin lesions in hands. Thus, transmission through skin lesions of the udder is not a neglectable source of infection. In addition, it is considered that dairy animals are subjected to more stress conditions on farms, leading to a higher susceptibility to brucellosis infection [135]. The persistence of the infection of the udder and supramammary lymph nodes leads to a constant or intermittent excretion in milk in successive lactations. This fact constitutes an important source of infection for humans and for the young animals [136].

Animal purchase has been considered as a risk for brucellosis. Purchasing in larger herds has usually been associated with more animal movements on and off the farm, and this practice

Factors described	Reference
Absence of calving paddock	[14,43]
Age	[75,77]
Breed	[39,77]
Cleaning and disinfection	[40,112,114,130]
Climatology	[79]
Commingling with other animals	[14,88,114,131]
Communal pastures	[36,43,112,130]
Contact with wildlife	[36,74,104]
Education	[40,42,80]
Handling of aborted material	[43,80]
Intensive management	[104,132,133]
Herd size	[36,40,75,77,88]
Lending males	[112]
Main animal production (beef /dairy)	[76]
Milking procedures	[80]
Purchase/entrance of new animals	[39,112]
Sex	[77]
Specie	[114]
Stocking rate	[14,77,125]
Transhumance	[104]
Veterinary services	[43,104,112,117,131]
Water sources	[40,125,130]
Handling of aborted material	[43,80,134]

Table 3. Risk factors of brucellosis infection in animals

increases the risk of introducing an infected animal into a herd [81]. Introduction of animals from market fairs also presents a higher risk of infection. The majority of infections or reinfection in disease-free herds starts through buying infected animals of unknown status [128]. This has a higher importance in those endemic areas or countries where there is an absence of control programmes. However, in countries with test-and-slaughter control programmes, the movement of cattle are subjected to a compulsory pre-movement test that consists in the serological brucellosis diagnostics before an animal leaves the farm [42]. Moreover, animal movement restriction measures are applied in brucellosis positive herds to avoid spreading the disease [34].

The proximity to other infected herds or flocks has also been described an infection risk, although, small ruminant contact with other flocks was reported to have no impact on *Brucella* seropositivity in Spain [137].

The influence of the agro-ecological zone has been also referred to as a brucellosis risk factor, having a higher prevalence in dry zones [132]. Since pasture areas are scarce in dry zones, animals must seek pastures over large areas implying an unrestricted animal-to-animal contact with potential transmission as previously described. In addition, transmission due to aerosol inhalation of contaminated dust from foetal discharges or abortions is possible [138]. In contrast, a lower prevalence of brucellosis in these areas has been proposed by other authors [139] due to lower survival of *Brucella* spp. in aborted material in dry-zones.

Larger herds might be expected to be associated with intensive management practices that are typically more difficult to control and allow for closer contact between animals and their environment, which increases the potential for exposure to infectious excretions [130]. In addition, the stressful conditions of animals subjected to intensive production may make them more susceptible to the infection, as previously described. On the other hand, extensive management may also imply a risk of brucellosis and higher prevalence has been reported in small ruminants. Although difficult to explain, it could be associated with controlling abortions, observation of sick animals or contact with animals, among others [86]. Since extensive management implies rearing a large number of animals in large areas and/or sharing communal pastures, the contamination of pastures with placentas or abortions is a source of infection to other animals in the herds, as we described previously in the risk factors of brucellosis by the herd size.

Animal handling and environmental conditions are risk factors which influence the transmission of infection, such as births and breeding in semi-dark settings, confinement in closed spaces and high animal densities [130]. Another risk of intensive systems could be associated with airborne dust transmission indoors [138].

The season also has an impact on herd management and animal nutrition, mainly in production systems involving transhumance or nomadic practices [114]. Rainfall affects the development and the nutritional state of the pasture. These factors influence the reproduction of animals kept in extensive systems and thus the time of delivery/miscarriages. In intensive systems, isolation of post-parturient animals in maternity facilities reduces the spread of infection to the rest of the herd or flock [128].

Cleaning and disinfection of farm facilities and proper manure removal have been described as a protective factor against brucellosis infection [114,118,130]. This fact is associated with the low resistance of *Brucella* spp. to most disinfectant agents [115] although their effectiveness is based on the previous elimination of organic material since it decreases the bactericidal effect of the disinfectant [140]. A similar risk of brucellosis was reported in kennels [119,120]. Kennels with improper management of excrement and built with materials such as tile, wood and earthern floors were considered to have a higher risk for infection since they maintain exposure to urine, faeces, or reproductive secretions [120].

Insect rodents on dogs could act as a mechanical vector of brucellosis. Blood-sucking insects have been reported as disseminators of brucellosis. *Brucella* was isolated from the stomach contents of *Stomoxys calcitrans, Ornithodoros* and *Musca autumnalis* (stable fly). The stable fly is dipterous in contact with ruminants. The female lays eggs in the faeces of these animals and feeds on their blood, tears and placental secretions. It is thought that these insects and ticks contribute to disease transmission [92,138]. As mentioned earlier, dogs intermingling with large and small ruminants in farms have presented an important role in the epidemiology of brucellosis. However, stray dogs which remain free on the streets and travel long distances also act as disseminators of the agent and provide chances for infection of other animals and humans through environmental contamination [141].

Environmental factors that affect the ability of *Brucella* to survive outside mammalian hosts need to be considered in the epidemiology of brucellosis. High humidity, low temperatures and absence of direct sun light may favour the survival of *Brucella* for several months in water, aborted foetuses, placental membranes, liquid manure, hay, buildings, equipment and clothes [129].

The survival of *Brucella* outside a mammalian host is relatively persistent compared to other non-sporulating pathogenic bacteria in similar circumstances [142]. Favourable conditions are pH>4, low temperatures, absence of direct sunlight and high humidity. *Brucella* can persist for several months in water, aborted placentas, faeces, manure, wool, facilities, equipment and clothes [143]. *Brucella* can survive for 40 days in dry soil and 60 days in moist soils, 144 days at 20 °C and 40% relative humidity, for several months in drinking water at 4 °C to 8 °C and two and a half years at 0 °C, 30 days in urine, 75 days in aborted foetuses, more than 200 days in uterine secretions and several years in frozen tissues or culture media. *Brucella* resistance to different environmental conditions increases in the presence of abundant organic matter. The spread of the disease via waterways is not frequent and can only be effective over short distances [129].

2.5. Other factors associated with brucellosis

The role of farmers' knowledge about brucellosis has been discussed in the literature. It was noted that knowledge ages equal to or older than 55 years was a protective factor for brucellosis prevention [40,42]. This observation is difficult to explain and may be due to younger farmers' lack of experience. Older farmers have more familiarity with recognizing the clinical signs of the disease or the main route of transmission and can be more aware of the importance of preventive measures [67,144,145]. Farmers who had previously experienced brucellosis in their herds had a higher probability of having greater knowledge of bovine brucellosis, which is consistent with having experience with the disease. Producer's associations, education and veterinary support have been recognized as protective factors [42,118]. Farmer's lack of awareness about brucellosis, improper handling of aborted materials and the habit of consuming raw milk, among other factors, might contribute to further spread of brucellosis in their livestock and expose the community to a public health hazard [80].

Keypoint - Risk factors associated with farm management and environment

The risk factors of brucellosis associated with the herd are size and the number of animal species. The higher prevalence of brucellosis in large herds could be explained by the higher odds of detecting at least one seropositive animal, the increase of the transmission of the disease by contact among them, utilization of communal pasture areas or improper cleaning and disinfection procedures in large farms. Farming several species in the same herd has been described as a risk of infection due to multiple sources of infection. Thus, presence of dogs in large herds may spread *Brucella* spp. by both mechanical carriers or by the spread of the organisms into the environment through urine, vaginal secretions, aborted foetuses or faeces.

Dairy animals have a much greater chance of not only contracting brucellosis but also of spreading it faster than beef animals. Because animals that live in concentrated smaller areas come into close contact when they are grazing and when they are milked. In addition, it is considered that dairy animals (intensive production) are subjected to more stress conditions on farms, leading to a higher susceptibility to brucellosis infection. Purchasing in larger herds has usually been associated with more animal movements on and off the farm, and this practice increases the risk of introducing an infected animal of unknown status with special importance in areas with absence of control programmes.

Also the influence of the agro-ecological zone has been also referred as a brucellosis risk factor. High humidity, low temperatures and absence of direct sun light may favour the survival of *Brucella* for several months in the environment. In addition, cleaning and disinfection of farm facilities and proper manure removal have been described as a protective factor against brucellosis infection. This fact could be explained to the low resistance of *Brucella* spp. to the disinfectant agents.

2.6. Brucellosis in wild animals — A threat to farm animals

Brucella abortus and *B. suis* have been isolated worldwide from a great variety of wildlife species [15]. Some general risk factors, which can be identified in most of the wildlife diseases are wildlife overabundance, movements of wild and domestic animals and fomites [146]. Artificial management of wild species, including fencing, feeding and translocation, can also increase the risk of transmission of infectious brucellosis. [147] The risk of infection increases dramatically with increasing wildlife density and their exposure to *Bucella abortus* around feeding grounds [148]. Wild ruminants have been suggested as brucellosis carriers, but they are probably not true reservoirs [146,148]. Other works showed that wild ruminants do not play a relevant role in the maintenance of *B. abortus* and *B. melitensis* infections since limited cases of brucellosis have been reported in wild ruminants [79,149,150]. Only weak evidence for a direct relationship between brucellosis and size/density of the population of wild animals has been reported [151]. However, a potential risk for brucellosis infection of livestock by wild animals could be associated when artificial management such as winter feeding increases aggregation [146,151]. Thus, wild animals are often at risk as a consequence of contact with infected livestock, particularly in extensive breeding systems [79].

With regards to elk and bison, artificial feeding management during winter results in significant congregations in the feeding grounds and increases the risk of elk being exposed to *B.*

abortus [15]. A possible risk factor for bison in the USA is environmental contamination by the RB51 vaccine strain, which is a rifampicin resistant strain released in the environment [15].

Rangiferine brucellosis (brucellosis in reindeer and caribou) is caused by *B. suis* biovar 4 in the Arctic regions of Siberia, Canada and Alaska, constituting a serious zoonosis. *B. suis* may also infect moose (*Alces alces*) and occasionally various carnivores [15]. In European wild boar *B. suis* biovar 2 was observed in all age categories [152,153].

2.7. Brucellosis in marine mammals — New threat?

Brucella was detected in free-ranging pinnipeds and cetaceans from America, Europe, Japan, New Zealand, the Solomon Islands and the Antarctic, as well as in captive bottlenose dolphin (*Tursiops truncates)* [154-157].

Brucella ceti and *B. pinnipedialis* prefer cetaceans and seal hosts respectively [157, 158]. Epidemiological studies of risk factors for *Brucella* infection in cetaceans and pinnipeds have not yet been performed, and the role of environmental factors in the emergence of marine mammal brucellosis is still unknown [157]. It seems unlikely that *B. ceti* could survive for long periods outside marine mammals.

The transmission of brucellosis in marine mammals is not totally understood [158]. The dilution of the agent in sea water may make transmission difficult due to a low infecting dose. It is likely that the mode of transmission is through close contact between hosts, such as sexual intercourse or maternal feeding, contact with aborted foetuses and placental tissues or through fish or helminth reservoirs [159]. A second alternative corresponds to vertical transmission from mother to foetus, which is feasible since foetuses and placenta from infected animals have been found to contain large quantities of *Brucella* [156]. In addition, the behaviour of assisting the births observed in several cetaceans could be a risk due to the close contact with foetal tissues and discharges [27]. This hypothesis should be considered since *B. ceti* have been found in aborted foetuses and the reproductive organs of captive bottlenose dolphins [156] and in the uterus of a stranded striped dolphin with placentitis [160]. *B. ceti* has been also associated with mastitis and endometritis in cetaceans [161]. Both *B. ceti* and *B. pinnipedialis* have also been isolated from the testes, uterus and mammary glands of cetaceans and pinnipeds without any apparent pathology [162-164]. A potential risk factor could be the infection through ingestion of *Brucella* contaminated fish or helminth vectors [165]. *B. ceti* and *B. pinnipedialis* have been isolated from lungworms (*Pseudalius inflexus*) in the lungs of cetaceans and pinnipeds and these parasites can be a reservoir and vector for *Brucella* in these animals [165].

2.8. Animal brucellosis and zoonotic risk

In endemic regions without brucellosis eradication programmes, zoonotic risk still represents an important public health threat [166]. Infection happens due to contact with infected animals or consumption of their products, mostly unpasteurized milk and milk products of sheep and goats [167]. It presents special importance in those regions where trading of raw milk and raw milk products is a common practice among farmers [168]. The survival of *Brucella* in milk and dairy products is related with curing methods, humidity, temperature and/or changes in pH.

For milk, *Brucella* survival is inversely proportional to the pH [169]. *Brucella* can be responsible for milk-borne diseases, particularly since the appearance and taste of the milk are rarely affected by the presence of the bacteria [170]. Boiling or heating of milk at 80–85 ºC [176–185 ºF] for several minutes [approximately 10 minutes] will destroy the bacteria [30]. Bacteria cannot survive if the cheese is cured longer than 3 months [171]. In acidified soft cheeses and dry cheese, their survival is greater. Thus, European legislation requires that all cheeses made from raw milk be submitted to a cure period of not less than 60 days [172]. Survival time in meat is lower, except in frozen meat where the microorganism can survive for several years [173].

Although zoonotic brucellosis is mainly associated with farmers in high prevalence areas, even in low prevalence countries brucellosis represents an important threat as a work-acquired infection among dairy farmers, butchers, veterinary practitioners, meat inspectors, slaughterhouse personnel or artificial inseminators who do not take adequate biosafety precautions while performing their jobs [174-176]. In addition, brucellosis vaccines such as Rev-1 and RB51 are live dried living vaccines. Thus, needlestick accidents during their preparation or administration could also be a risk factor for human infection. Close contact with animals may occur when farmers or veterinarians assist animals during parturition or abortion or handling of stillbirth. In some parts of the world it is also common practice for farmers to separate the placenta manually, thereby increasing their exposition to tissues infected with *Brucella* [168].

Dairy farmers who milk with bare hands have a greater chance of becoming infected from *Brucella* infected animals [177] as do farmers or slaughterhouse workers who have skin lesions which provide an entry point for the bacteria [128]. Also, inhalation of *Brucella* has been previously reported in slaughterhouse workers where the concentration of *Brucella* can be high due to aerosol generation [129].

Zoonotic brucellosis from marine mammal includes individuals in traditional communities where products from whales and seals are still an important part of their diet [16]. In addition, occupational acquired infection in people handling stranded marine mammals, whale and seal hunters, marine researchers and other people handling raw products from the ocean could be exposed [25,178]. Also, it is suggested that marine avian species may harbour *Brucella* by eating infected fish and thus become vectors of zoonotic infections [158]. Tourists who swim and interact closely with captive dolphins can be at risk when *Brucella* spp. could be circulating in these colonies [163].

Keypoint: Emerging risk factors for brucellosis

Wild animals have been referred as reservoir of brucellosis and represent an important risk of infection to farm animals, particularly in extensive breeding systems.

The prevalence of brucellosis in wildlife varies worldwide and several species such as bison, reindeer, caribou or wild boar have been described as potential source of infection of livestock. However, their role as risk factors of infection is still discussed since the microbiological isolation of *Brucella* spp. has been reported in wild ruminants. The zoonotical potential of *Brucella* spp. still represents an important public health threat not only in areas without eradication control programmes but as a work-acquired infection among dairy farmers, veterinarians or meat inspectors among others while performing their jobs. The discovery of brucellosis in marine mammals also represents a public health threat with special interest in occupational acquired infection in people handling stranded marine mammals.

Foodborne brucellosis is an important biological hazard associated with dairy products. However, the presence of *Brucella* spp. in marine animals indicates that fish-borne brucellosis could be a future hazard to be considered.

3. Conclusions

Brucella spp. is responsible for a contagious disease that results in reproductive failure and has an important economic impact, not only in animal health but also in public health because of its zoonotic characteristics. To achieve the control and eradication of brucellosis, the identification of all potential risks is necessary. Given the important role of domestic and wild animals as potential sources of *Brucella* infection, further risk assessment will require more complete and reliable data on the infection prevalence. Several risk factors have been described for brucellosis infection, although the herd or flock size, species and age have been cited as the most important. Brucellosis has traditionally been associated with farm animals, however, risks of brucellosis associated with wildlife and marine mammals could be a new threat and further epidemiological studies are necessary. In addition to animal sanitary measures, complementary measures such as good farm practices, biosecurity, training and education are necessary to control this old disease that is still of concern today.

Acknowledgements

The work was supported by the strategic research project PEst-OE/AGR/UI0772/2014 financed by the Foundation for Science and Technology [FCT]. This study was supported by the Foundation for Science and Technology of Portuguese Ministry of Education and Science [FCT - Fundação para a Ciência e Tecnologia do Ministério Português para a Educação e Ciência] by a research grant SFRH/BD/85118/2012 given to the author J. García Díez.

Author details

Ana Cláudia Coelho[1*], Juan García Díez[1] and Adosinda Maria Coelho[2]

*Address all correspondence to: accoelho@utad.pt

1 Animal and Veterinary Research Centre (CECAV). Univ. of Trás-os-Montes and Alto Douro, Portugal

2 National Authority of Food and Veterinary, North Regional Services of the National Authority of Food and Veterinary, Portugal

References

[1] Olsen S, Bellaire B. Brucella. In: McVey DS, Kennedy M, Chengappa MM, editors. Veterinary Microbiology. 3º ed. Willey-Blackwell. New Jersey; 2013.

[2] Edmondson MA, Roberts JF, Baird AN, Bychawski S, Pugh DG. Theriogenology of sheep and goats. In: Pugh DG, Baird NN, editors. Sheep & Goat Medicine. Elsevier Health Sciences. Missouri; 2012. p. 150-230.

[3] Neta AVC, Mol JP, Xavier MN, Paixão TA, Lage AP, Santos RL. Pathogenesis of bovine brucellosis. The Veterinary Journal. 2010;184:146-155.

[4] Seleem MN, Boyle SM, Sriranganathan N. Brucellosis: a re-emerging zoonosis. Veterinary Microbiology. 2010;140:392-398.

[5] McDermott J, Grace D, Zinsstag J. Economics of brucellosis impact and control in low-income countries. Revue Scientifique et Technique (International Office of Epizootics). 2013;32:249-261.

[6] Banai M, Corbel M. Taxonomy of *Brucella*. Open Veterinary Science Journal. 2010;4:85-101.

[7] Scholz HC, Nöckler K, Göllner C, Bahn P, Vergnaud G, Tomaso H, Al Dahouk S, Kämpfer P, Cloeckaert A, Maquart M, Zygmunt MS, Whatmore AM, Pfeffer M, Huber B, Busse HJ, De BK. *Brucella inopinata* sp. nov., isolated from a breast implant infection. International Journal of Systematic and Evolutionary Microbiology. 2010;60:801-808.

[8] López-Olvera JR, Vidal D, Vicente J, Pérez M, Luján L, Gortázar C. Serological survey of selected infectious diseases in mouflon (*Ovis aries musimon*) from south-central Spain. European Journal of Wildlife Research. 2009;55:75-79.

[9] Baek BK, Lim CW, Rahman MS, Kim CH, Oluoch A, Kakoma I. *Brucella abortus* infection in indigenous Korean dogs. Canadian Journal of Veterinary Research. 2003;67:312.

[10] Aznar MN, Samartino LE, Humblet MF, Saegerman C. Bovine brucellosis in Argentina and bordering countries: update. Transboundary and Emerging Diseases. 2014;61:121-133.

[11] Cvetnić Z, Spicić S, Toncić J, Majnarić D, Benić M, Albert D, Thiébaud M, Garin-Bastuji B. *Brucella suis* infection in domestic pigs and wild boar in Croatia. Revue scientifique et technique (International Office of Epizootics). 2009;28:1057-1067.

[12] Fosgate GT, Adesiyun AA, Hird DW, Hietala SK, Ryan J. Isolation of *Brucella abortus* biovar 1 from cattle and water buffaloes on Trinidad. Veterinary Record. 2002;151:272-273.

[13] Gul ST, Khan A, Ahmad M, Hussain I. Seroprevalence of brucellosis and associated hemato-biochemical changes in Pakistani horses. Pakistan Journal of Agricultural Sciences. 2013;50:745-750.

[14] Omer MK, Skjerve E, Woldehiwet Z, Holstad G. Risk factors for *Brucella* spp. infection in dairy cattle farms in Asmara, State of Eritrea. Preventive Veterinary Medicine. 2000;46:257-265.

[15] Godfroid J. Brucellosis in wildlife. Revue Scientifique et Technique-Office International des Epizooties. 2002;21:277-286.

[16] Tryland M, Nesbakken T, Robertson L, Grahek-Ogden D, Lunestad BT. Human pathogens in marine mammal meat–a northern perspective. Zoonoses and Public Health. 2014;61:377-394.

[17] Tiller RV, Gee JE, Frace MA, Taylor TK, Setubal JC, Hoffmaster AR, De BK. Characterization of novel *Brucella* strains originating from wild native rodent species in North Queensland, Australia. Applied and Environmental Microbiology. 2010;76:5837-5845.

[18] Teshome H, Molla B, Tibbo M. A seroprevalence study of camel brucellosis in three camel-rearing regions of Ethiopia. Tropical Animal Health and Production. 2003;35:381-390.

[19] Gyuranecz M, Erdélyi K, Makrai L, Fodor L, Szépe B, Mészáros AR, Dán A, Dencso L, Fassang E, Szeredi L. Brucellosis of the European brown hare (*Lepus europaeus*). Journal of Comparative Pathology. 2011;145:1-5.

[20] Her M, Cho DH, Kang SI, Lim JS, Kim HJ, Cho YS, Hwang IY, Lee T, Jung SC, Yoo HS. Outbreak of brucellosis in domestic elk in Korea. Zoonoses and Public Health. 2010;57:155-161.

[21] Cvetnic Z, Mitak M, Ocepek M, Lojkic M, Terzic S, Jemersic L, Humski A, Habrun B, Sostaric B, Brstilo, Krt B, Garin-Bastuji B. Wild boars (*Sus scrofa*) as reservoirs of *Brucella suis* biovar 2 in Croatia. Acta Veterinaria Hungarica. 2003;51:465-473.

[22] Eisenberg T, Hamann HP, Kaim U, Schlez K, Seeger H, Schauerte N, Melzer F, Tomaso H, Scholz HC, Koylass MS, Whatmore AM, Zschöck M. Isolation of potentially novel *Brucella* spp. from frogs. Applied and Environmental Microbiology. 2012;78:3753-3755.

[23] Junaidu AU, Salihu MD, Ahmed F, Ambursa MA, Gulumbe ML. Brucellosis in local chickens in North Western Nigeria. International Journal of Poultry Science. 2006;5:547-549.

[24] Kudi AC, Kalla DJU, Kudi MC, Yusuf H. Serological survey of brucellosis in traditionally managed domestic fowl in northern Guinea savannah, Nigeria. World's Poultry Science Journal. 1997;53:287-289.

[25] Nymo IH, Tryland M, Godfroid J. A review of *Brucella* infection in marine mammals, with special emphasis on *Brucella pinnipedialis* in the hooded seal (*Cystophora cristata*). Veterinary Research. 2011;42:1-14.

[26] Rich KM, Perry BD. The economic and poverty impacts of animal diseases in developing countries: new roles, new demands for economics and epidemiology. Preventive Veterinary Medicine. 2011;101:133-147.

[27] Guzmán-Verri C, González-Barrientos R, Hernández-Mora G, Morales JA, Baquero-Calvo E, Chaves-Olarte E, Moreno E. *Brucella ceti* and brucellosis in cetaceans. Frontiers in Cellular and Infection Microbiology. 2012;2.

[28] Bourg G, O'Callaghan D, Boschiroli ML. The genomic structure of *Brucella* strains isolated from marine mammals gives clues to evolutionary history within the genus. Veterinary Microbiology. 2007;125:375-380.

[29] Dawson CE, Perrett LL, Stubberfield EJ, Stack JA, Farrelly SSJ, Cooley WA, Davison NJ, Quinney S. Isolation and characterization of *Brucella* from the lungworms of a harbor porpoise (*Phocoena phocoena*). Journal of Wildlife Diseases. 2008;44:237-246.

[30] Blasco JM, Molina-Flores B. Control and eradication of *Brucella melitensis* infection in sheep and goats. Veterinary Clinics of North America: Food Animal Practice. 2011;27:95-104.

[31] Olsen S, Tatum F. Bovine brucellosis. Veterinary Clinics of North America: Food Animal Practice. 2010;26:15-27.

[32] Greece. Brucellosis program in 2011. Ministry of Rural Development and Food. 2012. http://ec.europa.eu/food/committees/regulatory/scfcah/animal_health/docs/0304072012_brucellosis_greece.pdf

[33] MAGRAMA – Ministério de Agricultura Alimentación y Médio Amniente. Programa Nacional de erradicación de la brucelosis ovina y caprina (*B. melitensis*) peresentado para su cofinanciación en 2013. España.

[34] Portugal. Brucelose dos pequenos ruminantes. Programa de erradicação para o ano 2012. Direção Geral de Veterinária. Lisboa. 2012.

[35] SANCO. Relazione su un audit condotto in Italia dal 7 al 15 ottobre 2013 al fine di valutare i programmi di eradicazione della brucellosi di bovini, ovini e caprini. 2013.

[36] Cowie CE, Marreos N, Gortázar C, Jaroso R, White PCL, Balseiro A. Shared risk factors for multiple livestock diseases: a case study of bovine tuberculosis and brucellosis. Research in Veterinary Science. 2014;97:491-497.

[37] Holt HR, Eltholth MM, Hegazy YM, El-Tras WF, Tayel AA, Guitian J. *Brucella* spp. infection in large ruminants in an endemic area of Egypt: cross-sectional study investigating seroprevalence, risk factors and livestock owner's knowledge, attitudes and practices (KAPs). BMC Public Health. 2011;11:341.

[38] Musallam II, Shehada MA, Omar M, Guitian J. Cross-sectional study of brucellosis in Jordan: prevalence, risk factors and spatial distribution in small ruminants and cattle. Preventive Veterinary Medicine. 2015;118:387-396.

[39] Mikolon AB, Gardner IA, De Anda JH, Hietala SK. Risk factors for brucellosis seropositivity of goat herds in the Mexicali Valley of Baja California, Mexico. Preventive Veterinary Medicine. 1998;37:185-195.

[40] Coelho AM, Coelho AC, Roboredo M, Rodrigues J. A case–control study of risk factors for brucellosis seropositivity in Portuguese small ruminants herds. Preventive Veterinary Medicine. 2007;82:291-301.

[41] Coelho AM, Coelho AC, Góis J, Pinto ML, Rodrigues J. Multifactorial correspondence analysis of risk factors for sheep and goat brucellosis seroprevalence. Small Ruminant Research. 2008;78:181-185.

[42] Díez JG, Coelho AC. An evaluation of cattle farmers' knowledge of bovine brucellosis in northeast Portugal. Journal of Infection and Public Health. 2013;6:363-369.

[43] Borba MR, Stevenson MA, Goncalves VSP, Neto JF, Ferreira F, Amaku M, Telles EO, Santana, SS, Ferreira JCA, Lobo JR, Figueiredo VCF, Dias RA. Prevalence and risk-mapping of bovine brucellosis in Maranhao State, Brazil. Preventive Veterinary Medicine. 2013;110:169-176.

[44] Ahmed MO, Elmeshri SE, Abuzweda AR, Blauo M, Abouzeed YM, Ibrahim A, Salem H, Alzwam F, Abid S, Elfahem A, Elrais A. Seroprevalence of brucellosis in animals and human populations in the western mountains region in Libya, December 2006–January 2008. Eurosurveillance. 2010;15:19625-19628.

[45] Rahman MS, Faruk MO, Her M, Kim JY, Kang SI, Jung SC. Prevalence of brucellosis in ruminants in Bangladesh. Veterinarni Medicina. 2011;56:379-385.

[46] Mai HM, Irons PC, Kabir J, Thompson PN. A large seroprevalence survey of brucellosis in cattle herds under diverse production systems in northern Nigeria. BMC Veterinary Research. 2012;8:144.

[47] Trangadia B, Rana SK, Mukherjee F, Srinivasan VA. Prevalence of brucellosis and infectious bovine rhinotracheitis in organized dairy farms in India. Tropical Animal Health and Production. 2010;42:203-207.

[48] Miller R, Nakavuma JL, Ssajjakambwe P, Vudriko P, Musisi N, Kaneene JB. The prevalence of brucellosis in cattle, goats and humans in rural Uganda: a comparative study. Transboundary and Emerging Diseases. 2015:1-5

[49] Bertu WJ, Ajogi I, Bale JOO, Kwaga JKP, Ocholi RA. Sero-epidemiology of brucellosis in small ruminants in Plateau State, Nigeria. African Journal of Microbiology Research. 2010;4:1935-1938.

[50] Bonfoh B, Kasymbekov J, Dürr S, Toktobaev N, Doherr MG, Schueth T, Zinsstag J, Schuelling E. Representative Seroprevalences of Brucellosis in Humans and Livestock in Kyrgyzstan. EcoHealth. 2011;9:132-138.

[51] Tahamtan Y, Namavari MM, Mohammadi G, Jula GM. Prevalence of brucellosis in horse north-east of Iran. Journal of Equine Veterinary Science. 2010;30:376-378.

[52] Ehizibolo DO, Gusi AM, Ehizibolo PO. Serologic prevalence of brucellosis in horse stables in two northern states of Nigeria. Journal of Equine Science. 2011;22:17.

[53] Wadood F, Ahmad M, Khan A, Gul ST, Rehman N. Seroprevalence of brucellosis in horses in and around Faisalabad. Pakistan Veterinary Journal. 2009;29:196-198.

[54] Mosallanejad B, Najafabadi MG, Avizeh R, Mohammadian N. A serological survey on *Brucella canis* in companion dogs in Ahvaz. Iranian Journal of Veterinary Research. 2009;10:383-386.

[55] López G, Ayala SM, Efron AM, Gómez CF, Lucero NE. A serological and bacteriological survey of dogs to detect *Brucella* infection in Lomas de Zamora, Buenos Aires province. Revista Argentina de Microbiologia. 2009;41:97-101.

[56] Cadmus SIB, Adesokan HK, Ajala OO, Odetokun WO, Perrett LL, Stack JA. Seroprevalence of *Brucella abortus* and *B. canis* in household dogs in southwestern Nigeria: a preliminary report: short communication. Journal of the South African Veterinary Association. 2011;82:56-57.

[57] Adesiyun AA, Abdullahi SU, Adeyanju JB. Prevalence of *Brucella abortus* and *Brucella canis* antibodies in dogs in Nigeria. Journal of Small Animal Practice. 1986;27:31-37.

[58] Behzadi MA, Mogheiseh A. Epidemiological survey of *Brucella canis* infection in different breeds of dogs in Fars province, Iran. Pakistan Veterinary Journal. 2011;31:140.

[59] Davis DS, Boeer WJ, Mims JP, Heck FC, Adams LG. *Brucella abortus* in coyotes I. A serologic and bacteriologic survey eastern Texas. Journal of Wildlife Diseases. 1979;15:367-372.

[60] Leuenberger R, Boujon P, Thür B, Miserez R, Garin-Bastuji B, Rüfenacht J, Stärk KD. Prevalence of classical swine fever, Aujeszky's disease and brucellosis in a population of wild boar in Switzerland. The Veterinary Record. 2007;160:362-368.

[61] Van Der Leek ML, Becker HN, Humphrey P, Adams CL, Belden RC, Frankenberger WB, Nicoletti PL. Prevalence of *Brucella* sp. antibodies in feral swine in Florida. Journal of Wildlife Diseases. 1993;29:410-415.

[62] Nielsen O, Stewart RE, Nielsen K, Measures L, Duignan P. Serologic survey of *Brucella* spp. antibodies in some marine mammals of North America. Journal of Wildlife Diseases. 2001;37:89.

[63] Tryland M, Sørensen KK, Godfroid J. Prevalence of *Brucella pinnipediae* in healthy hooded seals (*Cystophora cristata*) from the North Atlantic Ocean and ringed seals (*Phoca hispida*) from Svalbard. Veterinary Microbiology. 2005;105:103.

[64] Garín-Bastuji B. Brucelloses bovine, ovine et caprine: contrôle et prevention. Point Vet. 1993;25:15-22.

[65] Estein SM, Cassataro J, Vizcaíno N, Zygmunt M, Cloeckaert A, Bowden RA. The recombinant Omp31 from *Brucella melitensis* alone or associated with rough lipopolysaccharide induces protection against *Brucella ovis* infection in BALB/c mice. Microbes and Infection. 2003;5:85-93.

[66] OIE World Organisation for Animal Health. Porcine brucellosis. Chapter 2.8.5. OIE Terrestrial Manual. 2009. p. 1-7, Office International des Épizooties.

[67] Memish Z. Brucellosis control in Saudi Arabia: prospects and challenges. Journal of Chemotherapy. 2001;13:11-17.

[68] Paolicchi FA, Terzolo HR, Campero CM. Isolation of *Brucella suis* from the semen of a ram. Veterinary Record. 1993;132:67.

[69] Metcalf HE, Luchsinger DW, Ray WC. Brucellosis. In: Beran GW, Steele JH, editors. Handbook of Zoonoses: Section A. Bacterial, Rickettsial, Chlamydial, and Mycotic. Florida: CRC Press; 1994. p. 9-38.

[70] AHAW – Scientific Opinion of the Panel on Animal Health and Welfare (AHAW) on a request from the Commission on porcine brucellosis (*Brucella suis*). The EFSA Journal. 2009;1144:1-112.

[71] Acha PN, Szyfres B, editors. Brucellosis. Zoonoses and Communicable Diseases Common to Man and Animals: Bacterioses and Mycoses. 3rd ed. Pan American Sanitary Bureau. Pan American Health Organization. Washington. 2001. p. 40-66.

[72] Alton GG. *Brucella melitensis*. In: Nielsen K, Duncan JR, editors. Animal Brucellosis. Florida: CRC Press; 1990.

[73] Ashagrie T, Deneke Y, Tolosa T. Seroprevalence of caprine brucellosis and associated risk factors in South Omo Zone of Southern Ethiopia. African Journal of Microbiological Research. 2011;5:1682-1685.

[74] Muma JB, Samui KL, Siamudaala VM, Oloya J, Matop G, Omer MK, Munyeme M, Mubita C, Skjerve E. Prevalence of antibodies to *Brucella* spp. and individual risk factors of infection in traditional cattle, goats and sheep reared in livestock–wildlife interface areas of Zambia. Tropical Animal Health and Production. 2006;38:195-206.

[75] Sanogo M, Abatih E, Thys E, Fretin D, Berkvens D, Saegerman C. Risk factors associated with brucellosis seropositivity among cattle in the central savannah-forest area of Ivory Coast. Preventive Veterinary Medicine. 2012;107:51-56.

[76] Stringer LA, Guitian FJ, Abernethy DA, Honhold NH, Menzies FD. Risk associated with animals moved from herds infected with brucellosis in Northern Ireland. Preventive Veterinary Medicine. 2008;84:72-84.

[77] Solorio-Rivera JL, Segura-Correa JC, Sánchez-Gil LG. Seroprevalence of and risk factors for brucellosis of goats in herds of Michoacan, Mexico. Preventive Veterinary Medicine. 2007;82:282-290.

[78] Al-Majali AM, Al-Qudah KM, Al-Tarazi YH, Al-Rawashdeh OF. Risk factors associated with camel brucellosis in Jordan. Tropical Animal Health and Production. 2008;40:193-200.

[79] Muñoz PM, Boadella M, Arnal M, de Miguel MJ, Revilla M, Martínez D, Vicente J, Acevedo P, Oleaga A, Ruiz-Fons F, Marín CM, Prieto JM, de la Fuente J, Barral M, Barberán M, de Luco DF, Blasco JM, Gortázar C. Spatial distribution and risk factors of Brucellosis in Iberian wild ungulates. BMC Infectious Diseases. 2010;10:46.

[80] Bekele M, Mohammed H, Tefera M, Tolosa T. Small ruminant brucellosis and community perception in Jijiga district, Somali Regional State, eastern Ethiopia. Tropical Animal Health and Production. 2011;43:893-898.

[81] Matope G, Bhebhe E, Muma JB, Oloya J, Madekurozwa RL, Lund A, Skjerve E. Seroprevalence of brucellosis and its associated risk factors in cattle from smallholder dairy farms in Zimbabwe. Tropical Animal Health and Production. 2011;43:975-982.

[82] Petersen E, Rajashekara G, Sanakkayala N, Eskra L, Harms J, Splitter G. Erythritol triggers expression of virulence traits in *Brucella melitensis*. Microbes and Infection. 2013;15:440-449.

[83] Alavi-Shoushtari SM, Zeinali A. Responses of female lambs to Rev-1 vaccination. Preventive Veterinary Medicine. 1995;21:289-297.

[84] Megersa B, Biffa D, Abunna F, Regassa A, Godfroid J, Skjerve E. Seroprevalence of brucellosis and its contribution to abortion in cattle, camel, and goat kept under pastoral management in Borana, Ethiopia. Tropical Animal Health and Production, 2011;43:651-656.

[85] Talukder BC, Samad MA, Rahman AKMA. Comparative evaluation of commercial serodiagnostic tests for the seroprevalence study of brucellosis in stray dogs in Bangladesh. Bangladesh Journal of Veterinary Medicine. 2012;9:79-83.

[86] Coelho AM, Díez JG, Coelho AC. Brucelosis en pequeños rumiantes: efecto de la aplicación de un programa especial de vacunación en masa con REV-1. REDVET. Revista Electrónica de Veterinaria. 2013;14:1-16.

[87] León F. Brucellosis ovina y caprina. Ed. Office International des Epizooties – OIE. Francia; 1993.451p

[88] Jackson R, Pite L, Kennard R, Ward D, Stack J, Domi X, Rami A, Dedushaj I. Survey of the seroprevalence of brucellosis in ruminants in Kosovo. Veterinary Record. 2004;154:747-751.

[89] Musallam II, Shehada MA, Omar M, Guitian J. Cross-sectional study of brucellosis in Jordan: prevalence, risk factors and spatial distribution in small ruminants and cattle. Preventive Veterinary Medicine. 2015;118:387-396.

[90] OIE World Organisation for Animal Health. Caprine and Ovine brucellosis. In: Manual of Diagnostic Test and Vaccines for Terrestrial Animals; 2008. p. 974-982.

[91] Blasco JM. Control and eradication programmes of brucellosis in small ruminants and cattle. Implementation of Control and Eradication Programs in Animals. Zaragoza; Curso de Epidemiologia; 2001.

[92] Ferreira A, Ferreira C. Doenças infecto-contagiosas dos animais domésticos. Lisboa: Fundação Calouste Gulbenkian; 1990. p. 125-142.

[93] Louzã AC. Brucelose - Modelo de zoonose de impacto sócio-económico. Parte I. Veterinária Técnica. 1993;43:21-28.

[94] Young EJ. *Brucella* species. In: Mandell GL, Bennet JE, Dolin R, editors. Principles and Practice of Infectious Diseases. New York: Churchill Livingstone; 1995. p. 2053-2060.

[95] Boadella M, Carta T, Oleaga Á, Pajares G, Muñoz M, Gortázar C. Serosurvey for selected pathogens in Iberian roe deer. BMC Veterinary Research. 2010;6:51.

[96] Grégoire F, Mousset B, Hanrez D, Michaux C, Walravens K, Linden A. A serological and bacteriological survey of brucellosis in wild boar (*Sus scrofa*) in Belgium. BMC Veterinary Research. 2012;8:80.

[97] Higgins J, Stuber T, Quance C, Edwards WH, Tiller RV, Linfield T, Rhyan J, Berte A, Harris B. Molecular epidemiology of *Brucella abortus* isolates from cattle, elk, and bison in the United States, 1998 to 2011. Applied and Environmental Microbiology. 2012;78:3674-3684.

[98] Meng XJ, Lindsay DS, Sriranganathan N. Wild boars as sources for infectious diseases in livestock and humans. Philosophical Transactions of the Royal Society B: Biological Sciences. 2009;364:2697-2707.

[99] Ahmed RA, Munir MA. Epidemiological investigations of brucellosis in horses, dogs, cats and poultry. Pakistan Veterinary Journal. 1995;15:85-88.

[100] Sharma VD, Sethi MS, Yadav MP, Dube DC. Sero-epidemiologic investigations on brucellosis in the states of Uttar Pradesh (U.P.) and Delhi (India). International Journal of Zoonoses. 1979;6:75-81.

[101] Grilló MJ, Barberán M, Blasco JM. Transmission of *Brucella melitensis* from sheep to lambs. Veterinary Record. 1997;140:602-605.

[102] Edmondson MA, Roberts JF, Baird AN, Bychawski S, Pugh DG. Theriogenology of sheep and goats. In: Pugh DG, Baird AN, editors. Sheep and Goat Medicine. Missouri: Elsevier; 2012. p. 158-238.

[103] Díaz AE. Epidemiology of brucellosis in domestic animals caused by Brucella melitensis, *Brucella suis* and *Brucella abortus*. Revue scientifique et technique (International Office of Epizootics). 2013;32:43-51.

[104] Muma JB, Samui KL, Oloya J, Munyeme M, Skjerve E. Risk factors for brucellosis in indigenous cattle reared in livestock–wildlife interface areas of Zambia. Preventive Veterinary Medicine. 2007;80:306-317.

[105] Nahar A, Ahmed MU. Sero-prevalence study of brucellosis in cattle and contact human in Mymensingh district. Bangladesh Journal of Veterinary Medicine. 2009;7:269-274.

[106] Corbel MJ, Brinley-Morgan WJ. Genus *Brucella*. In: Krieg NR, Holt JG, editors. Bergey's Manual of Systemic Bacteriology. London: Williams e Wilkins; 1994. p. 377-388.

[107] Xiang F, Xia Z, Wu Q, Chen Y, Yu J, Wan J. Seroepidemiology of canine brucellosis in Beijing, China. Turkish Journal of Veterinary and Animal Sciences. 2013;37:28-42.

[108] Cameron HS, Hughes EH, Gregory PW. Genetic resistance to brucellosis in swine. Journal of Animal Science. 1942;1:106-110.

[109] Lovejoy GS, Carver HD, Moseley IK, Hicks M. Serosurvey of dogs for *Brucella canis* infection in Memphis, Tennessee. American Journal of Public Health. 1976;66:175-176.

[110] Ibrahim N, Belihu K, Lobago F, Bekana M. Sero-prevalence of bovine brucellosis and its risk factors in Jimma zone of Oromia Region, South-western Ethiopia. Tropical Animal Health and Production. 2010;42:35-40.

[111] Teklue T, Tolosa T, Tuli G, Beyene B, Hailu B. Sero-prevalence and risk factors study of brucellosis in small ruminants in Southern Zone of Tigray Region, Northern Ethiopia. Tropical Animal Health and Production. 2013;45:1809-1815.

[112] Al-Majali AM, Majok AA, Amarin NM, Al-Rawashdeh OF. Prevalence of, and risk factors for, brucellosis in Awassi sheep in Southern Jordan. Small Ruminant Research. 2007;73:300-303.

[113] Al-Majali AM. Seroepidemiology of caprine brucellosis in Jordan. Small Ruminant Research. 2005;58:13-18.

[114] Reviriego FJ, Moreno MA, Domínguez L. Risk factors for brucellosis seroprevalence of sheep and goat flocks in Spain. Preventive Veterinary Medicine. 2000;44:167-173.

[115] CFSPH-Center for Food Security and Public Health. Brucellosis, 2009. www.cfsph.iastate.edu/Factsheets/pdfs/brucellosis.pdf

[116] Godfroid J, Scholz HC, Barbier T, Nicolas C, Wattiau P, Fretin D, Whatmore AM, Cloeckaert A, Blasco JM, Moriyon I, Saegerman C, Muma JB, Al Dahouk S, Neubauer H, Letesson JJ. Brucellosis at the animal/ecosystem/human interface at the beginning of the 21st century. Preventive Veterinary Journal. 2011;102:118–131.

[117] Mainar-Jaime RC, Vázquez-Boland JA. Associations of veterinary services and farmer characteristics with the prevalences of brucellosis and border disease in small ruminants in Spain. Preventive Veterinary Medicine. 1999;40:193-205.

[118] Blasco JM. A review of the use of *B. melitensis* Rev. 1 vaccine in adult sheep and goats. Preventive Veterinary Medicine. 1997;31:275-283.

[119] Ramírez H, Calle E, Echevarría C, Morales C. Prevalencia de brucelosis canina en dos distritos de la Provincia Constitucional del Callao. Revista de Investigaciones Veterinarias del Perú. 2006;17:39-43.

[120] Castrillón-Salazar L, Giraldo-Echeverri CA, Sánchez-Jiménez MM, Olivera-Angel M. Factors associated with *Brucella canis* seropositivity in kennels of two regions of Antioquia, Colombia. Cadernos de Saúde Pública. 2013;29:1955-1973.

[121] Hollett RB. Canine brucellosis: outbreaks and compliance. Theriogenology. 2006;66:575-587.

[122] Garin-Bastuji B, Hars J, Drapeau A, Cherfa MA, Game Y, Le Horgne JM, Rautureau S, Maucci E, Pasquier JJ, Jay M, Mick V. Reemergence of *Brucella melitensis* infection in wildlife, France. Emerging Infectious Diseases. 2014;20:1570.

[123] Cvetnic Z, Spicic S, Curic S, Jukic B, Lojkic M, Albert D, Thiébaud M, Garin-Bastuji B. Isolation of *Brucella suis* biovar 3 from horses in Croatia. Veterinary Record-English Edition. 2005;156:584-585.

[124] Corbel MJ. Brucellosis: an overview. Emerging Infectious Disease. 1997;3:213-221.

[125] Aguiar DM, Cavalcante GT, Labruna MB, Vasconcellos SA, Rodrigues AAR, Morais ZM, Camargo LMA, Gennari SM. Risk factors and seroprevalence of *Brucella* spp. in cattle from western Amazon, Brazil. Arquivos do Instituto Biologico, Sao Paulo. 2007;74:301-305.

[126] Fretin D, Mori M, Czaplicki G, Quinet C, Maquet B, Godfroid J, Saegerman C. Unexpected *Brucella suis* biovar 2 infection in a dairy cow, Belgium. Emerging Infectious Diseases. 2013;19:2053.

[127] Al-Majali AM, Talafha AQ, Ababneh MM, Ababneh MM. Seroprevalence and risk factors for bovine brucellosis in Jordan. Journal of Veterinary Science. 2009;10:61-65.

[128] Islam MA, Khatun MM, Werre SR, Sriranganathan N, Boyle SM. A review of *Brucella* seroprevalence among humans and animals in Bangladesh with special emphasis on epidemiology, risk factors and control opportunities. Veterinary Microbiology. 2013;166:317-326.

[129] Sammartino LE, Gil A, Elzer P. Capacity building for surveillance and control of bovine and caprine brucellosis. In: FAO Animal Production and Health Proceedings - AO/WHO/OIE Expert and Technical Consultation. Rome. 2006; 7:55

[130] Al-Talafhah AH, Lafi SQ, Al-Tarazi Y. Epidemiology of ovine brucellosis in Awassi sheep in Northern Jordan. Preventive Veterinary Medicine. 2003;60:297-306.

[131] Kabagambe EK, Elzer PH, Geaghan JP, Opuda-Asibo J, Scholl DT, Miller JE. Risk factors for *Brucella* seropositivity in goat herds in Eastern and Western Uganda. Preventive Veterinary Medicine. 2001;52:91-108.

[132] Silva I, Dangolla A, Kulachelvy K. Seroepidemiology of *Brucella abortus* infection in bovids in Sri Lanka. Preventive Veterinary Medicine. 2000; 46:51-59.

[133] Mekonnen H, Kalayou S, Kyule M. Serological survey of bovine brucellosis in barka and arado breeds (*Bos indicus*) of Western Tigray, Ethiopia. Preventive Veterinary Medicine. 2010;94:28-35.

[134] Makita K, Fèvre EM, Waiswa C, Eisler MC, Thrusfield M, Welburn SC. Herd prevalence of bovine brucellosis and analysis of risk factors in cattle in urban and peri-urban areas of the Kampala economic zone, Uganda. BMC Veterinary Research. 2011;7:60.

[135] Kataria AK, Gahlot AK. Evaluation of oxidative stress in *Brucella* infected cows. Journal of Stress Physiology and Biochemistry. 2010;6:2.

[136] Henriques HS. Epidemiologia da brucelose em pequenos ruminantes. Sociedade Portuguesa de Ovinotecnia e Caprinotecnia. Proceeding of II Jornadas sobre Sanidade Ovina e Caprina. Bragança. 1990;21-28.

[137] Izquierdo de la Hoya S, Villanueva M. Transmisión de la brucelosis entre explotaciones ovinas próximas. Proceedings of the XXI Jornadas Científicas de la Sociedad Española de Ovinotecnia y Caprinotecnia (SEOC). Logroño, España 1996; 101-105.

[138] Crespo-León F. Brucellosis ovina y caprina. Paris: OIE. 1994; p. 451.

[139] Wickramasuriya UGJS, Peiris GS, Kendaragama KMT, Karunadasa WM. A survey on the incidence of bovine brucellosis in three districts in Sri Lanka. Sri Lanka Veterinary Journal. 1983;31:27-31.

[140] Quinn PJ, Markey BK. Disinfection and disease prevention in veterinary medicine. In: Block SS, editor. Disinfection, Sterilization and Preservation. 5th ed. Philadelphia: Lippincott Williams and Wilkins; 2001. p. 1069-1104.

[141] de Paula Dreer MK, Gonçalves DD, da Silva Caetano IC, Gerônimo E, Menegas PH, Bergo D, Lopes-Mori FM, Benitez A, Freitas JC, Evers F, Navarro I, Almeida Martins L. Toxoplasmosis, leptospirosis and brucellosis in stray dogs housed at the shelter in Umuarama municipality, Paraná, Brazil. Journal of Venomous Animals and Toxins including Tropical Diseases. 2013;19:23.

[142] Garín-Bastuji B. Le dépistage de la brucellose des ruminants et ses difficultés. Les cas des sérologies atypiques en brucellose bovine. Point Veterinaire 1993;25:23-32.

[143] Ferron A. Bactériologie Médicale à l'usage des étudients en médecine. La Madeleine Editions. 989.

[144] Godfroid J, Käsbohrer A. Brucellosis in the European Union and Norway at the turn of the twenty-first century. Veterinary Microbiology. 2002;90:135-145.

[145] Renukaradhya GJ, Isloor S, Rajasekhar M. Epidemiology, zoonotic aspects, vaccination and control/eradication of brucellosis in India. Veterinary Microbiology. 2002;90:183-195.

[146] Gortázar C, Ferroglio E, Höfle U, Frölich K, Vicente J. Diseases shared between wildlife and livestock: a European perspective. European Journal of Wildlife Research. 2007;53:241-256.

[147] Gortázar C, Acevedo P, Ruiz-Fons F, Vicente J. Disease risks and overabundance of game species. European Journal of Wildlife Research. 2006;2:81-87.

[148] Godfroid J, Garin Bastuji B, Saegerman C, Blasco Martínez, JM. Brucellosis in terrestrial wildlife. Revue Scientifique et Technique. 2013;32:27-42.

[149] Godfroid J, Cloeckaert A, Liautard JP, Kohler S, Fretin D, Walravens K, Garín Bastuji B, Letesson JJ. From the discovery of the Malta fever's agent to the discovery of a marine mammal reservoir, brucellosis has continuously been a re-emerging zoonosis. Veterinary Research. 2005;36:313-326.

[150] Garin-Bastuji B, Hars J, Drapeau A, Cherfa MA, Game Y, Le Horgne JM, Rautureau S, Maucci E, Pasquier JJ, Jay M, Mick V. Reemergence of *Brucella melitensis* in wildlife, France. Emerging Infectious Disease. 2014;20:157-1571.

[151] Conner MM, Ebinger MR, Blanchong JA, Cross PC. Infectious disease in cervids of North America. Annals of the New York Academy of Sciences. 2008;1134:146-172.

[152] Godfroid J. Brucellosis in wildlife. Revue Scientifique et Technique-Office International des Épizooties. 2002;21:277-286.

[153] Godfroid J, Michel P, Uytterhaegen L, Desmedt C, Rasseneur F, Boelaert F, Saegerman C, Patigny X. Brucellose enzootique a Brucella suis biotype 2 chez le sanglier (Sus scrofa) en Belgique, 1994.

[154] Ross HM, Foster G, Reid RJ, Jahans KL, MacMillan AP. *Brucella* species infection in sea-mammals. Veterinary Record. 1994;134:359-359.

[155] Tachibana M, Watanabe K, Kim S, Omata Y, Murata K, Hammond T, Watarai M. Antibodies to Brucella spp. in Pacific bottlenose dolphins from the Solomon Islands. Journal of Wildlife Diseases. 2006;42:412-414.

[156] Hernández-Mora G, González-Barrientos R, Morales JA, Chaves-Olarte E, Guzmán-Verri C, Baquero-Calvo E, De-Miguel MJ, Marín, CM, Blasco JM, Moreno E. Neuro-

brucellosis in stranded dolphins, Costa Rica. Emerging Infectious Diseases. 2008;14:1430.

[157] Van Bressem MF, Raga JA, Di Guardo G, Jepson PD, Duignan PJ, Siebert U, Barrett T, Santos MC, Moreno IB, Siciliano S, Aguilar A, Van Waerebeek K. Emerging infectious diseases in cetaceans worldwide and the possible role of environmental stressors. Diseases of Aquatic Organisms. 2009;86:143-157.

[158] Thakur SD, Vaid RK, Panda AK, Saini Y. Marine mammal brucellosis: a new dimension to an old zoonosis. Current Science. 2012;103:902-910.

[159] Ewalt DR, Payeur JB, Rhyan JC, Geer PL. *Brucella suis* biovar 1 in naturally infected cattle: a bacteriological, serological, and histological study. Journal of Veterinary Research. 1997;53:405-410.

[160] González-Barrientos R, Morales JA, Hernández-Mora G, Barquero-Calvo E, Guzmán-Verri C, Chaves-Olarte E, Moreno E. Pathology of striped dolphins (*Stenella coeruleoalba*) infected with *Brucella ceti*. Journal of Comparative Pathology. 2010;142:347-352.

[161] Foster G, MacMillan AP, Godfroid J, Howie F, Ross HM, Cloeckaert A, Reid RJ, Brew S, Patterson IAP. A review of *Brucella* sp. infection of sea mammals with particular emphasis on isolates from Scotland. Veterinary Microbiology. 2002;90:563-580.

[162] Foster G, Jahans KL, Reid RJ, Ross HM. Isolation of *Brucella* species from cetaceans, seals and an otter. Veterinary Record. 1996;138:583-586.

[163] Muñoz PM, García-Castrillo G, López-García P, González-Cueli JC, De Miguel MJ, Marín CM, Barberán M, Blasco JM. Isolation of *Brucella* species from a live-stranded striped dolphin (*Stenella coeruleoalba*) in Spain. Veterinary Record. 2006;158:450.

[164] Ross HM, Jahans KL, MacMillan AP, Reid RJ, Thompson PM, Foster G. *Brucella* species infection in North Sea seal and cetacean populations. Veterinary Record. 1996;138:647-648.

[165] Dawson CE, Perrett LL, Stubberfield EJ, Stack JA, Farrelly SSJ, Cooley WA, Davison NJ, Quinney S. Isolation and characterization of *Brucella* from the lungworms of a harbor porpoise (*Phocoena phocoena*). Journal of Wildlife Diseases. 2008;44:237-246.

[166] Moreno E. Retrospective and prospective perspectives on zoonotic brucellosis. Frontiers in Microbiology. 2014;5:213.

[167] Tabak F, Hakko E, Mete B, Ozaras R, Mert A, Ozturk R. Is family screening necessary in brucellosis?. Infection. 2008;36:575-577.

[168] Lindahl E, Sattorov N, Boqvist S, Sattori I, Magnusson U. Seropositivity and risk factors for *Brucella* in dairy cows in urban and peri-urban small-scale farming in Tajikistan. Tropical Animal Health and Production. 2014;46:563-569.

[169] El-Daher N, Na'Was T, Al-Qaderi S. The effect of the pH of various dairy products on the survival and growth of *Brucella melitensis*. Annals of Tropical Medicine and Parasitology. 1990;84:523-528.

[170] Dhanashekar R, Akkinepalli S, Nellutla A. Milk-borne infections. An analysis of their potential effect on the milk industry. Germs. 2012;2:101.

[171] Nicoletti P. Relationship between animal and human disease. In: Young EJ, Corbel MJ, editors. Brucellosis: Clinical and Laboratory Aspects. Boca Raton: CRC Press; 1989.

[172] Regulation (EC) Nº 853/2004 of the European Parliament and the Council of 29 April 2004 laying down specific hygiene rules for food of animal origin. Official Journal of the European Union. 2004; L 39.

[173] Pessegueiro P, Barata C, Correia J. Brucelose-uma revisão sistematizada. Medicina Interna. 2003;10:91-100.

[174] Ali S, Ali Q, Neubauer H, Melzer F, Elschner M, Khan I, Nji Abatih E, Ullah N, Irfan M, Akhter M. Seroprevalence and risk factors associated with brucellosis as a professional hazard in Pakistan. Foodborne Pathogens and Disease. 2013;10:500-505.

[175] Luce R, Snow J, Gross D, Murphy T, Grandpre J, Daley WR, Brudvig JM, Ari MD, Harris L, Clark TA. Brucellosis seroprevalence among workers in at-risk professions: Northwestern Wyoming, 2005 to 2006. Journal of Occupational and Environmental Medicine. 2012;54:1557-1560.

[176] Traxler RM, Lehman MW, Bosserman EA, Guerra MA, Smith TL. A literature review of laboratory-acquired brucellosis. Journal of Clinical Microbiology. 2013;51:3055-3062.

[177] Lachapelle JM. Biologic causes of occupational dermatoses. In: Kanerva's Occupational Dermatology. Berlin: Springer; 2012. p. 231-245.

[178] Waltzek TB, Cortés-Hinojosa G, Wellehan Jr JFX, Gray GC. Marine mammal zoonoses: a review of disease manifestations. Zoonoses and Public Health. 2012;59:521-535.

Chapter 2

Brucellosis at the Wildlife/Livestock/Human Interface

Calvin Gomo

Additional information is available at the end of the chapter

http://dx.doi.org/10.5772/61212

Abstract

There are a number of bacterial, viral, and parasitic diseases present at the Wildlife/livestock/human interface. Brucellosis is a zoonotic disease of importance and highly prevalent in sub-Saharan Africa. The important *Brucella* species at the wildlife/livestock/human interface are *Brucella arbortus, Brucella suis*, and *Brucella melitensis*. These species have been isolated from humans, livestock (cattle and goats), and wildlife (African buffalo and giraffe). A lot of studies indicated that density, herd size, age of cow, reduced veterinary services like vaccination programs, and geographical area are associated with *Brucella* prevalence. Studies in developing countries have indicated that the disease is more prominent in the both commercial and communal farming sectors. Access and consumption of contaminated foods and/or occupational exposure remain the significant source of infection to humans. The pathogen transmission of brucellosis is bidirectional in nature; hence, for control efforts to be successful, cooperation is required between livestock owners, animal health officials, and wildlife managers. Globally, trend is moving toward focusing on "one health," which recognizes that human, animal (both domestic and wild), and ecosystems are tightly linked. The successful management of disease requires an integrated approach where efforts are focused in concert across these domains. Climate change, increased human populations, and increased interaction at wildlife/livestock/human interface have resulted in the change of brucellosis dynamics.

Keywords: Brucellosis, wildlife/livestock/human interface, emerging diseases, zoonotic diseases, surveillance, disease management

1. Introduction

Interest in the epidemiology of emerging diseases of humans and livestock as they relate to wildlife has increased greatly over the past several decades [1]. The importance of wildlife in the emergence of livestock and human brucellosis is due to multiple changes occurring within wildlife, livestock, and human populations [1]. The epidemiology of infections and diseases is highly dependent on several factors within, or in the interfaces between, human, livestock, or wildlife populations. Land use changes being speared by humans, which include encroachment into wildlife habitat, continue to increase, along with more intensified livestock production practices. This scenario is favorable to the spread of brucellosis. The alteration of wildlife population demographics bring in a new dimension in the epidemiology of brucellosis, e.g., increasing African buffalo population in Southern Africa, which in turn increases the chances of potential for contact and *Brucella* species transmission at the wildlife/livestock interface.

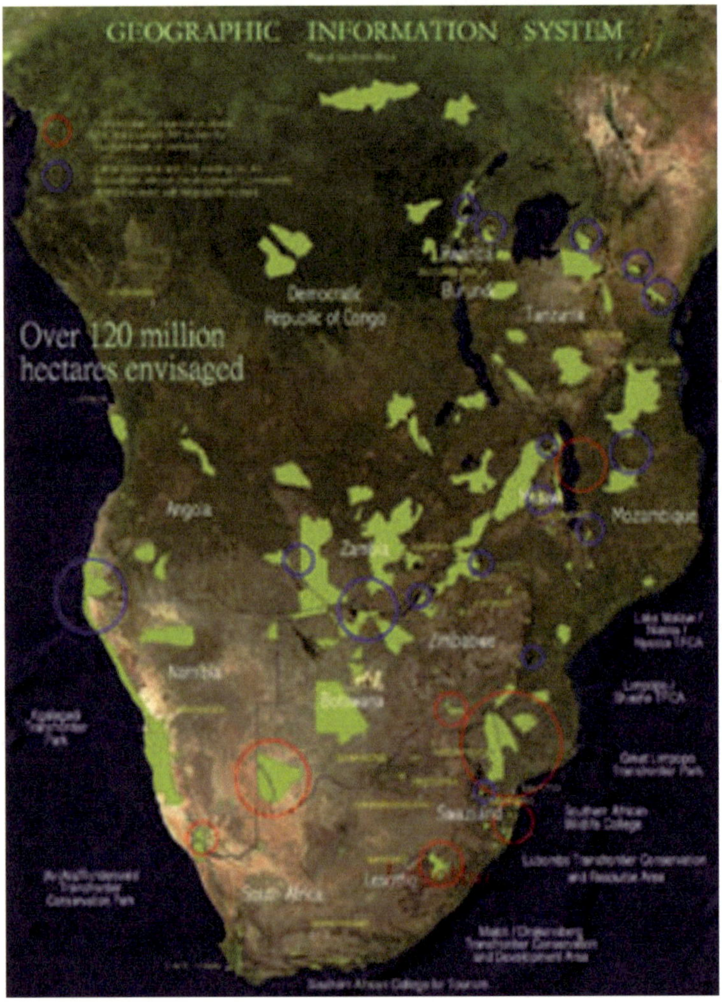

Figure 1. Map of proposed TFCAs in Africa.

Human and animal health populations are pivotal and important for economic development, prosperity, and stability. Infectious diseases like brucellosis affect health and reproductivity of livestock, thereby greatly reducing its value and opportunities for trade. Brucellosis is a zoonosis and a disease of veterinary and public health significance worldwide. It is a disease

http://dx.doi.org/10.5772/61212

that infects multiple species even in marine ecosystem, and it is also found in many continents. The incidences and prevalence of the disease vary widely from country to country. Brucellosis prevalence is relatively high in Africa, Latin American, and Asian countries. It is the disease of sexually matured animals with predilection for placentas, fetal fluids, and testes of male animals (OIE 2014). It is caused by bacteria of the genus *Brucella*. In sub-Saharan Africa, the bacterium *Brucella abortus* has been identified in several free-ranging wildlife species. *Brucella* antibodies have been detected in various wildlife species, including waterbuck (*Kobus ellipsiprymnus*), African buffalo (*Syncerus caffer*), eland (*Taurotragus oryx*), giraffe (*Giraffa camelopardalis*), and impala (*Aepyceros melampus*) in Zimbabwe and South Africa. The importance of brucellosis is reflected by its widespread distribution and impact on multiple animal species, including cattle, sheep, goats, and pigs [2]. The livestock sector is dominated by ruminants, and they are prone to brucellosis. This makes the disease economically important.

Interface spaces allow people, livestock, and wildlife to share space and resources in semi-arid landscapes, especially transfrontier conservation areas (TFCAs) in Africa (see Figure 1). The coexistence of domestic herbivores and wild animals has its advantages and disadvantages, for example, ecotourism, but one of the major consequences is the risk of pathogen transmission. The risk at the interface threatens local livelihoods depending on animal production, ecotourism, public health in the case of brucellosis, national economies in the context of transboundary animal diseases, and the success of integrated conservation and development initiatives [3]. Globally, the role of wildlife in livestock diseases is expected to increase [4] in conjunction with human population growth, which is expected to reach 9 billion by 2030. Increased demand for animal protein will further increase potentially infectious contacts between livestock and wildlife, leading to an increased potential for zoonotic diseases (brucellosis) to emerge. The changes in the dynamics will result in challenges that will require an improved understanding of the ecology of pathogens at the wildlife/livestock/human interface along with the development of tools and mitigations to manage these pathogens.

2. Brucella species associated with the interface

The members of the genus *Brucella* are aerobic bacteria that multiply within macrophages and cause infections in animals and humans [5]. The most relevant species from an economical and public health perspective are *B. abortus*, *B. suis*, and *B. melitensis*. The three *Brucella* species are the ones prevalent at the interfaces. The major cause of bovine brucellosis is *B. abortus;* however, *B. suis* or *B. melitensis* have been occasionally implicated in some cattle herds. The following species have been currently recognized: *B. abortus* (8 biovars), *B. melitensis* (3 biovars), *B. suis* (5 biovars), *B. ovis*, *B. canis*, *B. neotomae* [6], *B. pinnipedialis* [7], *B. ceti* [7], *B. microti* [8], and *B. inopinata* (wound fluid from human) [9, 10]. Little research has been done with regard to *B. canis* and *B. ovis* as far as their dynamics and importance at the wildlife/livestock/human interface. The traditional and current classification of *Brucella* species is largely based on its preferred host, pathogenicity, and phenotypic laboratory tests (biotyping) [11]. Bovine brucellosis is caused by *B. abortus* (8 biovars), which principally affects cattle and other Bovidae, e.g., African buffalo and grater kudu. *B. abortus* biovar (bv.) 1 is the most frequently isolated biotype worldwide and the major cause of brucellosis in cattle. Mainly *B. abortus* bv 1 has been isolated from aborted fetuses and milk from cattle [12] and to a lesser extent *B. abortus* bv 2 in commercial and communal farms in Zimbabwe [12].

B. melitensis (3 biovars) affects goats but can also infect sheep and cattle. *B. melitensis* has a global distribution but does not occur in North America, Australia, and New Zealand. Apart from affecting goats and sheep, it also affects camels (*Camelus dromedarius*), alpacas (*Vicugna pacos*), and llamas (*Lama glama*) [13]. *B. melitensis* is rarely reported in wildlife with a few cases reported in Europe in chamois and ibex in the Alps [13]. This is an area that needs more research since very few studies have been done on the seroprevalence of brucellosis in wild ungulates, which share interface with domestic animals.

The causative agent of brucellosis in swine, hares (*Lepus*), reindeer (*Rangifer tarandus*), and other no primary hosts like dogs, horses, humans, and cattle is *B. suis* [6]. *B. suis* is currently divided into 5 biovars. Biovars 1–3 infect Suidae of which bv. 1 and 3 may cause severe disease in humans and require high biosafety laboratory precautions. *B. suis* bv. 4 infects reindeers and caribous (*R. tarandus*) throughout the Arctic region and can be transmitted to cattle, Canidae, and occasionally to humans [13], whereas *B. suis* bv. 5 has been reported from rodents. *B. abortus* and *B. suis* have also been isolated worldwide from variety of wildlife species, namely, African buffalo, eland, wild boar (*Sus scrofa*), and water buck [13]. In South American countries, *B suis* biovar 1 has become established in cattle, and in some areas, cattle are now more important than pigs as source of human infections. In sub-Saharan TFCAs, little work has been done on brucellosis in wild pigs and warthogs. Information is not available on the dynamics of the epidemiology of brucellosis in a scenario where wild pigs and warthogs are infected with *B. suis* and interact with other wildlife especially other bovines.

3. Epidemiology of brucellosis at the interface

Areas with high population density result in increased infections in humans, while transmission from livestock to humans is more likely in areas with high human and herd/farm density, especially where humans and livestock live in close proximity, as is often the case in developing countries [1]. The discovery of strains in marine animals has increased the complexity of interactions between humans and other animals due to the fact that each type of species discovered has distinctive epidemiological features. This overall affects the epidemiology of brucellosis. The epidemiology of brucellosis is influenced by several factors, such as livestock production type, herd size, interaction with wildlife, ecological, and socioeconomic factors [14]. A lot of work done indicated that density, herd size, age of cow, reduced veterinary services like vaccination programs, and geographical area are associated with high *Brucella* prevalence. Seroprevalence studies in developing countries indicated that the disease is more prominent in the commercial than communal farming sector. In cases where commercial farms share an interface with wildlife, there is usually physical barrier to separate cattle and wildlife. In cases of communal farms, there is usually no physical barrier and animals share grazing space, thereby facilitating the transmission of *Brucella* pathogens. The dissemination of *Brucella*

http://dx.doi.org/10.5772/61212

can be by direct or indirect contact with infectious animals. The major source of exposure to *B. abortus* is the infected cattle. Sheep and goats are mainly infected by *B. melitensis* through aborted fetuses, placenta, and post abortion uterine fluid. *Brucella* infection is principally transmitted through contact with fetal membranes, lochia, post parturient discharges, and milk [15]. Milk and vaginal secretions represent important potential routes of animal-to-animal transmission following close contact. Venereal transmissions of brucellosis are common in swine, ovine, and canines (dogs). Most of the *Brucella* organisms are shed by animals in their blood at the early stages of the infection.

Access and consumption of contaminated foods and/or occupational exposure remains the significant source of infection to humans. Infection occurs through the skin (intact or abraded), inhalation, or conjunctiva. The main source of infection for the public is through the ingestion of contaminated dairy product, especially raw milk, in developing countries. The bacteria can also be transmitted in raw or undercooked meat from infected animals. This factor poses a greater threat at TFCAs since communities have access to game meat through illegal means, e.g., poaching. Abortion and infertility are the predominant clinical signs in ruminants [16]

B. suis typically causes chronic inflammatory lesions in the reproductive organs of susceptible animals that may extend to joints and other organs. The most prominent clinical sign is abortion at any stage of gestation [17]. *B. suis* biovar 1 infections have been reported in cattle but have partial induced pathology and no induction of abortion despite the excretion of organisms in the milk [13]. Evidence indicates the transmission of *B. suis* biovar 1 to cattle by feral swine in USA [18]. *B. suis* infection in wild boars is of widespread occurrence but with a generally low prevalence, while in domestic pigs, it is considered as a reemerging disease in some countries as a consequence of spillover from wild boars to outdoor-reared pigs.

Studies in the mid-1990s found *Brucella* antibodies in sera of Zimbabwean wildlife in national parks, hunting areas, and game ranches collected in 2009–2011. In most of the wildlife studies, African buffalo is found to have the highest seroprevalence, followed by eland, and impala had the lowest seroprevalence. Studies by Gomo et al. (2011) established low prevalence in giraffe. Studies in the United States of America found out that of the 86 avian, ruminant, swine, poultry, and lagomorph diseases that are reportable to the World Organization for Animal Health (OIE), 53 are present in the United States; 42 (79%) of these have a putative wildlife component associated with the transmission, maintenance, or life cycle of the pathogen; and 21 (40%) are known to be zoonotic [1]. Brucellosis has a wildlife reservoir that is a recognized impediment to eradication in domestic populations [1]. A recent example of effects of changes of the ecology at the interface is the transmission and introduction of bovine brucellosis from livestock to native wood bison (*Bison bison athabascae*) populations in Canada, which has created a conservation challenge for the species. Another well-publicized example is the introduction of brucellosis into native bison and elk populations of the Yellowstone ecosystem in 1917 [19]. This resulted in a wildlife management challenge due to conflicts between livestock and bison. Spillover events from livestock into wildlife impact conservation of species of concern. Transmission between livestock and wildlife is more likely to occur if the animal population density is high and if livestock and wildlife are allowed to come into contact, as in free-range systems. Characterization of the environmental conditions associated with disease and disease outbreaks is an important part to the understanding for the epidemiology of brucellosis in wildlife. A very good example will be that of bison. They calve with other herd members in close proximity, and calving events attract the attention of other cows and calves, with licking and sniffing of the fetal membranes and neonate around parturition. This behavior is especially marked early in the calving season and diminishes later after most animals have calved. This behavior has contributed significantly in the spread of brucellosis in bison populations and explains the maintenance host role of bison. In the elk, it is a different scenario because they usually calve in seclusion, consume the placenta, and clean the calves soon after birth. Elks keep the calf isolated from the herd for several days or weeks following parturition. This behavior explains the absence of brucellosis in most elk populations in North America [1].

4. Brucellosis in human at the interface

About 58% of the infectious diseases of humans are estimated to be zoonoses, and they comprise almost three-quarters of emerging infectious diseases [1]. Brucellosis is directly and indirectly transmitted from animals to humans. Human-to-human transmissions are rare, and small ruminants are the main reservoir for human cases. Humans can be infected directly by contact with the conjunctival or oronasal mucosae of infected animals, or indirectly by the ingestion of contaminated animal products (mainly dairy products) [16]. Naturally acquired brucellosis in humans almost always comes from the animal reservoirs, although very few cases of human to human transmission have been reported [11]. Brucellosis is considered an occupational disease of adults, but there are now several reports of childhood brucellosis in literature [20]. Human brucellosis is predominantly an occupational disease; professions in direct contact with livestock (farmers, butchers, veterinarians, laboratory personnel, etc.) are those at higher risk. In humans, both acute and chronic forms of the disease with variable clinical manifestations were found. Disease can occur at any age and affect any organ system [21].

Low reporting figures and lack of resources have resulted in the global incidence of human brucellosis not being accurately recorded. Hence, great variations exist between different geographic areas even within the same country. Although the reported incidence in most developed countries where infection is present is generally smaller than 1 case per 100,000 inhabitants, in endemic areas, such as some Arab countries, reports reach up to 200 cases per 100,000 inhabitants. However, because of the deficiencies in health services of many countries where brucellosis is endemic, there are no reliable data on the global status of the human disease [16].This is one of the reasons why exact impact of human brucellosis at the interface is not known. At present, there is no fully reliable method of preventing human brucellosis. To safeguard people, attention has been directed toward effectively controlling the disease in animals especially at wildlife/livestock/human interface. Sheep and goats are the main reservoirs of infection for humans; in some countries, bovines, buffalos, yaks (*Bos grunniens*), and camels can also be implicated. Unfortunately, there is a lack of knowledge on the alternatives for controlling *B melitensis* infection in these species. Globally, there is growing recognition that more integrated determinants of health approach will be required to make further gains in managing wildlife diseases like brucellosis, especially those at the wildlife, human, and domestic animal interface [22]. *Brucella has* been isolated from milk and blood (indicating that some animals are bacteremic). It is crucial that public awareness should be strengthened to reduce the risk of human exposure to *Brucella* infection.

5. Preventions and control of brucellosis at the interface

The control of brucellosis shared with wildlife requires the development of strategies that will reduce pathogen transmission between wildlife, both domestic animals and human beings. *B. abortus* is adapted to cattle as its primary host, and control strategies have focused on elimination of the disease from cattle populations. Best available methods to control brucellosis include comprehensive surveillance before and after import testing [23]. The control of brucellosis is usually based on vaccination, serology testing, and culling. These methods are not very successful at the interface due to the complexity of interactions and cost involved. Most framers in developing countries cannot afford the test and slaughter policy in cattle, and the situation will be far worse if it involves wildlife. The eradication of brucellosis in livestock is an expensive and a labor- and diagnostic-intensive process. One of the reasons why many countries have failed to successively eradicate brucellosis is poor animal health management conditions/programs. Brucellosis control strategies in developed and developing countries are based on calf hood vaccination with the S19 vaccine, test, and slaughter techniques. In countries like Zimbabwe, vaccination with S19 was compulsory for commercial herds and optional in the communal areas since the 1980s [14], and this strategy managed to reduce prevalence of brucellosis in cattle. Bovine brucellosis has been successfully eradicated in many developed countries after significant investment and many years of vaccinating and culling. A figure of 500,000 new cases per year is usually accepted as a global estimate [16]. There is a substantial economic burden of brucellosis reflected by the costs of attaining and maintaining disease free status, or the cost of disease in terms of loss of productivity and control costs [24]

In order to improve and succeed, governments need to improve on the quality of the national veterinary services and administrative organizations involved. The prevention and control of brucellosis in sub-Saharan Africa is hampered by low veterinary coverage and use of outdated diagnostic techniques [25]. Furthermore, clinical diagnosis is complicated by variable incubation periods. Testing of livestock is cumbersome when dealing with farms located in remote areas or with animals from nomadic populations and migratory farmers. The identification of genus, species of field isolates, and molecular epidemiology of strains will benefit brucellosis eradication programs [18] since correct vaccination and control management will be possible. Many countries have implemented eradication programs resulting in the reduction or elimination of the disease, but the disease remains enzootic in many regions of the world. In those countries where the disease has been eradicated or strictly controlled, continued surveillance is essential to preventing the reemergence of the disease. Microbial genome typing or DNA fingerprinting is important for the delineation of outbreaks of infectious diseases and for the universal tracing of virulent or multi resistant pathogens [26]. It is now of paramount importance to determine by epidemiological trace-back analysis where the infection originated, how it was spread, and what measures are needed to prevent additional spread of the disease from this primary source. The information will be vital at the interface since it will confirm the source of pathogen; hence, control and prevention efforts will be targeted at source. Knowledge of the spread and prevalence of the infection is essential when planning control measures.

It is generally recognized that the prevention of human brucellosis is best achieved by the control or eradication of the disease in animals, but this strategy is not relevant for protection against a bioterrorist attack on military or civilian populations. A human vaccine could possibly be an effective countermeasure for prevention of naturally occurring or deliberately induced human infections [23]. Currently, three vaccine strains (*B. abortus* S19 and RB51 and *B. melitensis* Rev1) are recommended by the World Organization for Animal Health (Office International des Epizooties [OIE]) for use in the control of brucellosis in livestock [27]. It is generally acknowledged that all of the available brucellosis vaccines are only effective in specific hosts, and cross-protection is not readily achieved [23]. At present, no effective vaccine is available for the protection of swine from brucellosis [28]. The vaccination of sheep is by smooth *B. melitensis* Rev1 vaccine, but it does not provide 100% protection, and it interferes with common serological test use in sheep (rose bengal test (RBT) and complement fixation test (CFT). *B. melitensis* Rev1 is one of the most commonly used attenuated live vaccines against caprine brucellosis and induces high level of protection in goat. Rev1 vaccine has suffered from a lack of coordinated standardization in production methods, leading to considerable variability in efficiency of different preparations [29], and carries resistance to streptomycin, an antibiotic that is therapeutically useful in man. Despite the availability of two smooth live vaccine strains, *B. abortus* S19 for cattle and *B. melitensis* Rev1 for small ruminants, and a further rough attenuated strain, *B. abortus* RB51 for cattle, the search for improved vaccines and vaccine for human continues. Vaccination now has only a small role in the prevention of human disease. *B. abortus* strain 19 still appears to be as effective as the method of prevention of *B. abortus* infection in cattle. The RB51 strain of *B. abortus*, an R mutant used as a live vaccine, has been licensed in some countries, for example, the United States of America. RB51 does not interfere with diagnostic serologic tests, and during laboratory trials, efficacy appeared well compared with that of strain 19 [68]. Currently, *rfb* mutants of *B. melitensis* and *B. suis are* under development for the prevention of ovine/caprine and porcine brucellosis. The current vaccine strains can cause abortion when administered to pregnant animals, and they are virulent. Currently, they are no vaccines for pigs and wildlife and no satisfactory vaccines against human brucellosis.

The control of brucellosis at wildlife/livestock/human interface requires improved collaboration between public health and veterinary services; this can be enhanced through the reinforcement or the establishment of national zoonoses committees, in which the relevant producer and consumer organizations should be also represented. As long as the national veterinary service organization is adequate, the prevalence of disease and economic resources will dictate the approach. Test- and slaughter-based programs are often unfeasible in developing countries because of the economic cost. In addition, countries that have successfully eradicated *B melitensis* offer monetary compensation to affected shepherds, which are not possible in poor resource developing countries. When veterinary service organizations, farmers' involvement, and economic resources are adequate, the final technical elements to select a proper strategy should be the prevalence of disease and the definition of the minimal epidemiologic unit(s) of intervention. A survey should identify the percentage of infected flocks/herds, understanding that differences in prevalence would be expected between different regions placed in the same epidemiologic unit of intervention. Calculating mean prevalence figures for the whole country or particular region considered is a frequent error of decision makers, as those figures may not reflect local conditions. Taking generalist sanitary measures will result in failure of brucellosis control and eradication, but decision makers should apply different strategies adequate to each of the different epidemiologic situations identified. The minimal epidemiologic unit of intervention should be a given territorial extension with similar epidemiologic situation. In some cases, this can be a couple of isolated flocks/herds in a village and in others, the whole flocks/herds of a given county, but frequently, all flocks/herds in a region or country. The implementation of any brucellosis sanitary strategies requires considerable technical training and an awareness campaign aimed at the farmers and general population. Once all these elements have been properly defined, two possible alternatives exist to fight *B melitensis* infection in small ruminants: [1] control based on mass (whole flock/herd) vaccination or [2] eradication based on test and slaughter with or without vaccination. In both cases, the use of adequate vaccination procedures and diagnostic tests is of paramount importance.

Successful disease control may be dependent on accurate detection in wildlife reservoirs, including African buffalo (*S. caffer*). Nishi et al. (2006) stated that it was important to understand the ecologic, socioeconomic, and political factors that affect the wildlife–human–agriculture interface. It is equally important to having technically sound information when developing management plans for disease control. For the sake of public, livestock, and wildlife health, a holistic approach beyond conventional human and veterinary medicine must be taken. This approach must include ecosystem health as well as social/cultural aspects. The success of disease control in wildlife depends on many factors, including disease ecology, natural history, and the characteristics of the pathogen, the availability of suitable diagnostic tools, the characteristics of the domestic and wildlife host(s) and vectors, the geographical spread of the problem, the scale of the control effort, and the attitude of stakeholders. The successful management or eradication of these diseases will require the development of cross-discipline and institutional collaborations. The complex nature of these systems highlights the need to understand the role of wildlife in the epidemiology, transmission, and maintenance of infectious diseases of livestock [1]. Despite social and policy challenges, there remain opportunities to develop new collaborations and new technologies to mitigate the risks posed at the wildlife/livestock interface.[1]. The need to develop comprehensive surveillance systems that integrate livestock, wildlife, and human components has been suggested. Robust surveillance systems in wildlife and at the livestock–wildlife interface to provide early detection of brucellosis or spill over and spillback of pathogens between livestock and wildlife is essential. Diseases that arise from the wildlife/livestock interface are of paramount importance and must be an area of focus for animal health authorities [4].There are many barriers in preventing, detecting, monitoring, and managing brucellosis. These may include political and legal hurdles, lack of knowledge about brucellosis of wildlife, absence of basic data on wildlife populations, difficulties with surveillance, and logistical constraints. Once a pathogen is identified at the wildlife/livestock interface, active management and control of the disease agent is often the only method for reducing impacts to human health, agriculture, and recreational hunting industries [30].

Acknowledgements

This work has been possible thanks to progressive collaboration between Chinhoyi University of Technology and other technical institutions, particularly the Department of Livestock production and Veterinary services, Zimbabwe and CIRAD Zimbabwe.

Author details

Calvin Gomo*

Address all correspondence to: drcalvingomo@yahoo.com

Department of Animal production and Technology, Chinhoyi University of Technology, off Harare-Chirundu road, Chinhoyi, Zimbabwe

References

[1] Miller RS, Farnsworth ML, Malmberg JL. Diseases at the livestock–wildlife interface: status, challenges, and opportunities in the United States. Preventive Veterinary Medicine. 2013;110(2):119–32.

[2] McDermott JJ, Arimi SM. Brucellosis in sub-Saharan Africa: epidemiology, control and impact. Veterinary Microbiology. 2002;90(1–4):111–34.

[3] Caron A, Miguel E, Gomo C, Makaya P, Pfukenyi DM, Foggin C, et al. Relationship between burden of infection in ungulate populations and wildlife/livestock interfaces. Epidemiology and Infection. 2013;141(Special Issue 07):1522–35.

[4] Siembieda JL, Kock RA, McCracken TA, Newman SH. The role of wildlife in transboundary animal diseases. Animal Health Research Reviews. 2011;12(01):95–111.

[5] Moreno E, Cloeckaert A, Moriyon I. *Brucella* evolution and taxonomy. Veterinary Microbiology. 2002;90:209–27.

[6] Whatmore A. Current understanding of the genetic diversity of *Brucella*, an expanding genus of zoonotic pathogens. Infection, Genetics and Evolution. 2009;9:1168–84.

[7] Foster G, Osterman BS, Godfroid J, Jacques I, Cloeckaert A. *Brucella ceti* sp. nov. and *Brucella pinnipedialis* sp. nov. for *Brucella* strains with cetaceans and seals as their preferred hosts. International Journal of Systematic and Evolutionary Microbiology. 2007;57(Pt 11):2688–93.

[8] Scholz H, Hubalek Z, Sedlacek I, Vergnaud G, Tomaso H, Al Dahouk S, et al. *Brucella microti* sp. nov., isolated from the common vole *Microtus arvalis*. International Journal of Systematic and Evolutionary Microbiology. 2008;58:375–82.

[9] Bricker B, Ewalt D, MacMillan A, Foster G, Brew S. Molecular characterization of *Brucella* strains isolated from marine mammals. Journal of Clinical Microbiology. 2000;38:1258–62.

[10] Scholz H, Nockler K, Gollner C, Bahn P, Vergnaud G, Tomaso H, et al. *Brucella inopinata* sp. nov., isolated from a breast implant infection. International Journal of Systematic and Evolutionary Microbiology. 2010;60:801–8.

[11] Godfroid J, Scholz HC, Barbier T, Nicolas C, Wattiau P, Fretin D, et al. Brucellosis at the animal/ecosystem/human interface at the beginning of the 21st century. Preventive Veterinary Medicine. 2011;102(2):118–31.

[12] Matope G, Muma JB, Toft N, Gori E, Lund A, Nielsen K, et al. Evaluation of sensitivity and specificity of RBT, c-ELISA and fluorescence polarisation assay for diagnosis of brucellosis in cattle using latent class analysis. Veterinary Immunology and Immunopathology. 2011;141(1–2):58–63.

[13] Godfroid J, Saegerman C, Wellemans V, Walravens K, Letesson J-J, Tibor A, et al. How to substantiate eradication of bovine brucellosis when aspecific serological reactions occur in the course of brucellosis testing. Veterinary Microbiology. 2002;90(1–4): 461–77.

[14] Matope G, Bhebhe E, Muma JB, Lund A, Skjerve E. Herd-level factors for *Brucella* seropositivity in cattle reared in smallholder dairy farms of Zimbabwe. Preventive Veterinary Medicine. 2010;94(3–4):213–21.

[15] Gorvel J-P. *Brucella*: a Mr "Hide" converted into Dr Jekyll. Microbes and Infection. 2008;10(9):1010–3.

[16] Blasco JM, Molina-Flores B. Control and eradication of *Brucella melitensis* infection in sheep and goats. Veterinary Clinics of North America: Food Animal Practice. 2011;27(1):95–104.

[17] Godfroid J, Cloeckaert A, Liautard J, Kohler S, Fretin D, Walravens K, et al. From the discovery of the Malta fevers agent to the discovery of a marine mammal reservoir, brucellosis has continuously been a re-emerging zoonosis. Veterinary Research. 2005;36:313–26.

[18] Halling S, Tatum F, Bricker B. Sequence and characterization of an insertion sequence, IS711, from *Brucella ovis*. Gene. 1993;133:123–7.

[19] Meagher M, Meyer ME. On the origin of Brucellosis in bison of Yellowstone National Park: a review. Conservation Biology. 1994;8(3):645–53.

[20] Akhvlediani T, Clark D, Chubabria G, Zenaishvili O, Hepburn M. The changing pattern of human brucellosis: clinical manifestations, epidemiology, and treatment outcomes over three decades in Georgia. BMC Infectious Diseases. 2010;10(1):346.

[21] Pappas G, Akritidis N, Bosilkovski M, Tsianos E. Brucellosis. New England Journal of Medicine. 2005;352:2325–36.

[22] Cutler SJ. Bacterial zoonoses: an overview. In: Schwartzman Y-WTSLP, editor. Molecular Medical Microbiology (second edition). Boston: Academic Press; 2015. pp. 1771–80.

[23] Corbel M. Brucellosis: an overview. Emerging Infectious Diseases. 1997;3:213–21.

[24] Whatmore AM. Current understanding of the genetic diversity of *Brucella*, an expanding genus of zoonotic pathogens. Infection, Genetics and Evolution. 2009;9(6): 1168–84.

[25] Muma JB, Munyeme M, Matope G, Siamudaala VM, Munang'andu HM, Matandiko W, et al. *Brucella* seroprevalence of the Kafue lechwe (*Kobus leche kafuensis*) and Black lechwe (*Kobus leche smithemani*): exposure associated to contact with cattle. Preventive Veterinary Medicine. 2011;100(3–4):256–60.

[26] Van Belkum A. High-throughput epidemiologic typing in clinical microbiology. Clinical Microbiology and Infection. 2003;9(2):86–100.

[27] Martins H, Garin-Bastuji B, Lima F, Flor L, Fonseca AP, Boinas F. Reply to letter to the editor by Blasco and Moriyon (2009) concerning the manuscript "Eradication of bovine brucellosis (BB) in the Azores, Portugal—outcome of a 5-year programme (2002–2007) based on test-and-slaughter and RB51 vaccination" by H. Martins et al. (2009). Preventive Veterinary Medicine. 2010;94(1–2):158–62.

[28] Cutler SJ, Whatmore AM, Commander NJ. Brucellosis—new aspects of an old disease. Journal of Applied Microbiology. 2005;98(6):1270–81.

[29] López-Goñi I, García-Yoldi D, Marín CM, de Miguel MJ, Barquero-Calvo E, Guzmán-Verri C, et al. New Bruce-ladder multiplex PCR assay for the biovar typing of *Brucella suis* and the discrimination of *Brucella suis* and *Brucella canis*. Veterinary Microbiology. 2011;154(1–2):152–5.

[30] Gortazar C, Diez-Delgado I, Barasona JA, Vicente J, de la Fuente J, Boadella M. The wild side of disease control at the wildlife–livestock–human interface: a review. Frontiers in Veterinary Science. 2015;1.

Chapter 3

The Interaction Between Brucella and the Host Cell in Phagocytosis

Suk Kim

Additional information is available at the end of the chapter

http://dx.doi.org/10.5772/61463

Abstract

Brucella spp. are facultative intracellular parasitic pathogens that can survive and multiply in professional and nonprofessional phagocytes. These pathogens are responsible for brucellosis, which can cause abortion in domestic animals and undulant fever in humans. *Brucella* spp. can survive in a variety of cells and their virulence and chronic infections are thought to be due to their ability to evade the killing mechanisms within host cells, one of which is the inhibition of phagosome-lysosome fusion. Lipid raft-associated molecules, such as GPI-anchored proteins, GM1 ganglioside, and cholesterol, are selectively integrated into *Brucella*-containing macropinosomes following the internalization of *Brucella* into macrophages, continuously sustaining a dynamic state of the phagosomal membrane. Toll-like receptors (TLRs) are important systems that detect microbial invasion via recognition of microbial components that triggers signaling pathways to promote the expression of genes and regulate innate immune responses. Recent several studies have revealed the importance between TLRs-*Brucella* interactions to control *Brucella* infection. Here, we reviewed selected aspects of lipid raft-associated molecules and TLRs-*Brucella* interaction, which may help to understand the mechanism of *Brucella* pathogenesis.

Keywords: *Brucella*, phagocytes, lipid-rafts associated molecules, TLRs, intracellular survival

1. Introduction

Brucellosis is a major zoonotic disease worldwide that causes a serious debilitating disorder in humans known as undulant fever, and abortion and sterility in domestic animals.

Brucella spp. are gram-negative and facultative intracellular bacteria that can survive and replicate within professional and nonprofessional phagocytes [1, 2]. Six well-recognized species of *Brucella* are known according to host preference: *B. melitensis* (sheep and goats), *B. abortus* (cattle), *B. suis* (hogs), *B. ovis* (sheep), *B. canis* (dogs), and *B. neotomae* (wood rats) [3]. In the past few years, *Brucella* has been recovered from several marine mammals, including cetaceans and pinnipeds, that belong to two potential new species, *B. pinnipedialis* and *B. ceti* [4]. Recently, a new species of *Brucella, B. microti,* was isolated from wild common voles suffering from a systemic disease [5, 6]. *B. melitensis, B. abortus,* and *B. suis* strains cause abortion and infertility in their natural hosts, goats and sheep, cattle and swine, respectively. Humans can also acquire Brucellosis in a form of a severe, debilitating febrile illness as a result of contact with infected animals or their products [7]. *B. ovis* is a natural pathogen of sheep where it primarily causes epididymitis and infertility in rams [8].

B. canis infection causes abortion and infertility in dogs [9]. Although *B. ovis* and *B. canis* are important in animals, human infection with *B. canis* is rare [10], and human infection with *B. ovis* has not been reported. *B. neotomae,* which infects only desert wood rats, is not known to be associated with clinical disease in any host species.

Brucella species, in contrast to other intracellular pathogens, do not produce exotoxins, antiphagocytic capsules or thick cell walls, resistance forms, or fimbriae and do not show antigenic variation [11]. The key aspect of the virulence of *Brucella* is thought to be due to their ability to avoid the killing mechanisms within macrophages [12, 13].

The most common points of entry of *Brucella* are the respiratory, digestive, and genital tracts of both animals and humans. *Brucella* enters the phagocytic cells in an unknown cellular site and spreads throughout the body by the regional lymph nodes. *Brucella* shows high tropism in macrophages, especially monocytes in the liver, spleen, mammary glands, and reproductive tracts. Chronic brucellosis mainly leads to bacterial resistance to host immune response and host debilitated health status [14].

A tenth of the total *Brucella* will survive to avoid phagocytosis and penetrate cell membrane for intracellular growth; macrophages are the most important for a successful infection. During the infection, *Brucella* can interfere with the macrophage function, particularly the inhibition of IFN-γ [15] and TNF-α expression [16], and the reduction of antigen presentation and subsequent T cell activation [17]. *Brucella* inside dendritic cells (DC) contributes to the chronic infection and induced low levels of pro-inflammatory cytokines and increased MHC II expression [18]. Placental trophoblasts produce erythritol during the last trimester and increases carbon source for *Brucella* and this pathogen caused abortion or stillbirth of the infected fetus by inducing placental damage [19] and targeting giant trophoblasts [20]. *Brucella* has also been reported in other cell types and are studied with cell models and lines such as human pulmonary epithelial cells, caprine uterine epithelial cells, human osteoblastic cell lines, murine neurons, bovine and human polymorphonuclear, and many other cells lines. Surprisingly, extracellular brucellae were observed on the 21st day post infection [21–26].

Phagocytosis is a critical step for a successful immune reaction against microbial pathogens that provokes both degradation of pathogens and the subsequent presentation of pathogen peptide antigens. Ligation of various phagocytic receptors, including Fc gamma receptors and complement receptor 3, activates a series of intracellular signal transductions that induce dynamic and rapid rearrangement of the actin cytoskeleton essential for phagocytic uptake [27]. Several host cells such as M cells, macrophages, and neutrophils ingest *Brucella* by zipper-like phagocytosis [28]. In addition, *Brucella* invades macrophages through lipid raft microdomains [29]. Phagocytosis of *Brucella* in both epithelial cells and macrophages requires F-actin polymerization [30, 31].

Toll-like receptors (TLRs) are the best characterized pattern recognition receptors (PRRs) of host cells. Receptor-ligand interaction via TLRs leads to the production of antimicrobial peptides and proinflammatory cytokines through NF-κB, mitogen-activated protein kinase (MAPK), and other various signaling pathways [32]. As a result, TLR signaling is crucial to develop host innate immune response, including recruitment of DCs and T effector cells, upregulation of MHC I and II on antigen presenting cells (APCs), and extension of adaptive immunity against infection. In Brucellosis, many studies have reported that TLRs play important roles in controlling *Brucella* infection. When unopsonized *B. melitensis, B. abortus,* and *B. suis* strains internalize into macrophages and epithelial cells, the *Brucella*-containing vacuoles (BCVs) enter into an intracellular trafficking pathway that results in the development of specialized membrane-bound compartments [33–38] known as replicative phagosomes or brucellosomes [39]. Interactions between the O-chain of *Brucella* smooth LPS and the lipid rafts on the surface of macrophages have been shown to be important for mediating entry into host cells in a manner that leads to the development of replicative phagosome [40]. During the initial stages of intracellular trafficking of the BCVs, these compartments suffer temporary interactions with lysosomes [41] which results in their acidification [34, 42] and initiate extensive interaction with the endoplasmic reticulum [33]. Eventually, intracellular pH rises to a level that allows intracellular replication of the *Brucella*. In epithelial cells, the BCVs during development of the replicative phagosome acquire properties resembling autophagosomes [37], which does not appear to be the case in macrophages [33]. Studies employing the human monocytic cell line THP-1 and *B. abortus* strains opsonized with hyperimmune IgG have also shown that when the *Brucella* internalizes host macrophages in this manner, the resulting BCVs also undergo temporary association with the lysosomal compartment and become acidified but do not interact extensively with the ER [43]. This altered intracellular trafficking limits the fusion of the BCVs with lysosomes, which minimizes the exposure of these bacteria to the bactericidal proteins that reside in these intracellular compartments [43].

In this section, we will discuss the key roles of several receptors for *Brucella* including immune response, signal transduction cascade, and phagocytic pathway for *Brucella* infection within host cells.

2. The roles of lipid rafts on Brucella infection

Brucella proliferates within professional and nonprofessional phagocytic host cells including macrophages, epitheloid HeLa cells, fibroblasts NIH3T3, Vero cells, MDBK cells, etc., and successfully bypasses the bactericidal effects of phagocytes [13]. The macrophage response to infection has important consequences for both the survival of phagocytized bacteria and the further development of host immunity. For many bacterial pathogens, adherence to the host tissue is believed to be essential for virulence, and the microbial characteristics that promote adherence to receptors on a host cell surface are considered to be attributes of virulence [44]. For intracellular pathogens, including *Brucella*, the nature of the interaction with the host cell will have important consequences for pathogen survival, proliferation, and dissemination, as well as the development of specific immunity [45]. Lipid rafts are specialized membrane microdomains rich in cholesterol, glycosylphosphatidylinositol (GPI)-anchored proteins, and GM1 gangliosides [46]. Evidence regarding the potential role of lipid rafts in host-pathogen interactions has been continuously accumulated, and lipid rafts have been implicated as portals of entry for intracellular pathogens [47]. Several studies have implicated the involvement of lipid rafts in the entry and endocytic pathway of *B. abortus* in host cells. These studies indicated that lipid raft-associated molecules, such as GPI-anchored proteins, GM1 ganglioside, and cholesterol, are selectively integrated into *Brucella*-containing macropinosomes following the internalization of *Brucella* into macrophages, continuously sustaining a dynamic state of the phagosomal membrane [48]. Moreover, the internalization route of *Brucella* into phagocytic cells determines the intracellular fate of these bacteria, and this event is modulated by lipid rafts [48].

2.1. Roles of lipid rafts-associated molecules in Brucella infection

Time-lapse videomicroscopy has been used to follow the internalization of *B. abortus* strains by mouse bone marrow-derived macrophages [35]. After contact of macrophages with wild-type *B. abortus*, the bacteria move around from the site of initial contact and swim on the macrophage surface, which often lasts up to several minutes; ruffling of the generalized plasma membrane occurs before the eventual enclosure in large vacuoles. In contrast, contact of the virB4 mutant of *B. abortus* with the target macrophage results in a much smaller ruffling restricted to the area near the bacteria and uptake is more rapid than for the wild-type strain. If the bacteria are deposited onto macrophages by centrifugation, generalized actin polymerization around the site of bacterial binding was observed in the wild-type strain when stained with phalloidin to detect actin filament formation by using fluorescence microscopy, which can also be observed by phase-contrast microscopy and the virB4 mutant shows primarily small regions of phalloidin staining at the sites of binding. Therefore, *B. abortus* appears to promote events on the macrophage cell surface that are dependent on the presence of the VirB system. In case of *B. abortus*, macropinocytosis occurs within minutes of attachment to bacteria on the surface of the macrophage. During bacterial contact, effector molecule(s) are translocated by the VirB system to the target cell, which initiates the process that leads to formation of the macropinosome [29, 35]. These macropinosomes are induced transiently and shrink rapidly, with the majority of vacuoles appearing tightly apposed against the bacterial surface within 20 minutes after their initial appearance. In addition, macropinosomes are probed with other components associated with lipid raft-associated molecules, such as GM1 gangliosides and cholesterol, by incubating *B. abortus* and biotin-labeled cholera toxin B subunit (CTB), which binds GM1-gangliosides, simultaneously with macrophages. CTB localizes around the

http://dx.doi.org/10.5772/61463

internalized wild-type strain with kinetics of association similar to those for aerolysin-labeled GPI-anchored proteins. In contrast, colocalization of CTB with the virB4 mutant was much less pronounced, suggesting that the formation of the VirB-dependent macropinosome includes a sorting process that allows transient association of lipid raft-associated components with macropinosomes containing *B. abortus*.

2.2. Roles of cellular prion protein in Brucella infection

In addition to membrane sorting for brucella infection, key roles have been made in describing bacterial entry where it has been shown that these bacteria penetrate into the macrophage through a particular structure found in eukaryotic cells, lipid rafts, or lipid microdomains [48]. In order to interact with lipid rafts, *Brucella* requires smooth LPS to avoid the bactericidal arsenal of macrophages that strains with rough LPS (without an O-side chain) encounter [40]. Moreover, a report has proposed that *Brucella* interacts with the cellular prion protein of macrophages (Prp^C), a protein anchored by a GPI-link in lipid rafts. This interaction was found to be mediated by the membrane expression of *Brucella* HSP60 [49].

2.3. Roles of clathrin in Brucella infection

Lipid raft-associated clathrin is essential for host-pathogen interactions in infectious processes. The focus of a recent study was to elucidate the clathrin-mediated phagocytic mechanisms of *Brucella* [50]. From that study, the clathrin dependency of *Brucella* infection in HeLa cells was investigated with an infection assay and immunofluorescence microscopy. The redistribution of clathrin in the membrane and phagosomes was detected through sucrose gradient fractions of lipid rafts and the isolation of *Brucella*-containing vacuoles (BCVs), respectively (Fig. 1). Clathrin and dynamin were concentrated into lipid rafts upon *Brucella* infection, and the entry and intracellular survival of *Brucella* were abrogated by clathrin inhibition in HeLa cells. Clathrin disruption decreased actin polymerization and the colocalization of BCVs with clathrin and Rab5 but not LAMP-1. Consequently, our data verified that clathrin plays a fundamental role in the entry and intracellular survival of *Brucella* via the interaction with lipid rafts and actin rearrangement, which determines the early intracellular trafficking of *Brucella* to its advantage.

3. General aspects of toll-like receptors

Toll-like receptors (TLRs) are single-pass type I transmembrane-spanning proteins with a single intracellular Toll/interleukin-1 (IL-1) receptor (TIR) domain and multiple extracellular leucine-rich repeats (LRRs) responsible for binding to ligands that recognize and are activated by a small collection of microbe-derived molecules [51]. Through studies of targeted mutants among 13 paralogous TLRs, 10 in humans and 12 in mice, the diverse mode of ligands recognition of individual TLRs were determined, except for TLR8, TLR10 (only present in humans), and TLR11–13 (only present in mice). TLR2 is activated by lipopeptides and other gram-positive bacterial components in conjunction with either TLR1 or TLR6; TLR4 detects

LPS, which requires accessory protein MD-2; TLR5 detects flagellin; TLR3 detects poly I:C, a double-stranded RNA (dsRNA) analog; TLR9 detects unmethylated DNA and CpG-oligodeoxynucleotides (CpG-DNA) proposed to be delivered by Granulin and high mobility group (HMG) B proteins through an ability to bind simultaneously to both CpG-DNA and TLR9; and TLR7 is activated by single-stranded RNA and its synthetic analogs such as resiquimod, imiquimod, and loxoribine. All known TLR dimer structures display the same arrangement with the two carboxy-terminal tails closely juxtaposed and the amino termini at opposite ends but each varies in modes of ligand recognition [51–54]. This conformation may be required to bring the intracellular TIR domains into close proximity to initiate signaling. TLR activation can induce cell-intrinsic antimicrobial activity such as activation of TLR2 and TLR4 can recruit NADPH oxidase assembly and mitochondria to bacteria-containing phagosome, which lead to a burst of reactive oxygen and nitrogen species within this compartment [55–57]. Evidence suggests that possibly through recruitment of vacuolar-ATPase subunits to the phagosomal membrane, TLR signaling can cause a rapid acidification of the phagosome in which TLR signaling has occurred [53, 54, 58, 59]. These activities increase the antimicrobial capacity of the phagosome, although some bacteria have actually cooped these signals to regulate their virulence programs. Expression and secretion of antimicrobial peptides (AMPs) such as β-defensins and cathelicidin can also be induced by TLRs upon detection of microbial ligands, which further supports the role of TLR-mediated detection in cell-intrinsic antimicrobial activity [60–62]. However, pathogens have evolved a variety of strategies to avoid TLR signaling such as altering their surface structures, interfering with TLR signaling pathways, and inhibiting, escaping, or subverting phagocytosis [52]. *Brucella* spp. are recognized by TLR2, TLR4, and TLR9, which identifies lipopolysaccharide (LPS), lipoproteins, and bacterial DNA, respectively [63].

3.1. TLRs and Brucella infection

The involvement of TLR2 and TLR4 in recognizing *Brucella* was reported in several studies. TLR2 was proposed to induce secretion of TNF-α, IL-6, IL-12, and IL-10 in peritoneal macrophages stimulated by *B. abortus* lipoproteins, such as Omp16 and Omp19 [64], responsible for pro-inflammatory response, but no role was observed in controlling the pathogen in vivo [63]. TLR4, in cooperation with TLR9, was demonstrated in *B. melitensis* resistance [65]. The interaction of TLR4 with non-canonical *Brucella* LPS induces activation of NF-κB, and its interaction with *Brucella* spp. lumazine synthase stimulates maturation of dendritic cells [66] followed by increased expression of co-stimulatory molecules and major histocompatibility class II, as well as the production of IL-6, TNF-α, and IL-12p70 [63].

Maturation of dendritic cells and production of IL-12 and TNF-α in macrophages and dentritic cells are impaired [67], and levels of inflammatory chemokines RANTES (CCL5), MCP-1 (CCL2) and MIP-1α (CCL) are reduced in the absence of MyD88 protein during *Brucella* infection [65]. MyD88 molecule is required for the development of IFN-γ producing T cells and control of brucellosis [65], suggesting that induction of Th1 response during the infection is regulated by a MyD88-dependent pathway [63]. Furthermore, this molecule is used by other inflammatory signaling pathways that include IL-1 and IL-18 [58]. However, IL-18 was observed to have no role in controlling murine brucellosis [63].

Brucella appears to interfere in TLR signaling by producing inhibitory homologues of Toll/interleukin-1 receptor (TIR) domain, such as *B. abortus* Btp1, which targets TLR2 signaling down-modulating maturation of infected dendritic cells and secretion of pro-inflammatory cytokines [18], and *B. melitensis* TcpB that interacts with MyD88 in vitro impeding TLR2 and TLR4 activation pathway and secretion of pro-inflammatory cytokines [68].

3.2. Roles of individual TLRs in Brucella infection

3.2.1. TLR2

The role of TLR2 in *Brucella* infection remains controversial. Some studies suggest that TLR2 is not required to control *Brucella* infection in the mouse [67, 69, 70]. However, other studies indicate that TLR2 is important for clearance of *Brucella* from the lung following aerosol exposure [71], cytokine production such as TNFα and IL-12 [64, 65, 67, 72, 73], MHC-II expression [74], and down regulation of the type I receptor for the Fc portion of IgG (FcγRI, CD64) [15].

3.2.2. TLR4

The role of TLR4 in *Brucella* infection also remains disputed. Some studies suggest that TLR4 is required to control *Brucella* replication in the mouse [65, 69, 70], others reveal that TLR4 is not involved [67, 75]. Lee et al. [76] reported that TLR4-associated Janus kinase 2 (JAK2) activation in the early cellular signaling events plays an essential role in *B. abortus*-induced phagocytosis by macrophages (Fig. 2), implying the significance of JAK2 in pathogenesis of *Brucella* [65]. TLR2, TLR4, and MyD88 play diverse roles in *Brucella* antigen specific antibody production and antibody class switching [71].

3.3. TLR6

TLR6 is an important component that triggers an innate immune response against *B. abortus*. TLR6 is recruited to the macrophage phagosome and recognizes bacterial peptidoglycan and lipoproteins [77]. TLR6 also plays a role in bacterial diacylated lipopeptides recognition such as MALP2, but is not essential for cytokine production in response to triacylated lipopeptides. TLR6, in cooperation with TLR2, recognizes *Brucella* and further activates NF-κB signaling in vitro and is required for the efficient control of *B. abortus* infection in vivo [78].

3.4. TLR9

TLR9 plays a role in controlling *B. abortus* infection in mice [65, 67]. Furthermore, TLR9 partially mediates the expression of IL-12 by dendritic cells in response to heat-killed *B. abortus* [79]. TLR9 plays a significant role in preventing *B. ovis* replication in vivo, but only MyD88 is required for wild type levels of inflammation [80].

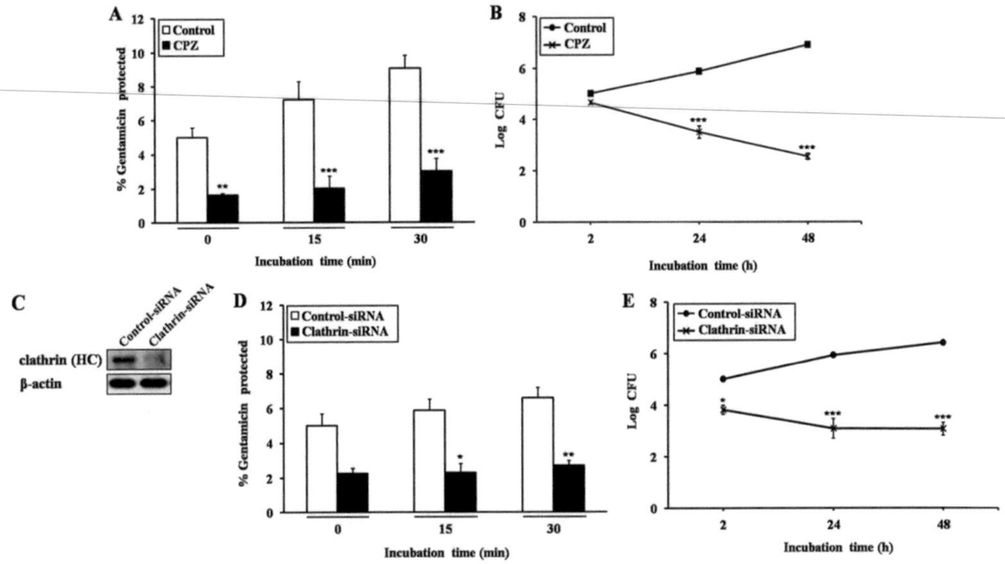

Figure 1. The role of clathrin in the entry and intracellular survival of *B. abortus* in non-professional phagocytes. A and B: HeLa cells were pretreated with 12.5 μM CPZ, a clathrin inhibitor, for 45 minutes prior to infection with *B. abortus* at an MOI of 10 for the indicated times. C–E: HeLa cells were transiently transfected with control or clathrin siRNA, whose optimal conditions were evaluated by Western blotting (C), and subsequently infected according to the procedure described above (D and E). Bacterial internalization and intracellular survival efficiency were determined by evaluating the protection of internalized bacteria from gentamicin killing and calculating the log10 CFU, respectively. The data represent the mean ± S.D. of triplicate trials from three independent experiments. Differences that were statistically significant compared with untreated samples are indicated. *, $p < 0.05$; **, $p < 0.01$; ***, $p < 0.001$ [50].

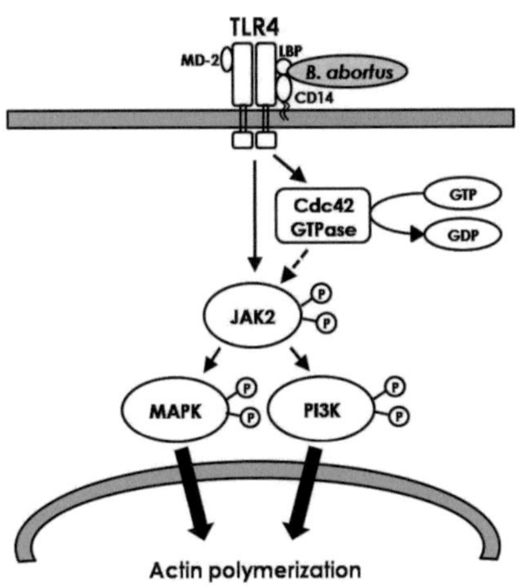

Figure 2. Diagram illustrating the phagocytic signaling pathway initiated by TLR4-linked JAK2 activation during the internalization of *B. abortus* into macrophage. The interaction of *B. abortus* with TLR4 induces the activation of Cdc42 GTPase and JAK2, and the subsequent activation of PI3K and MAPKs promotes actin polymerization. This event contributes to the phagocytosis of *B. abortus* by macrophage. Lines with arrows denote an activating reaction and dotted lines denote uncertainty of the reaction [76].

http://dx.doi.org/10.5772/61463

4. Conclusion

Throughout this chapter, we described the interaction between *Brucella* and lipid rafts-associated molecules and TLRs, including interacting specific molecules (ligands), immune response, signal cascade, and controlling strategies. This review may help to understand the pathogenic and defense mechanisms of Brucellosis. Furthermore, the understanding of lipid rafts-associated molecules and TLRs-mediated controlling of intracellular parasitic bacterial infection would be helpful to eradicate these diseases.

Abbreviation

IFN-γ	Interferon gamma
TNF-α	Tumor necrosis factor alpha
DC	Dendritic cell
MHC II	Major histocompatibility complex
TLR	Toll-like receptor
PRRs	Pattern recognition receptors
NF-κB	Nuclear factor kappa-light-chain-enhancer of activated B cells
MAPK	Mitogen-activated protein kinase
APCs	Antigen-presenting cells
BCVs	*Brucella*-containing vacuoles
LPS	Lipopolysaccharide
IgG	Immunoglobulin
ER	Endoplasmic reticulum
GPI	Glycosylphosphatidylinositol
GM1	Monosialotetrahexosylganglioside
CTB	Cholera toxin B
Prp^C	Cellular prion protein
HSP60	Heat shock protein 60
LAMP-1	Lysosomal-associated membrane protein 1
IL	Intracellular Toll/interleukin
TIR	Intracellular Toll/interleukin receptor
LRRs	Leucine-rich repeats

HMG	High mobility group
NADPH	Nicotinamide adenine dinucleotide phosphate
AMPs	Antimicrobial peptides
Omp	Outer membrane protein
RANTES	Regulated on activation, normal T cell expressed and secreted
MCP-1	Monocyte chemotactic protein 1
MIP-1α	Macrophage inflammatory protein 1 alpha
Th	T helper
JAK2	Janus kinase 2
MALP-2	Macrophage-activating lipopeptide-2

Author details

Suk Kim*

Address all correspondence to: kimsuk@gnu.ac.kr

Institute of Animal Medicine, College of Veterinary Medicine, Gyeongsang National University, Jinju, Republic of Korea

References

[1] Detilleux PG, Deyoe BL, Cheville NF. Entry and intracellular localization of *Brucella* spp. in Vero cells: Fluorescence and electron microscopy. Vet Pathol. 1990; 27: 317-328.

[2] Detilleux PG, Deyoe BL, Cheville NF. Penetration and intracellular growth of *Brucella abortus* in nonphagocytic cells in vitro. Infect Immun. 1990; 58: 2320-2328.

[3] Ko J, Splitter GA. Molecular host-pathogen interaction in brucellosis: Current understanding and future approaches to vaccine development for mice and humans. Clin Microbiol Rev. 2003; 16: 65-78.

[4] Foster G, Osterman BS, Godfroid J, Jacques I, Cloeckaert A. *Brucella ceti* sp. nov. and *Brucella pinnipedialis* sp. nov. for *Brucella* strains with cetaceans and seals as their preferred hosts. Int J Syst Evol Microbiol. 2007; 57: 2688-2693.

[5] Hubalek Z, Scholz HC, Sedlacek I, Melzer F, Sanogo YO, Nesvadbova J. Brucellosis of the common vole (Microtus arvalis). Vector Borne Zoonotic Dis. 2007; 7: 679-687.

[6] Scholz HC, Hubalek Z, Sedlacek I, Vergnaud G, Tomaso H, Al Dahouk S, Melzer F, Kampfer P, Neubauer H, Cloeckaert A, Maquart M, Zygmunt MS, Whatmore AM, Falsen E, Bahn P, Gollner C, Pfeffer M, Huber B, Busse HJ, Nockler K. *Brucella microti* sp. nov., isolated from the common vole *Microtus arvalis*. Int J Syst Evol Microbiol. 2008; 58: 375-382.

[7] Pappas G, Papadimitriou P, Akritidis N, Christou L, Tsianos EV. The new global map of human brucellosis. Lancet Infect Dis. 2006; 6: 91-99.

[8] Buckrell BC, McEwen SA, Johnson WH, Savage NC. Epididymitis Caused by *Brucella ovis* in a Southern Ontario Sheep Flock. Can Vet J. 1985; 26: 293-296.

[9] Wanke MM. Canine brucellosis. Anim Reprod Sci. 2004; 82: 195-207.

[10] Corbel MJ. Brucellosis: An overview. Emerg Infect Dis. 1997; 3: 213-221.

[11] Finlay BB, Falkow S. Common themes in microbial pathogenicity revisited. Microbiol Mol Biol Rev. 1997; 61: 136-169.

[12] Sangari FJ, Aguero J. Molecular basis of *Brucella* pathogenicity: An update. Microbiologia. 1996; 12: 207-218.

[13] Ugalde RA. Intracellular lifestyle of *Brucella* spp. Common genes with other animal pathogens, plant pathogens, and endosymbionts. Microbes Infect. 1999; 1: 1211-1219.

[14] Martirosyan A, Moreno E, Gorvel JP. An evolutionary strategy for a stealthy intracellular *Brucella* pathogen. Immunol Rev. 2011; 240: 211-234.

[15] Barrionuevo P, Delpino MV, Velasquez LN, Garcia Samartino C, Coria LM, Ibanez AE, Rodriguez ME, Cassataro J, Giambartolomei GH. *Brucella abortus* inhibits IFN-gamma-induced Fc gamma RI expression and Fc gamma RI-restricted phagocytosis via toll-like receptor 2 on human monocytes/macrophages. Microbes Infect. 2011; 13: 239-250.

[16] Caron E, Gross A, Liautard JP, Dornand J. *Brucella* species release a specific, protease-sensitive, inhibitor of TNF-alpha expression, active on human macrophage-like cells. J Immunol. 1996; 156: 2885-2893.

[17] Forestier C, Deleuil F, Lapaque N, Moreno E, Gorvel JP. *Brucella abortus* lipopolysaccharide in murine peritoneal macrophages acts as a down-regulator of T cell activation. J Immunol. 2000; 165: 5202-5210.

[18] Salcedo SP, Marchesini MI, Lelouard H, Fugier E, Jolly G, Balor S, Muller A, Lapaque N, Demaria O, Alexopoulou L, Comerci DJ, Ugalde RA, Pierre P, Gorvel JP. *Brucella* control of dendritic cell maturation is dependent on the TIR-containing protein Btp1. PLoS Pathog. 2008; 4: e21.

[19] Tobias L, Cordes DO, Schurig GG. Placental pathology of the pregnant mouse inoculated with *Brucella abortus* strain 2308. Vet Pathol. 1993; 30: 119-129.

[20] Kim S, Lee DS, Watanabe K, Furuoka H, Suzuki H, Watarai M. Interferon-gamma promotes abortion due to *Brucella* infection in pregnant mice. BMC Microbiol. 2005; 5: 22.

[21] Ferrero MC, Fossati CA, Baldi PC. Smooth *Brucella* strains invade and replicate in human lung epithelial cells without inducing cell death. Microbes Infect. 2009; 11: 476-483.

[22] Meador VP, Hagemoser WA, Deyoe BL. Histopathologic findings in *Brucella abortus*-infected, pregnant goats. Am J Vet Res. 1988; 49: 274-280.

[23] Delpino MV, Fossati CA, Baldi PC. Proinflammatory response of human osteoblastic cell lines and osteoblast-monocyte interaction upon infection with *Brucella* spp. Infect Immun. 2009; 77: 984-995.

[24] Garcia Samartino C, Delpino MV, Pott Godoy C, Di Genaro MS, Pasquevich KA, Zwerdling A, Barrionuevo P, Mathieu P, Cassataro J, Pitossi F, Giambartolomei GH. *Brucella abortus* induces the secretion of proinflammatory mediators from glial cells leading to astrocyte apoptosis. Am J Pathol. 2010; 176: 1323-1338.

[25] Iyankan L, Singh DK. The effect of *Brucella abortus* on hydrogen peroxide and nitric oxide production by bovine polymorphonuclear cells. Vet Res Commun. 2002; 26: 93-102.

[26] Rolan HG, Xavier MN, Santos RL, Tsolis RM. Natural antibody contributes to host defense against an attenuated *Brucella abortus* virB mutant. Infect Immun. 2009; 77: 3004-3013.

[27] Gruenheid S, Finlay BB. Microbial pathogenesis and cytoskeletal function. Nature. 2003; 422: 775-781.

[28] Ackermann MR, Cheville NF, Deyoe BL. Bovine ileal dome lymphoepithelial cells: Endocytosis and transport of *Brucella abortus* strain 19. Vet Pathol. 1998; 25: 28-35.

[29] Watarai M, Makino S, Fujii Y, Okamoto K, Shirahata T. Modulation of *Brucella*-induced macropinocytosis by lipid rafts mediates intracellular replication. Cell Microbiol. 2002; 4: 341-355.

[30] Guzman-Verri C, Chaves-Olarte E, von Eichel-Streiber C, Lopez-Goni I, Thelestam M, Arvidson S, Gorvel JP, Moreno E. GTPases of the Rho subfamily are required for *Brucella abortus* internalization in nonprofessional phagocytes: Direct activation of Cdc42. J Biol Chem. 2001; 276: 44435-44443.

[31] Kusumawati A, Cazevieille C, Porte F, Bettache S, Liautard JP, Sri Widada J. Early events and implication of F-actin and annexin I associated structures in the phagocyt-

ic uptake of *Brucella suis* by the J-774A.1 murine cell line and human monocytes. Microb Pathog. 2003; 28: 343-352.

[32] Kawai T, Akira S. TLR signaling. Cell Death Differ. 2006; 13: 816-825.

[33] Celli J, de Chastellier C, Franchini DM, Pizarro-Cerda J, Moreno E, Gorvel JP. *Brucella* evades macrophage killing via VirB-dependent sustained interactions with the endoplasmic reticulum. J Exp Med. 2003; 198: 545-556.

[34] Arenas GN, Staskevich AS, Aballay A, Mayorga LS. Intracellular trafficking of *Brucella abortus* in J774 macrophages. Infect Immun. 2000; 68: 4255-4263.

[35] Kim S, Watarai M, Makino S, Shirahata T. Membrane sorting during swimming internalization of *Brucella* is required for phagosome trafficking decisions. Microb Pathog. 2002; 33: 225-237.

[36] Naroeni A, Jouy N, Ouahrani-Bettache S, Liautard JP, Porte F. *Brucella suis*-impaired specific recognition of phagosomes by lysosomes due to phagosomal membrane modifications. Infect Immun. 2001; 69: 486-493.

[37] Pizarro-Cerda J, Meresse S, Parton RG, van der Goot G, Sola-Landa A, Lopez-Goni I, Moreno E, Gorvel JP. *Brucella abortus* transits through the autophagic pathway and replicates in the endoplasmic reticulum of nonprofessional phagocytes. Infect Immun. 1998; 66: 5711-5724.

[38] Rittig MG, Alvarez-Martinez MT, Porte F, Liautard JP, Rouot B. Intracellular survival of *Brucella* spp. in human monocytes involves conventional uptake but special phagosomes. Infect Immun. 2001; 69: 3995-4006.

[39] Kohler S, Michaux-Charachon S, Porte F, Ramuz M, Liautard JP. What is the nature of the replicative niche of a stealthy bug named *Brucella*? Trends Microbiol. 2003; 11: 215-219.

[40] F, Naroeni A, Ouahrani-Bettache S, Liautard JP. Role of the *Brucella suis* lipopolysaccharide O antigen in phagosomal genesis and in inhibition of phagosome-lysosome fusion in murine macrophages. Infect Immun. 2003; 71: 1481-1490.

[41] Starr T, Ng TW, Wehrly TD, Knodler LA, Celli J. *Brucella* intracellular replication requires trafficking through the late endosomal/lysosomal compartment. Traffic 2008; 9: 678-694.

[42] Porte F, Liautard JP, Kohler S. Early acidification of phagosomes containing *Brucella suis* is essential for intracellular survival in murine macrophages. Infect Immun. 1999; 67: 4041-4047.

[43] Bellaire BH, Roop RM, 2nd, Cardelli JA. Opsonized virulent *Brucella abortus* replicates within nonacidic, endoplasmic reticulum-negative, LAMP-1-positive phagosomes in human monocytes. Infect Immun. 2005; 73: 3702-3713.

[44] Casadevall A, Pirofski L. Host-pathogen interactions: The attributes of virulence. J Infec Dis. 2001;1884: 337-344.

[45] Jimenez de Bagues MP, Dudal S, Dornand J, Gross A. Cellular bioterrorism: How *Brucella* corrupts macrophage physiology to promote invasion and proliferation. Clin Immunol. 2005;114: 227-238.

[46] Brown DA, London E. Functions of lipid rafts in biological membranes. Annu Rev Cell Dev Biol. 1998; 14: 111-136

[47] Gatfield J, Pieters J. Essential role for cholesterol in entry of mycobacteria into macrophages. Science 2000; 288: 1647-1650.

[48] Naroeni A, Porte F. Role of cholesterol and the ganglioside GM(1) in entry and short-term survival of *Brucella suis* in murine macrophages. Infect Immun. 2002; 70: 1640-1644.

[49] Watarai M, Kim S, Erdenebaatar J, Makino S, Horiuchi M, Shirahata T, Sakaguchi S, Katamine S. Cellular prion protein promotes *Brucella* infection into macrophages. J Exp Med. 2003; 198: 5-17.

[50] Lee JJ, Kim DG, Kim DH, Simborio HL, Min W, Lee HJ, Her M, Jung SC, Watarai M, Kim S. Interplay between clathrin and Rab5 controls the early phagocytic trafficking and intracellular survival of *Brucella abortus* within HeLa cells. J Biol Chem. 2013; 288: 28049-28057.

[51] Moresco EM, LaVine D, Beutler B. Toll-like receptors. Curr Biol. 2011; 21: 488-493.

[52] Arpaia N, Barton GM. The impact of Toll-like receptors on bacterial virulence strategies. Curr Opin Microbiol. 2013; 16: 17-22.

[53] Blander JM, Medzhitov R. Regulation of phagosome maturation by signals from toll-like receptors. Science 2004; 304: 1014-1018.

[54] Blander JM, Medzhitov R. Toll-dependent selection of microbial antigens for presentation by dendritic cells. Nature. 2006; 440: 808-812.

[55] Lambeth JD. NOX enzymes and the biology of reactive oxygen. Nat Rev Immunol. 2004; 4: 181-189.

[56] Underhill DM, Ozinsky A. Phagocytosis of microbes: Complexity in action. Annu Rev Immunol. 2002; 20: 825-852.

[57] West AP, Brodsky IE, Rahner C, Woo DK, Erdjument-Bromage H, Tempst P, Walsh MC, Choi Y, Shadel GS, Ghosh S. TLR signalling augments macrophage bactericidal activity through mitochondrial ROS. Nature. 2011; 472: 476-480.

[58] Arpaia N, Godec J, Lau L, Sivick KE, McLaughlin LM, Jones MB, Dracheva T, Peterson SN, Monack DM, Barton GM. TLR signaling is required for *Salmonella typhimurium* virulence. Cell. 2011; 144: 675-688.

[59] Trombetta ES, Ebersold M, Garrett W, Pypaert M, Mellman I. Activation of lysosomal function during dendritic cell maturation. Science. 2003; 299: 1400-1403.

[60] Redfern RL, Reins RY, McDermott AM. Toll-like receptor activation modulates antimicrobial peptide expression by ocular surface cells. Exp Eye Res. 2011; 92: 209-220.

[61] Rodriguez-Martinez S, Cancino-Diaz ME, Cancino-Diaz JC. Expression of CRAMP via PGN-TLR-2 and of alpha-defensin-3 via CpG-ODN-TLR-9 in corneal fibroblasts. Br J Ophthalmol. 2006; 90: 378-382.

[62] Tauszig S, Jouanguy E, Hoffmann JA, Imler JL. Toll-related receptors and the control of antimicrobial peptide expression in Drosophila. Proc Natl Acad Sci. 2000; 97: 10520-10525.

[63] Oliveira SC, de Oliveira FS, Macedo GC, de Almeida LA, Carvalho NB. The role of innate immune receptors in the control of *Brucella abortus* infection: Toll-like receptors and beyond. Microbes Infect. 2008; 10: 1005-1009.

[64] Giambartolomei GH, Zwerdling A, Cassataro J, Bruno L, Fossati CA, Philipp MT. Lipoproteins, not lipopolysaccharide, are the key mediators of the proinflammatory response elicited by heat-killed *Brucella abortus*. J Immunol. 2004; 173: 4635-4642.

[65] Macedo GC, Magnani DM, Carvalho NB, Bruna-Romero O, Gazzinelli RT, Oliveira SC. Central role of MyD88-dependent dendritic cell maturation and proinflammatory cytokine production to control *Brucella abortus* infection. J Immunol. 2008; 180: 1080-1087.

[66] Berguer PM, Mundinano J, Piazzon I, Goldbaum FA. A polymeric bacterial protein activates dendritic cells via TLR4. J Immunol. 2006; 176: 2366-2372.

[67] Weiss DS, Takeda K, Akira S, Zychlinsky A, Moreno E. MyD88, but not toll-like receptors 4 and 2, is required for efficient clearance of *Brucella abortus*. Infect Immun. 2005; 73: 5137-5143.

[68] Cirl C, Wieser A, Yadav M, Duerr S, Schubert S, Fischer H, Stappert D, Wantia N, Rodriguez N, Wagner H, Svanborg C, Miethke T. Subversion of Toll-like receptor signaling by a unique family of bacterial Toll/interleukin-1 receptor domain-containing proteins. Nat Med. 2008; 14: 399-406.

[69] Campos MA, Rosinha GM, Almeida IC, Salgueiro XS, Jarvis BW, Splitter GA, Qureshi N, Bruna-Romero O, Gazzinelli RT, Oliveira SC. Role of Toll-like receptor 4 in induction of cell-mediated immunity and resistance to *Brucella abortus* infection in mice. Infect Immun. 2004; 72: 176-186.

[70] Copin R, De Baetselier P, Carlier Y, Letesson JJ, Muraille E. MyD88-dependent activation of B220-CD11b+LY-6C+ dendritic cells during *Brucella melitensis* infection. J Immunol. 2007; 178: 5182-5191.

[71] Pei J, Ding X, Fan Y, Rice-Ficht A, Ficht TA. Toll-like receptors are critical for clearance of *Brucella* and play different roles in development of adaptive immunity following aerosol challenge in mice. Front Cell Infect Microbiol. 2012; 2: 115.

[72] Huang LY, Aliberti J, Leifer CA, Segal DM, Sher A, Golenbock DT, Golding B. Heat-killed *Brucella abortus* induces TNF and IL-12p40 by distinct MyD88-dependent pathways: TNF, unlike IL-12p40 secretion, is Toll-like receptor 2 dependent. J Immunol. 2003; 171: 1441-1446.

[73] Zwerdling A, Delpino MV, Barrionuevo P, Cassataro J, Pasquevich KA, Garcia Samartino C, Fossati CA, Giambartolomei GH. *Brucella* lipoproteins mimic dendritic cell maturation induced by *Brucella abortus*. Microbes Infect. 2008; 10: 1346-1354.

[74] Barrionuevo P, Cassataro J, Delpino MV, Zwerdling A, Pasquevich KA, Garcia Samartino C, Wallach JC, Fossati CA, Giambartolomei GH. *Brucella abortus* inhibits major histocompatibility complex class II expression and antigen processing through interleukin-6 secretion via Toll-like receptor 2. Infect Immun. 2008; 76: 250-262.

[75] Barquero-Calvo E, Chaves-Olarte E, Weiss DS, Guzman-Verri C, Chacon-Diaz C, Rucavado A, Moriyon I, Moreno E. *Brucella abortus* uses a stealthy strategy to avoid activation of the innate immune system during the onset of infection. PLoS One 2007; 2: e631.

[76] Lee JJ, Kim DH, Kim DG, Lee HJ, Min W, Rhee MH, Cho JY, Watarai M, Kim S. Toll-like receptor 4-linked Janus kinase 2 signaling contributes to internalization of *Brucella abortus* by macrophages. Infect Immun. 2013; 81:2448-2458.

[77] Ozinsky A, Underhill DM, Fontenot JD, Hajjar AM, Smith KD, Wilson CB, Schroeder L, Aderem A. The repertoire for pattern recognition of pathogens by the innate immune system is defined by cooperation between toll-like receptors. Proc Natl Acad Sci. 2000; 97:13766-13771.

[78] de Almeida LA, Macedo GC, Marinho FA, Gomes MT, Corsetti PP, Silva AM, Cassataro J, Giambartolomei GH, Oliveira SC. Toll-like receptor 6 plays an important role in host innate resistance to *Brucella abortus* infection in mice. Infect Immun. 2013; 81:1654-1662.

[79] Huang LY, Ishii KJ, Akira S, Aliberti J, Golding B. Th1-like cytokine induction by heat-killed *Brucella abortus* is dependent on triggering of TLR9. J Immunol. 2005; 175: 3964-3970.

[80] Vieira AL, Silva TM, Mol JP, Oliveira SC, Santos RL, Paixao TA. MyD88 and TLR9 are required for early control of Brucella ovis infection in mice. Res Vet Sci. 2013; 94: 399-405.

Chapter 4

Brucella-induced Thrombocytopenia and Bleeding

Ali Akbar Heydari

Additional information is available at the end of the chapter

http://dx.doi.org/10.5772/61134

Abstract

Mild anemia and leukopenia are the most common hematologic problems of acute brucellosis. Mild thrombocytopenia also occurs, but severe cases are uncommon. Thrombocytopenia occurs because of bone marrow suppression, hypersplenisem, hemophagocytosis, and immunologic destruction of the cells or disseminated intravascular coagulation. In endemic areas, hemorrhagic fevers, hematologic malignancies, as well as idiopathic thrombocytopenic purpura should be considered as differential diagnoses for complicated brucellosis. Thrombocytopenia and bleeding can be improved with antibiotic and hematologic supportive therapy whereas in severe cases corticosteroid therapy or splenectomy might be necessary.

Keywords: Brucella, thrombocytopenia, fever, hemorrhage

1. Introduction

Although brucellosis is a treatable and non-severe disease, 5–10% of patients experience some complications [1]. Brucella plays an important role in infectious diseases, and can mimic many other infectious and non-infectious diseases. This mimicry can result in delayed diagnosis and increased mortality and morbidity. Almost all body systems can be affected by brucellosis, including the hematological system.

The most common hematological finding in brucellosis is an unchanged hemogram, including normal counts of platelets, white blood cells, and hemoglobin [2]. Hematological problems may occur and are most common in children with brucella infection, but sometimes occur in adults as well. Several blood disorders have been reported in brucellosis, including hemolytic anemia [3], thrombocytopenia, leukopenia [4], leukocytosis [5], thrombocytosis [6], and pancytopenia [7]. Mild anemia and leukopenia are the most common complications of acute infection. Mild thrombocytopenia also occurs in about 1–26% of the patients, while severe cases are uncommon [4].

Isolated thrombocytopenia or pancytopenia has been rarely reported. Severe thrombocytopenia with pancytopenia imitates hematologic diseases (Figure 1). Thrombocytopenia occurs less than leukopenia in brucellosis. We and others have several published [8–10] and unpublished papers regarding confirmed brucellosis cases presenting with severe hemorrhagic fever mimicking Crimean-Congo Hemorrhagic Fever (CCHF). These patients are usually isolated before an established diagnosis is reached.

Mild thrombocytopenia is more common than the severe form and the incidence of splenomegaly in thrombocytopenic cases is higher than that reported for uncomplicated brucellosis [11]. Thrombocytopenic purpura and microangiopathy may also occur in brucellosis [12, 13]. The latter event may be associated with thrombocytopenia, bleeding, hemolytic anemia, and impaired consciousness. Disseminated intravascular coagulation (DIC) is rarely seen [14]. DIC may occur in the patients suffering from gram-negative sepsis. Bacterial endotoxins activate the coagulation cascade. Microrhrombi are deposited in the wall of the vasculature, resulting in thrombiosis, bleeding, and Microangiopatic Hemolytic Anemia (MAHA). DIC and/or MAHA are rarely reported in association with brucellar endocarditis with the clinical presentation of mild disease to severe bleeding, thrombosis, and death [2].

Hence, brucellosis must be considered in the differential diagnosis of all those conditions leading to diverse hematologic disorders including pancytopenia, hemolytic anemia, leukopenia, thrombocytopenia, and disseminated intravascular coagulation in endemic areas [15, 16].

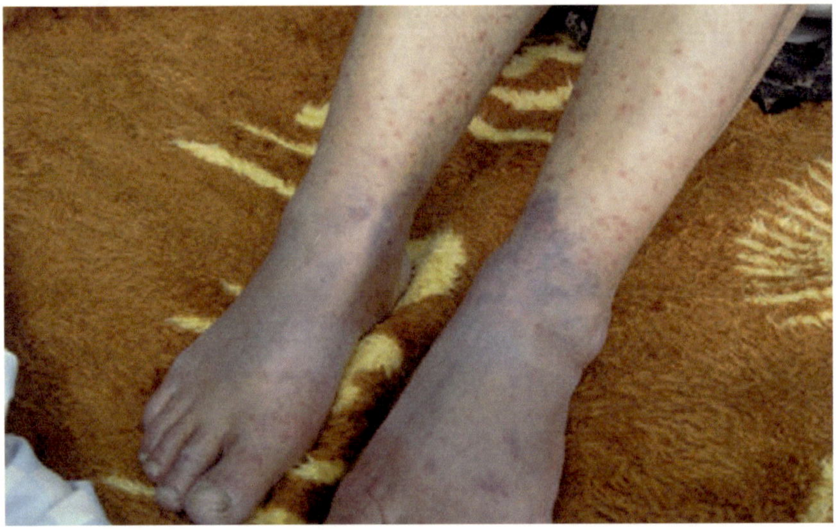

Figure 1. Ecchymosis of the lower limbs in a patient with brucella-induced hemophagocytosis.

The key point in the evaluation of thrombocytopenia is to prepare a peripheral blood smear to assess the morphology of the blood cells and to exclude pseudo-thrombocytopenia, especially in patients with an unexplained low platelet count. The latter condition is attributed to the use of certain anti-coagulants (such as ethylenediamine tetra-acetic) and subsequent platelet agglutination [17].

Although bone marrow smear and culture plays an important role in detecting infectious causes of thrombocytopenia, it is possible to find the etiology of thrombocytopenia with less invasive procedures such as blood smear and culture. In many cases, thrombocytopenia will disappear after antibiotic therapy within a few days. Therefore, in suspected infectious induced thrombocytopenia, there is often no need for bone marrow examination for confirmed diagnosis. It is a well-known fact that thrombocytosis may be a marker of inflammation, but low platelet count can be a significant alarming sign for severe infection and infection-induced immunosuppression [18]. Microbial endotoxin can cause endothelial damage, platelet adhesion and/or its removal from the bloodstream [19].

Thrombocytopenia may occur due to platelet destruction by the immune system. A positive Coombs test in most patients with brucella, response to corticosteroid, and detection of anti-platelet antibodies are the evidence of such mechanism [20].

In general, low platelet count may be due to the production failure in the bone marrow, being trapped in an enlarged spleen, or damaged in the peripheral circulation. Thrombocytopenia due to infectious diseases occurs because of bone marrow suppression, hypersplenism, hemophagocytosis, immunologic destruction of the cells, and DIC [21, 10].

Granuloma formation in the bone marrow is added to the etiologies of thrombocytopenia in brucellosis [22]. In one study [23], bone marrow biopsy revealed hypercellular marrow in 75% and granuloma formation in 41% of the samples. Seventy-five percent of the patients with both thrombocytopenia and hypercellular marrow had splenomegaly, as well. In hemophagocytosis phenomena, active histiocytes play an important role in erythrophagocytosis, leukophagocytosis, and platelet phagocytosis. Hemophagocytosis occurs not only during the course of brucellosis, but also in many infectious and noninfectious diseases including viral, fungal, bacterial, parasitic, malignant, and reumatological diseases [24].

Despite the existence of thrombocytopenia, the bone marrow may be hypercellular with sufficient megakaryocytes or hypocellular [25, 23]. Therefore, bone marrow suppression is not a good explanation for thrombocytopenia. Hence, other etiologies should be considered for this cytopenia. One of the significant causes of thrombocytopenia is stimulated autoimmune phenomena induced by brucella bacteria that may lead to bleeding, purpura, and hemolytic anemia [26]. Moreover, monoclonal hypergammaglobulinemia and cryoglobulinemia are rare complications of brucellosis [27].

Hemorrhagic fevers in endemic areas, hematologic malignancies, as well as idiopathic thrombocytopenic purpura (ITP) should be considered as the differential diagnosis of brucellosis, even if the patient is afebrile at the time of admission [28]. Brucellosis and CCHF are both common in rural areas of endemic regions. They affect farmers and shepherds. Both of these diseases cause fever, rigors, thrombocytopenia, and bleeding, sometimes without other signs and symptoms. However, the main difference is a significant reduction in incidence of Crimean-Congo in the winter due to inactivity of the carrier ticks [29] while brucellosis continues to occur. Severe thrombocytopenia and/or hemorrhage are characteristic clinical features of severe CCHF but they rarely occur in brucellosis. Finally, serologic tests, viral polymerase chain reaction, and obvious contact of CCHF patients with blood and tissues of sick animals or other affected patients, as well as history of tick bite will confirm the diagnosis of CCHF.

In case of brucella induced thrombocytopenia, severe thrombocytopenia and bleeding of the urinary tract, skin, gastrointestinal tract, as well as hemoptysis and hematemesis rarely occur [30]. As mentioned above, hematological changes are mild and subside with anti-brucella treatment, but even severe bleeding can be improved with antibiotic and hematologic supportive therapy [31]. In emergent cases with severe thrombocytopenia and bleeding, a short trial of intravenous immunoglobulin (IVIG) has been recommended to increase platelet count and to control bleeding. In the patients with platelets count of less than 10.000 mm^3, corticosteroid therapy would be effective [4, 32]. However, in rare cases of severe and refractory thrombocytopenia, splenectomy may be helpful [33]. In one study [34], among 19 patients with severe thrombocytopenia, 10 received corticosteroids for less than two months and responded well to the treatment. Seven patients received corticosteroid for more than two months, 4 of them recovered and 3 underwent splenectomy and finally recovered. Two out of 19 patients died.

2. Summary

Brucella induced severe thrombocytopenia and pancytopenia imitates several hematological diseases. Not only infectious disease specialists, but also other experts in other fields such as gynecology, gastroenterology, hematology, ENT, dermatology, and urology should be familiar with brucellosis and its uncommon clinical pictures including bleeding and thrombocytopenia. All physicians should be aware of infectious diseases such as brucellosis and CCHF, which may be presented with severe thrombocytopenia and have to include them in the differential diagnosis of any disorder with thrombocytopenia and bleeding, even in afebrile patients. In these conditions, the patient's occupation and/or a minor fever may provide important clues to the diagnosis of infectious diseases such as brucellosis.

Author details

Ali Akbar Heydari*

Address all correspondence to: heydariaa@mums.ac.ir

Research Center for Infection Control and Hand Hygiene, Imam Reza Hospital, Mashhad University of Medical Sciences, Mashhad, IR, Iran

References

[1] Citak EC, Citak FE, Tanyeri B, Arman D. Hematologic manifestations of brucellosis in children: 5 years experience of an anatolian center. J Pediatr Hematol Oncol. 2010;32:137-140. DOI: 10.1097/MPH.0b013e3181ced382.

[2] Madkour MM. Madkour's brucellosis. 2nd ed. New York: Springer-Verlag; 2001. 33-37 pp.

[3] Eskazan AE, Dal MS, Kaya S, Dal T, Ayyildiz O, Soysal T. Two cases of autoimmune hemolytic anemia secondary to brucellosis: A review of hemolytic disorders in patients with brucellosis. Intern Med. 2014;53:1153-1158.

[4] Guzel Tunccan O, Dizbay M, Senol E, Aki Z, Ozdemir K. Isolated Severe Immune Thrombocytopenia due to Acute Brucellosis. Indian J Hematol Blood Transfus. 2014;30:27-29. DOI: 10.1007/s12288-012-0222-3.

[5] Fanni F, Shahbaznejad L, Pourakbari B, Mahmoudi S, Mamishi S. Clinical manifestations, laboratory findings, and therapeutic regimen in hospitalized children with brucellosis in an Iranian Referral Children Medical Centre. J Health Popul Nutr. 2013;31:218-222.

[6] Sathyanarayanan V, Razak A, Saravu K, Ananthakrishna SB, MukhypranaPrabhu M, Vandana KE. Clinical profile of brucellosis from a tertiary care center in southern India. Asian Pac J Trop Med. 2011;4:397-400. DOI: 10.1016/S1995-7645(11)60111-9.

[7] El-Koumi MA, Afify M, Al-Zahrani SH. A prospective study of brucellosis in children: Relative frequency of pancytopenia. Mediterr J Hematol Infect Dis. 2013;5:e2013011. DOI: 10.4084/MJHID.2013.011.

[8] Heydari AA, Ahmadi F, Sarvghad MR, Safari H, Bajouri A, Saeidpour M. Hemophagocytosis and pulmonary involvement in brucellosis. Int J Infect Dis. 2007;11:89-90.

[9] Metin O, AydinTeke T, GayretliAydin ZG, Kaman A, Oz FN, Bayhan GI, Tanir G. A case of brucellosis mimicking Crimean-Congo hemorrhagic fever. J Infect Public Health. 2015;8:302-304. DOI: 10.1016/j.jiph.2014.09.008.

[10] Al Mousa AI. Epistaxis as the initial manifestation of brucellosis. Int J Health Sci (Qassim). 2008;2:157-162.

[11] Colmenero JD, Reguera JM, Martos F, Sánchez-De-Mora D, Delgado M, Causse M, Martín-Farfán A, Juárez C. Complications associated with Brucellamelitensis infection: A study of 530 cases. Medicine (Baltimore). 1996;75:195-211.

[12] Young EJ, Tarry A, Genta RM, Ayden N, Gotuzzo E. Thrombocytopenic purpura associated with brucellosis: Report of 2 cases and literature review. Clin Infect Dis. 2000;31:904-909.

[13] Altuntas F, Eser B, Sari I, Yildiz O, Cetin M, UnalA. Severe thrombotic microangiopathy associated with brucellosis: Successful treatment with plasmapheresis. Clin Appl Thromb Hemost. 2005;11:105-108.

[14] Turunc T, Demiroglu YZ, Kizilkilic E, Aliskan H, Boga C, Arslan H. A case of disseminated intravascular coagulation caused by Brucella melitensis. J Thromb Thrombolysis. 2008;26:71-73.

[15] Al-Eissa YA, Kambal AM, Al-Nasser MN, Al-Habib SA, Al-Fawaz IM, Al-Zamil FA. Childhood brucellosis: A study of 102 cases. Pediatric Infectious Disease Journal. 1990;9:74-79.

[16] Crosby E, Llosa L, Miro Quesada M, Carrillo C, Gotuzzo E. Hematologic changes in brucellosis. J Infect Dis. 1984;150:419-424.

[17] Schrezenmeier H, Müller H, Gunsilius E, Heimpel H, Seifried E. Anticoagulant-induced pseudothrombocytopenia and pseudoleucocytosis. Thromb Haemost. 1995;73:506-513.

[18] de Stoppelaar SF, van 't Veer C, Claushuis TA, Albersen BJ, Roelofs JJ, van der Poll T. Thrombocytopenia impairs host defense in gram-negative pneumonia-derived sepsis in mice. Blood. 2014;124:3781-3790. DOI: 10.1182/blood-2014-05-573915.

[19] McCuskey RS, Urbaschek R, Urbaschek B. The microcirculation during endotoxemia. Cardiovasc Res. 1996;32:752-763.

[20] Baldane S, Sivgin S, Alkan TS, Kurnaz F, Pala C, Keklik M, Karaman A, Kaynar L. An atypical presentation of brucellosis in a patient with isolated thrombocytopenia complicated with upper gastrointestinal tract bleeding. Case Rep Med. 2012;2012:473784. DOI: 10.1155/2012/473784

[21] Jonathan J. Wilson, Peter B. Neame, John G. Kelton infection-induced thrombocytopenia. Semin Thromb Hemost. 1982;8:217-233. DOI: 10.1055/s-2007-1005053.

[22] García P, Yrivarren JL, Argumans C, Crosby E, Carrillo C, Gotuzzo E. Evaluation of the bone marrow in patients with brucellosis. Clinico-pathological correlation. Enferm Infecc Microbiol Clin. 1990;8:19-24. (See comment in PubMed Commons below)

[23] Demir C, Karahocagil MK, Esen R, Atmaca M, Gönüllü H, Akdeniz H. Bone marrow biopsy findings in brucellosis patients with hematologic abnormalities. Chin Med J (Engl). 2012;125:1871-1876.

[24] George MR. Hemophagocytic lymphohistiocytosis: Review of etiologies and management. J Blood Med. 2014;69-86.

[25] Yildirmak Y, Palanduz A, Telhan L, Arapoglu M, Kayaalp N. Bone marrow hypoplasia during Brucella infection. J Pediatr Hematol Oncol. 2003;25:63-4.

[26] Pappas G, Kitsanou M, Christou L, TsianosE. Immune thrombocytopenia attributed to brucellosis and other mechanisms of Brucella-induced thrombocytopenia. Am J Hematol. 2004;75:139-141.

[27] Yrivarren JL, Lopez LR. Cryoglobulinemia and cutaneous vasculitiesin human brucellosis. J Clin Immunol. 1987;7:471-474.

[28] Sevinc A, Buyukberber N, Camci C, Buyukberber S, Karsligil T. Thrombocytopenia in brucellosis: Case report and literature review. J Natl Med Assoc. 2005;97:290-293.

[29] Köksal I, Yilmaz G, Iskender S, Arslan M, Yavuz I, Aksoy F. The first Crimean-Congo hemorrhagic fever case in the winter season from Turkey. Vatansever ZIntervirology. 2011;54:144-145. DOI: 10.1159/000319432.

[30] Akıncı E, Bodur H, Erbay C, Cevik MA, Erbay A, Colpan A. A case of brucellosis presenting with severe thrombocytopenia. Turk J Hematol. 2003;20:43-45.

[31] Karsen H, Duygu F, Yapıcı K, Baran Aİ, Taskıran H, Binicii̇. Severe thrombocytopenia and hemorrhagic diathesis due to brucellosis. Arch Iran Med. 2012;15:303-306.

[32] Elmas Dal S, Ersoy Y, Ali Erkurt M, Yetkin F, Kuzucu C, Akdogan O. An uncommon case of acute brucellosis presenting with severe thrombocytopenia. Intern Med. 2012;51:3291-3.

[33] Hussein I, Gokul BN, Paul A. Brucellosis associated with thrombocytopenia Saudi Medical Journal. 2000;21:877-879.

[34] Ulloa V, Rojas Otarola J, Gotuzzo E. Púrpura trombocitopénica asociada a brucelosis. Rev Med Hered. 1992;3:87-93.

Chapter 5

Ocular Manifestations of Brucellosis

Ozlem Sahin

Additional information is available at the end of the chapter

http://dx.doi.org/10.5772/61475

Abstract

Brucellosis is considered a zoonotic disease which is still an important health problem in endemic areas such as the Middle East, the Mediterranean, and Asia. Brucellosis is a systemic infection that might affect any organ or system in the body. Ocular involvement has been reported in 21% of brucellosis patients. The most common ocular manifestations of brucellosis were considered as anterior uveitis and choroiditis. The patients with anterior uveitis were reported to be usually in the acute stage and the patients with choroiditis, papilledema, and posterior uveitis were reported to be usually in the chronic stage of the disease. Ocular manifestations of brucellosis might also involve dacryoadenitis, conjunctivitis, episcleritis, scleritis, nummular keratitis, cataract, glaucoma, exudative retinal detachment, maculopathy, and neuro-ophthalmic defects including papilledema, papillitis, and cranial nerve paresis. Optic nerve involvement in brucellosis is considered secondary to meningeal inflammation, and it usually involves both optic nerves. Premacular hemorrhage related to *Brucella* endocarditis was reported as a rare ocular manifestation. Since ocular brucellosis has a wide spectrum of clinical manifestations, the diagnosis is considered to be mainly dependent on positive bacteriological and serological tests. Agglutinations and/or culture has been widely used for diagnosis of brucellosis. *Brucella* agglutination test over 1/160 titer and positive blood culture are considered as diagnostic factors for brucellosis. Early diagnosis and prompt treatment are considered to be effective for preventing blindness from severe ocular damage. Systemic antibiotics including streptomycine, rifampicin, doxycycline along with topical or systemic corticosteroid treatment have been recommended for at least 2 months. The purpose of this chapter is to describe the ocular manifestations of brucellosis, early diagnostic procedures, and treatment with reviewing the literature.

Keywords: brucella, uveitis, optic neuritis, preretinal hemorrhage

1. Introduction

Brucellosis is considered a common zoonotic disease that has been reported to cause more than 500,000 new human cases worldwide annually [1,2]. It is still more prevalent in some parts of the world, especially Middle East countries including Iran, Saudi Arabia, Kuwait, Turkey, the Mediterranean, Mexico, and Central and South America [3-6]. *Brucella melitensis* has been reported as the most common and virulent species in endemic countries [7]. *B. abortus* has been seen mostly in Europe and North America [7]. *B. canis* causes canine brucellosis with intraocular inflammation, and *B.* suis infects domestic pigs [7].

2. Ocular manifestations

Brucellosis has unusual clinical manifestations, and the clinical presentation might vary from asymptomatic infection to a full-blown clinical picture of fever, night sweats, and joint manifestations; rarely, there is hepatic, cardiac, ocular, or central nervous system involvement [8]. Since there is no pathognomonic sign of ocular involvement caused by brucellosis, it remains poorly recognized in areas where brucellosis is endemic [9]. In a large series including 1551 patients with brucellosis from Peru during a period of 26 years, 52 (3.3%) patients have been diagnosed with ocular brucellosis [10]. Both acute and chronic brucellosis have been reported to cause ocular involvement [10]. All the ocular structures might be affected by brucellosis [9,11]. However, the most frequent ocular presentation has been reported as uveitis [12,13]. Uveitis has been reported between 21 and 67% of patients with ocular brucellosis in the previous studies [12-14]. The following presentations of uveitis might be identified: anterior uveitis, including iritis, and iridocyclitis; intermediate uveitis, including pars planitis and vitritis; posterior uveitis, including choroiditis, chorioretinitis, retinitis, and neuroretinitis; and panuveitis, including inflammation of all 3 components of the uveal tract [11-15]. The most frequent presentation of uveitis in ocular brucellosis has been considered as posterior uveitis [16]. Patients with panuveitis had the worst visual prognosis [16,17]. In a case series, 8 of 9 patients with panuveitis were legally blind, including 5 patients with no light perception [17]. In a cohort study from Turkey including 132 patients with brucellosis, anterior uveitis was the most frequent manifestation with a frequency of 41%, followed by choroiditis (32%), panuveitis (9%), papilledema (9%), and retinal hemorrhages (9%) [12]. 41% of the patients with ocular involvement were found in the acute stage and 59% were in the chronic stage of brucellosis [12]. In this study, all the patients with anterior uveitis were reported to be in the acute stage, and all the other patients with choroiditis, papilledema, and retinal hemorrhages were reported to be in the chronic stage of the disease. [12] In another cohort study from Turkey including 147 patients with the diagnosis of brucellosis, 38 patients (26.0%) had ocular manifestations including conjunctivitis in 26 (17.7%), anterior uveitis in 6 (4.1%), posterior uveitis in 1 (0.7%), dacryoadenitis in 2 (1.4%), and episcleritis in 3 (2.1%) of patients [18]. Brucellosis might have unusual ocular manifestations [17,19,20] such as: recurrent episcleritis associated with brucellosis has been reported as a rare occurrence from Turkey and France [19,20]. A rare presentation of brucellosis has also been reported as bilateral optic nerve, right abducent nerve involvement, and endocarditis complicated by right premacular hemorrhage in a 28-year-old white female from Turkey [21]. Bilateral multifocal choroiditis with serous retinal detachment in a patient with *Brucella* infection has been reported from USA considering

Vogt-Koyanagi-Harada (VKH) syndrome, which is characterized by bilateral panuveitis associated with bilateral retinal detachments spontaneously resolving, as differential diagnosis [17].

3. Pathogenesis and diagnosis

The infection was rapidly controlled at the site of inoculation but resulted in a local and systemic dissemination of *Brucella* mainly in the pharyngeal tonsil, local and peripheral lymph nodes, and the spleen [24]. The control of the infection is considered to be associated with the induction of a specific immune response characterized by an increase in IgG producing B-cells, the production of IFN- gamma, and IL-10 by cells from draining parotid, retropharyngeal, and submaxillary lymph nodes, but also from more distant peripheral lymph nodes.[24] IFN-gamma is produced by CD4+, CD8+, and CD4(-)CD8(-) gamma delta(-) cells, and probably contributed to the control of both local and systemic infection [25]. Human brucellosis is diagnosed by clinical criteria, isolation of the causative agent from blood or tissue cultures with a positivity rate of 40-70%, or by using serologic techniques as complementary tools. Rose Bengal Plate Test (RBPT) and serum agglutination test (SAT) are the most widely used serologic tests [26]. The sensitivity of RBPT is considered high, but its specificity is low for testing individuals residing in an endemic area [26]. SAT is used to confirm RBPT results. It has limitations of lack of sensitivity as well as specificity [27-29]. Recently, molecular biology diagnostic techniques have been developed, intending to optimize the etiological confirmation [30]. Polymerase chain reaction (PCR) amplification-based methods are being used effectively in the detection of brucellosis [31]. They are considered safer than culture-based methods for the staff [31]. Intraocular serological tests are used to support the diagnosis of ocular brucellosis [14,32]. The Goldmann-Witmer coefficient, which is the ratio of intraocular to serum IgG production against the *Brucella* organism, is usually determined by analyzing the serum and intraocular fluid agglutinations for *Brucella* [14,33,34]. The diagnosis is usually confirmed with a high *Brucella* agglutination titer in the vitreous specimen [33]. The sensitivity of the Goldmann-Witmer analysis has been reported as 66.7% and the specificity was 100% [14].

4. Differential diagnosis

Ocular involvement of brucellosis should be differentially diagnosed from tuberculosis, syphilis, toxoplasmosis, toxocariasis, sarcoidosis, behcet's disease, Vogt-Koyanagi-Harada syndrome, and multifocal choroiditis [16,17,32]. No pathognomonic sign of ocular involvement of brucellosis has been reported. However, acute form of brucellosis is usually presented as fever, headache, sweating, lower back pain, and organomegaly [9]. Ocular involvement in acute form has been reported usually in the form of bilateral acute anterior uveitis, which might be associated with episcleritis and scleritis [10]. Posterior uveitis followed by panuveitis associated with papillitis and retinal hemorrhages were considered the most common ocular manifestations of chronic brucellosis [10]. Neuro-ophthalmologic signs, including the cranial nerves involved in ocular movements, were also reported to be more common in chronic brucellosis [34].

5. Complications

Ocular brucellosis might lead to blindness from severe ocular damage in patients having late diagnosis and improper treatment. The following complications have been reported: cataracts, glaucoma, maculopathy, vitreal alterations, phthisis bulbi, optic atrophy, neovascular retinal membrane, and tractional retinal detachment [18,32].

6. Treatment

Ophthalmic manifestations of brucellosis are usually treated with both antibiotics and steroids [35]. Cavallarro et al. reported a patient with papilledema due to brucellosis that was treated with sole anti-brucellosis treatment without steroid administration [36]. Abd Elrazak reported a case of bilateral optic neuritis caused by brucellosis that resolved following anti-brucellosis and steroid administration [37]. Sahin et al. reported the resolution of unilatreral papillitis and premacular hemorrhage with antibiotics and intravenous high-dose steroid followed by oral steroid administration for 3 months [21]. The tetracyclines remain the most active and clinically effective antibiotics for the treatment of brucellosis [38]. Doxycycline is now the preferred tetracycline analogue for treating human brucellosis [38]. The use of tetracyclines as monotherapy for human brucellosis is complicated by a relapse rate between 8 and 39% [38]. The high relapse rates are dramatically reduced when doxycycline is combined with other drugs, such as streptomycin (relapse rate 4.5%) or rifampicin (relapse rate 8.4%) [38]. Streptomycin in combination with tetracycline or doxycycline has been the "gold standard" for comparison of other antibiotic regimens for the treatment of human brucellosis [38]. A major drawback to the use of tetracyclines is the permanent staining of teeth in young children [39]. Consequently, tetracyclines are contraindicated for brucellosis in pregnant women and children under 8 years of age [39,40]. In this regard, doxycycline binds less to calcium than do other tetracyclines and may cause dental complications less frequently [41]. Cotrimoxazole is a useful alternative in the treatment of brucellosis when the use of tetracyclines is contraindicated [42,43]. Although, rifampin has been used as monotherapy in brucellosis relapses, and the emergence of rifampin-resistant strains have led to its use primarily in combination with other drugs [38]. Results have been generally disappointing in monotherapy with quinolones, which were used to treat human brucellosis [38]. In a study from Turkey, 21 patients received ofloxacin (200 mg twice daily) for varying periods of time; the relapse rate was 16% [44]. In contrast, a group of patients in Israel treated with ciprofloxacin (750 or 1000 mg twice daily) for 6 weeks had a relapse rate of 66% [45]. Similarly, another study from Turkey reported 12 patients treated with ciprofloxacin (500 mg thrice daily) for 3 to 6 weeks, with a relapse rate of 21% [46]. Consequently, monotherapy of brucellosis with quinolones is not recommended, and they should be used in combination with other antimicrobials [38, 47]. The combination of doxycycline for 6 weeks plus streptomycin for 2 to 3 weeks remains the most frequently used and most effective treatment for human brucellosis [47]. Most authorities consider that gentamicin (5 mg/kg/day) intravenously or intramuscularly as a single injection can be used in place of streptomycin; however, the duration of gentamicin administration is unclear [48]. Although 5- and 7- day regimens of gentamicin have been used, we advise no fewer than 10 days [48]. In summary, many clinicians prefer to administer rifampin (600-900 mg/day orally) for the remainder of the 6 weeks after discontinuing gentamicin, but this regimen has not been studied in comparative trials. The second-choice regimen consists of doxycycline (200 mg/day orally) plus rifampin (600-900 mg/day orally), with both drugs administered for 45 days.

7. Conclusions

Ocular involvement in acute or chronic brucellosis is still prevalent in endemic countries. A wide range of ocular manifestations have been described for brucellosis. However, uveitis and neuro-ophthalmic manifestations are the most common presentations. Diagnosis of ocular brucellosis mainly depends on culture and serology of blood and intraocular fluids. Early diagnosis and prompt treatment might restore the vision in ocular involvement.

Author details

Ozlem Sahin*

Address all correspondence to: ozlem1158@yahoo.com

Dunyagoz Hospital LTD., Department of Ophthalmology/Uveitis, Ankara, Turkey

References

[1] Corbel MJ. Brucellosis: an overview. *Emerg Infect Dis.* 1997;3(2):213-221.

[2] Pappas G, Papadimitriou P, Akritidis N, Christou L, Tsianos EV. The new global map of human brucellosis. *Lancet Infect Dis.* 2006;6(2):91-99.

[3] Ahmed MO, Abouzeed YM, Bennour EM, van Velkinburgh JC. Brucellosis update in Libya and regional prospective. *Pathog Glob Health.* 2015 Feb;109(1):39-40.

[4] Köse Ş, Serin Senger S, Akkoçlu G, Kuzucu L, Ulu Y, Ersan G, Oğuz F. Clinical manifestations, complications, and treatment of brucellosis: evaluation of 72 cases. *Turk J Med Sci.* 2014;44(2):220-3.

[5] Martínez P. Human brucellosis: epidemiological situation in Chile, 2001-2010. *Rev Chilena Infectol*. 2013 Dec;30(6):653-9.

[6] Beheshti S, Rezaian GR, Azad F, Faghiri Z, Taheri F. Seroprevalence of brucellosis and risk factors related to high risk occupational groups in Kazeroon, South of Iran. *Int J Occup Environ Med*. 2010 Apr;1(2):62-8.

[7] Mantur BG, Amarnath SK, Shinde RS. Review of clinical and laboratory features of human brucellosis. *Ind J Med Microbiol*. 2007 Jul;25(3):188-202.

[8] Rahil AI, Othman M, Ibrahim W, Mohamed MY. Brucellosis in Qatar: A retrospective cohort study. *Qatar Med J*. 2014 Jun 16;2014(1):25-30.

[9] Bazzazi N, Yavarikia A, Keramat F. Ocular involvement of brucellosis. Middle East Afr J Ophthalmol. 2013;20(1):95-7.

[10] Rolando I, Olarte L, Vilchez G, Lluncor M, Otero L, Paris M, Carrillo C, Gotuzzo E. Ocular manifestations associated with brucellosis: a 26-year experience in Peru. Clin Infect Dis. 2008;46(9):1338-45.

[11] Mesquida M, Llorenç V, Cervera C, Adán A. Ocular brucellosis. *Med Clin (Barc)*. 2013 Mar 16;140(6):284.

[12] Sungur GK, Hazirolan D, Gurbuz Y, Unlu N, Duran S, Duman S. Ocular involvement in brucellosis. *Can J Ophthalmol*. 2009;44(5):598-601.

[13] Ghasemi Barghi R, Meraat H, Pahlevan AA. A review on ophthalmic manifestations of brucellosis and reporting a case of ophthalmic brucellosis. *Iran Red Crescent Med J*. 2011;13(5):352-3.

[14] Rolando I, Vilchez G, Olarte L, Lluncor M, Carrillo C, Paris M, Guerra H, Gotuzzo E. *Brucella* uveitis: intraocular fluids and biopsy studies. *Int J Infect Dis*. 2009;13(5):e206-11.

[15] Rabinowitz R, Schneck M, Levy J, Lifshitz T. Bilateral multifocal choroiditis with serous retinal detachment in a patient with *Brucella* infection: case report and review of the literature. *Arch Ophthalmol*. 2005;123(1):116-8.

[16] Walker J, Sharma OP, Rao NA. Brucellosis and uveitis. *Am J Ophthalmol*. 1992 Sep 15;114(3):374-5.

[17] Goldstein DA, Tessler HH. Ocular brucellosis vs Vogt-Koyanagi-Harada syndrome. *Arch Ophthalmol*. 2006;124(4):608-9.

[18] Güngür K, Bekir NA, Namiduru M. Ocular complications associated with brucellosis in an endemic area. *Eur J Ophthalmol*. 2002;12(3):232-7.

[19] Güngör K, Bekir NA, Namiduru M. Recurrent episcleritis associated with brucellosis. *Acta Ophthalmol Scand*. 2001 Feb;79(1):76-8.

[20] Bourcier T, Cassoux N, Karmochkine M, Lehoang P. Episcleritis and brucellosis. Apropos of a case. J Fr Ophtalmol. 1998;21(2):126-7.

[21] Sahin OG, Pelit A, Turunc T, Akova YA Ophthalmoparesis, papillitis and premacular hemorrhage in a case with endocarditis: a rare presentation of Brucellosis. *Ind J Ophthalmol*. 2010;58(2):164-6.

[22] Namiduru M, Gungor K, Dikensoy O, Baydar I, Ekinci E, Karaoglan I, Bekir NA. Epidemiological, clinical and laboratory features of brucellosis: a prospective evaluation of 120 adult patients. *Int J Clin Pract*. 2003;57(1):20-4.

[23] Lyall M. Ocular brucellosis. *Trans Ophthalmol Soc U K*. 1973;93(0):689-97.

[24] Vitry MA, Hanot Mambres D, De Trez C, Akira S, Ryffel B, Letesson JJ, Muraille E. Humoral immunity and CD4+ Th1 cells are both necessary for a fully protective immune response upon secondary infection with Brucella *melitensis*. *J Immunol*. 2014;192(8):3740-52.

[25] Vitry MA, De Trez C, Goriely S, Dumoutier L, Akira S, Ryffel B, Carlier Y, Letesson JJ, Muraille E. Vitry MA, De Trez C, Goriely S, Dumoutier L, Akira S, Ryffel B, Carlier Y, Letesson JJ, Muraille E. *Infect Immun*. 2012;80(12):4271-80.

[26] Serra J, Viñas M. Laboratory diagnosis of brucellosis in a rural endemic area in Northeastern Spain. *Int Microbiol*. 2004;7:53-8.

[27] Gómez MC, Nieto JA, Rosa C, Geijo P, Escribano MA, Muñoz A, et al. Evaluation of seven tests for diagnosis of human brucellosis in an area where the disease is endemic. *Clin Vaccine Immunol*. 2008;15:1031-3.

[28] Clavijo E, Díaz R, Anguita A, García A, Pinedo A, Smits HL. Comparison of a dipstick assay for detection of *Brucella*-specific immunoglobulin M antibodies with other tests for serodiagnosis of human brucellosis. *Clin Diagn Lab Immunol*. 2003;10:612-5.

[29] Nielsen K, Yu WL. Serological diagnosis of brucellosis. *Sec Biol Med Sci*. 2010;XXXI/1:65-89.

[30] Morales-García MR, García-Méndez N, Regalado-Jacobo SD, López-Merino A, Contreras-Rodríguez A. Clinical, serological and polymerase chain reaction follow-up of a family with brucellosis. *Rev Chilena Infectol*. 2014 Aug;31(4):425-33.

[31] Jafar A. Qasem, Sabah AlMomin, Salwa A. Al-Mouqati, Vinod Kumar. Characterization and evaluation of an arbitrary primed Polymerase Chain Reaction (PCR) product for the specific detection of *Brucella* species. *Saudi J Biol Sci*. 2015; 22: 220-226.

[32] al-Kaff AS. Ocular brucellosis. *Int Ophthalmol Clin*. 1995 Summer;35(3):139-45.

[33] Akduman L, Or M, Hasanreisoğlu B, Kurtar K. A case of ocular brucellosis: importance of vitreous specimen. *Acta Ophthalmol (Copenh)*. 1993;71(1):130-2.

[34] Puig SM, Heatley J, Arenas F, Guerrero IG. Ocular complications in brucellosis. *Am J Ophthalmol.* 1953;36:675-89.

[35] Poletti J, Poletti A, Larmande A. Diagnostic and therapeutic problems in brucellosis uveitis. *Med Trop (Mars).* 1981;41(5):523-5.

[36] Cavallaro N, Randone A, La Rosa L, Muqhinin L. Bilateral papilledema in a patient with brucellosis. *Metab Pediatr Syst Ophthalmol.* 1990;13:115-8.

[37] Abd-Elrazak M. *Brucella* optic neuritis. *Arch Intern Med.* 1991;15:776-8.

[38] Hashemi SH, Gachkar L, Keramat F, Mamani M, Hajilooi M, Janbakhsh A, Majzoobi MM, Mahjub H. Comparison of doxycycline-streptomycin, doxycycline-rifampin, and ofloxacin-rifampin in the treatment of brucellosis: a randomized clinical trial. *Int J Infect Dis.* 2012;16:e247-51.

[39] Solera J. Update on brucellosis: therapeutic challenges. *Int J Antimic Agents.* 2010;36:S18-20.

[40] Gulsun S, Aslan S, Satıcı O, Gul T. Brucellosis in pregnancy. *Trop Doct.* 2011;41:82-4.

[41] Long SS. Good news about doxycycline and dental staining. *J Pediatr.* 2015;166:1101-4.

[42] Roushan MR, Amiri MJ. Update on childhood brucellosis. *Recent Pat Antiinfect Drug Discov.* 2013;8:42-6.

[43] Al-Tawfiq JA, Memish ZA. Pregnancy associated brucellosis. *Recent Pat Antiinfect Drug Discov.* 2013;8:47-50.

[44] Tanyel E, Coban AY, Koruk ST, Simsek H, Hepsert S, Cirit OS, Tulek N. Actual antibiotic resistance pattern of Brucella *melitensis* in central Anatolia. An update from an endemic region. *Saudi Med J* 2007;28:1239-42.

[45] Lang R, Raz R, Sacks T, Shapiro M. Failure of prolonged treatment with ciprofloxacin in acute infections due to Brucella *melitensis*. *J Antimicrob Chemother.* 1990;26:841-6.

[46] Denk A, Demirdag K, Kalkan A, Ozden M, Cetinkaya B, Kilic SS. *In vitro activity of* Brucella *melitensis isolates to various antimicrobials in* Turkey. *Infect Dis. 2015;24:1-6.*

[47] Sofian M, Velayati AA, Aghakhani A, McFarland W, Farazi AA, Banifazl M, Eslamifar A, Ramezani A. Comparison of two durations of triple-drug therapy in patients with uncomplicated brucellosis: A randomized controlled trial. *Scand J Infect Dis.* 2014;46:573-7.

[48] Maves RC, Castillo R, Guillen A, Espinosa B, Meza R, Espinoza N, Núñez G, Sánchez L, Chacaltana J, Cepeda D, González S, Hall ER. Antimicrobial susceptibility of Brucella melitensis isolates in Peru. Antimic Agents Chemother. 2011;55:1279-81.

Chapter 6

Neurobrucellosis

Farhad Abbasi and Soolmaz Korooni

Additional information is available at the end of the chapter

http://dx.doi.org/10.5772/61655

Abstract

Brucellosis is a multi-system infectious disease that presents with various clinical manifestations and complications. Neurobrucellosis is an uncommon but serious presentation of brucellosis that can be seen in all stages of the disease. Neurobrucellosis is a focal complication of brucellosis affecting both central and peripheral nervous system presenting varieties of signs and symptoms. The most reported manifestations are meningitis and meningoencephalitis. It is a rare presentation of brucellosis. The estimated mean incidence of neurobrucellosis is 1.7%–10%. The incidence is equal in males and females. Initial clinical manifestations consisted of meningoencephalitis, acute and subacute meningitis, intracranial hypertension, polyradiculoneuritis, cerebral and subarachnoid hemorrhage, transverse myelitis, lumbar epidural abscess with root involvement, and cranial nerve involvement. Other rare manifestation includes pseudotumor cerebri, intracranial granuloma, sagittal sinus thrombosis, spinal arachnoiditis, and intracranial vasculitis. High index of suspicion, especially in endemic areas is essential to prevent morbidity from this disease. Clinical suspicion and accurate evaluation of a patient's history is the most important clue in diagnosis and treatment. Neurobrucellosis can be diagnosed by isolation of microorganism from the CSF or detection of antibodies in the CSF. The CSF pattern in neurobrucellosis can be helpful for diagnosis; lymphocytic pleocytosis, increased protein, and decreased glucose levels in the CSF are in favor of neurobrucellosis. Imaging modalities, including CT scan or magnetic resonance imaging, may reveal information for diagnosis. Many laboratory procedures are usually employed in the diagnosis of neurobrucellosis. Even though the culture method is the gold standard, growth rate is low and time consuming. Coombs' test should be performed in both the CSF and serum. Different regimens are usually used based on ceftriaxone, doxycycline, cotrimoxasole, streptomycin, and rifampicin. Treatment with intravenous ceftriaxone and oral rifampicin, doxycycline, and trimethoprim–sulfamethoxazole resulted in a good clinical response. Patients with severe and persistent headache and other neurologic symptoms and signs should be considered for neurobrucellosis in endemic regions. Early diagnosis and treatment of neurobrucellosis will be helpful in decreasing the sequelae of this complication.

Keywords: Neurobrucellosis, clinical manifestation, diagnosis, treatment

1. Introduction

Brucellosis is a common zoonotic infection worldwide and is caused by Brucella species. Central nervous system (CNS) involvement is a serious complication of brucellosis with different clinical presentation [1]. Neurobrucellosis is a focal complication of brucellosis affecting both central and peripheral nervous system (PNS) presenting with a variety of signs and symptoms [2]. Neurologic involvement due to brucellosis was reported in 1.7%–10% of the patients with brucellosis [3, 4, 5]. Neurological complications of brucellosis are divided into two groups. The first are those that have a direct effect of microorganism on the CNS and PNS, and the second are those that have indirect effect of brucellosis on the CNS or PNS, e.g., toxic-febrile neurobrucellosis [6].

2. Clinical manifestations

Neurobrucellosis can affect any part of the nervous system and can mimic any neurological disease [7]. The most reported manifestations of neurobrucellosis are meningitis and meningoencephalitis [2]. Neurobrucellosis may also present as myelitis, myelopathy, stroke, paraplegia, radiculoneuritis, intracerebral abscess, epidural abscess, intradural abscess, demyelination, Guillain-Barré syndrome, polyneuritis, and cranial nerve involvement or any combination of these manifestations [3, 8, 9, 10]. Neurobrucellosis affects the second, third, sixth, seventh, and eighth cranial nerves. Involvement of the oculomotor nerves is a very rare complication in neurobrucellosis [11]. Optic neuritis due to neurobrucellosis has been reported [12]. Neurobrucellosis can cause hearing loss. It may affect the auditory pathway. Sensorineural hearing loss can be seen due to brucellosis. Cochlear implantation may be successful for treatment of patients with sensorineural hearing loss [13]. Neurobrucellosis may present rarely with communicating hydrocephalus with symptoms of headaches, nausea, vomiting, gait disturbance and signs of dysmmetry, ataxia, and sensorineural hearing loss [14]. Spastic paraparesis and the sensorineural involvement are rare manifestations [8]. Solitary intracranial mass lesions mimicking cerebral tumor are extremely rare presentations of neurobrucellosis [15]. It may also present as leukoencephalopathy [16]. Cerebral venous sinus thrombosis due to brucellosis is a rare form of stroke caused by thrombosis in venous sinuses of the brain [17]. Sagittal sinus thrombosis is one of the manifestations [18]. Neurobrucellosis is associated rarely with demyelination. It may involve the corpus callosum [19]. Spinal epidural abscess due to the Brucella species is usually associated with spondylodiscitis. Urgent surgical decompression should be performed in cases with moderate to severe neurological deficits particularly if progressive [20]. Quadriplegia and multiple brain abscesses have been reported as manifestations of neurobrucellosis [21]. There are reports of intramedullary brucellar granuloma as rare cases of neurobrucellosis. Nas et al. reported a patient presented with loss of strength of four extremities. An intramedullary mass lesion was detected in the cervical level and brucellar granuloma of the cervical spine was diagnosed finally [22]. In Asadipouya's study on neurobrucellosis, headache, fever, neck rigidity, fatigue, altered mental status, speech disturbances, nausea, and vomiting were the most common symptoms. Hearing loss, paraplegia, cerebellar ataxia, diplopia, photophobia, blurred vision, abnormal behavior, hypoesthesia, low back

http://dx.doi.org/10.5772/61655

pain, and right side weakness are categorized as less common clinical features [6]. An analytical study on several publications on neurobrucellosis demonstrated that the most frequent symptoms of neurobrucellosis are fever, headache, weight loss, sweating, and back pain; and the most frequent signs of neurobrucellosis are meningeal irritation, confusion, hypoesthesia, hepatomegaly, and splenomegaly. Crainial nerve involvement, polyneuropathy, polyradiculopathy, paraplegia, and abscess formation may occur during neurobrucellosis. Symptom duration may vary between one week and six months [23, 24]. Patients with neurobrucellosis may present with neuropsychiatric signs and symptoms including aphasia, diplopia, hemiparesis, facial paralysis, tremor, ataxia, depression, personality disorder, hallucinations, agitation, behavioral disorders, muscle weakness, and disorientation [25, 26]. Shehata's study demonstrated that CNS involvement (vascular stroke, meningeoencephalitis, and dementia) was seen in 33% of patients and PNS involvement (polyneuropathy, radiculoapathy, and polyradiculoneuropathy) was seen in 22% of patients. Depression was recorded in 29% of patients. Patients with neurobrucellosis reported highly significant impairment in some cognitive function measures (mental control, logical memory, visual reproduction) and higher scores on depressive symptoms compared with controls [27]. Brucellosis may infect ventriculoperitoneal shunt [28]. The mean duration of symptoms before admission is 8 weeks (range: 1 week–4 months) [6]. In neurobrucellosis, CNS invasion by bacteria results in an inflammatory disorder. During neurobrucellosis, migroglia and astrocytes may be involved. The results of these involvements are production of pro-inflammatory cytokines that are harmful for CNS. Matrix metalloproteinases (MMP) has been found in the inflammatory process of CNS. Pro-inflammatory cytokines cause increased production of MMP. During neurobrucellosis, astrogliosis occurs [29]. Inflammatory response elicited by Brucella in astrocytes would lead to the production of MMP-9 and that mitogen-activated protein kinases may play a role in this phenomenon. Mitogen-activated protein kinases inhibition may thus be considered as a strategy to control inflammation and CNS damage in neurobrucellosis [30]. Brucella lipoproteins could be key virulence factors in neurobrucellosis and that astrogliosis might contribute to neurobrucellosis pathogenesis [31].

3. Complications

Recovery of neurobrucellosis may accompany with sequela. Paraparesis, dementia, sphincter dysfunction, peripheral facial paralysis, and sensorineural hearing loss may occur [10, 25].

Communicating hydrocephalus has been reported as a complication of neurobrucellosis that may need external ventricular drainage [32]. Mild sequelae, including aphasia, hearing loss, and hemiparesis, may remain after successful treatment [33]. The mortality of neurobrucellosis can be up to 0.5% with suitable antibiotics [24].

4. Diagnosis

Clinical suspicion and accurate evaluation of a patient's history is the most important clue in the diagnosis and treatment of brucellosis [17]. Early detection and treatment is an important predictor of favorable outcome of neurobrucellosis [7]. Diagnosis requires a high index of suspicion in patients from endemic areas. Diagnosis is often based on neurological symptoms, serology, and suggestive brain imaging [34]. In patients with laboratory-confirmed brucellosis, the neurobrucellosis may be diagnosed with one of these criteria: first, signs and symptoms of neurobrucellosis include fever, headache, and cranial nerve palsies; second, CSF abnormality compatible with brucellosis including CSF lymphocytic pleocytosis, low glucose, and high protein levels of CSF detection of anti-Brucella antibodies in the CSF or isolation of Brucella from the CSF; third, imaging abnormality compatible with brucellosis especially in CT scan and MRI [25].

In a study on patients with neurobrucellosis, criteria for diagnosis was defined as: 1) neurobrucellosis clinical manifestation; 2) CSF abnormality (lymphocytosis, decreased glucose, increased protein); 3) positive anti-brucella antibody in the CSF or serum; 4) clinical response to empirical therapy; and 5) no other diagnosis compatible with signs and symptoms [6]. The sensitivity of tube agglutination in the CSF is 0.94, specificity 0.96, positive predictive value 0.94, and negative predictive value 0.96 [25].

In Erdem's study on 177 patients with neurobrucellosis mean values of the CSF, biochemical test results were as follows: CSF leucocyte count=215, CSF protein=330 mg/dL, CSF/blood-glucose ratio=0.35. The sensitivity of serum standard tube agglutination was 94%; CSF standard tube agglutination was 78%. Blood culture was positive for brucellosis in 37% by automated method and CSF culture was positive in 25% and 9% by automated and conventional CSF culture, respectively [35]. Another study showed the CSF WBC count to be between 6 cells/dl and 3600 cells/dl with mean count of 403 cells/dl. Most of the patients had CSF lymphocyte predominance and some had CSF polymorphonuclear predominance. Elevated CSF protein (>45 mg/dl) was detected in about 90% of the patients. CSF low glucose level (<40 mg/dl or CSF/Serum glucose ratio of <0.4) was seen in about half of the patients [6]. Yetkin's study demonstrated that the mean count of CSF WBC was 244 with high CSF protein level in all patients and low CSF glucose level in half of the patients [23]. Brucella bacteria may be isolated from CSF in only 15% of the patients. Brucella tube agglutination with Coombs test in the CSF is sensitive and specific [25]. Serum agglutination test is often used for screening and as a complement fixation test for confirmatory tests. Enzyme-linked immunosorbant assay (ELISA) for brucella is more sensitive and specific than other serological tests and it may replace other serological tests. ELISA may detect antibodies against brucella in the serum and CSF. A patient with neurobrucellosis may have negative serological markers of brucellosis in the CSF and serum. Serum anti-brucella immunoglobulin G (IgG) and immunoglobulin M (IgM) antibody may be checked using the ELISA method for patients who had negative Coomb's Wright agglutination tests results [6]. Adenosine deaminase (ADA) activity in the CSF of patients with brucella meningitis can be used for diagnosis. CSF ADA activity with cut-off value of 12.5 IU/L has a sensitivity of 92% and specificity of 88% for diagnosis of brucella meningitis [36]. When cerebrospinal fluid culture is negative, PCR may be an optimal alternative tool for an immediate and accurate diagnosis [37]. Imaging findings of neurobrucellosis is divided into four categories: (1) normal, (2) inflammation (recognized by granulomas, abnormal enhancement of the meninges, perivascular space, or lumbar nerve roots), (3) white matter changes, and (4) vascular changes [38]. Infarct in the anterior limb of the left internal capsule and putamenal infarctions has been reported due to brucellosis. The diagnosis of neurobrucellosis can be considered despite negative CSF culture and serology based on clinical response and resolution of CSF abnormality with anti-brucella treatment [6]. Tekin-Koruk reported a seronegative neurobrucellosis case with depression and diplopia. Results of agglutination tests for Brucella both in the serum and CSF were negative. Diagnosis was made only by positive culture of Brucella mellitensis with inoculation of the patient's cerebrospinal fluid in a BACTEC 9050 System [39].

5. Treatment

Neurobrucellosis is a treatable disease with a favorable outcome. Doxycycline, rifampicin, ceftriaxone, trimethoprim sulfamethoxazole, ciprofloxacin, and streptomycin have been found effective in neurobrucellosis [6]. An important challenge in treatment of brucellar meningitis or meningoencephalitis is that patients should be treated with oral antibiotics or whether an intravenous extended-spectrum cephalosporin, such as ceftriaxone, which does not accumulate in phagocytes, should be added to the regimen. Several different protocols have been used for treatment. Ceftriaxone, rifampin, and doxycycline or trimethoprim-sulfamethoxazole, rifampin, and doxycycline have been used for treatment. Ceftriaxone-based regimens are more successful and require shorter therapy than the oral treatment protocol [40]. Treatment protocol in Karsen's study consisted of ceftriaxone, rifampicin, and doxycyline for a period of four weeks, followed by rifampicin and doxycyline for an additional four weeks [26]. Duration of treatment will depend on the patient's condition. If rapid improvement occurs, we may shorten the duration of antibiotic therapy to 12 weeks and continue their treatment by clinical assessment. In the study by Bodur, all patients received antibiotic therapy with ceftriaxone, rifampicin, and doxycycline initially and after one month they were continued with rifampicin and doxycycline up to four months. Oral Doxycycline and rifampin with intravenously ceftriaxone are the most common antibiotics in the treatment of neurobrucellosis [6]. Gul's study demonstrated that parenteral ceftriaxone should be used as an initial alternative in the management of neurobrucellosis [41]. Duration of treatment varies in different studies ranging from several weeks to several months. In Ceran's study, duration of treatment varied between 3 and 12 months according to the CSF response [33]. According to Gul's study, it is recommended that the duration of therapy should be a minimum of six months with suitable antibiotics, although the therapy should be individualized [41]. In contrast, in Asasipouya's study in Iran, duration of treatment was as short as eight weeks in about half of the patients. Short course treatment in neurobrucellosis is possible in patients with meningoencephalitis who do not have any focal neurologic deficit or have minimal deficit. Other patients need treatment for a long duration according to neurologic manifestations [6].

6. Conclusion

Patients with severe and persistent headache and other neurologic symptoms and signs should be considered for neurobrucellosis in endemic regions [25]. It should be included in differential diagnosis for any patient presenting with central or peripheral neurological manifestations especially in endemic areas [7]. With early diagnosis and treatment, neurobrucellosis has a good outcome with no or minimal neurologic complications. The duration of disease and the time between starting symptoms and starting antibiotic influences the prognosis [6].

Author details

Farhad Abbasi* and Soolmaz Korooni

*Address all correspondence to: f_abbasi55@yahoo.com

Bushehr University of Medical Sciences, Bushehr, Iran

References

[1] Kanik-Yuksek S, Gulhan B, Ozkaya-Parlakay A, Tezer H. A case of childhood Brucellosis with neurological involvement and epididymo-orchitis. J Infect Dev Ctries. 2014;8(12):1636-8.

[2] Tajdini M, Akbarloo S, Hosseini SM, Parvizi B, Baghani S, Aghamollaii V, Tafakhori A. From a simple chronic headache to neurobrucellosis: A case report. Med J Islam Repub Iran. 2014;28:12.

[3] Elzein FE, Mursi M. Brucella induced Guillain-Barré syndrome. Am J Trop Med Hyg. 2014;91(6):1179-80.

[4] Baykal T, Baygutalp F, Senel K, Levent A, Erdal A, Ugur M, Ozgocmen S. Spastic paraparesis and sensorineural hearing loss in a patient with neurobrucellosis. J Back Musculoskelet Rehabil. 2012;25(3):157-9.

[5] Ozkavukcu E, Tuncay Z, Selçuk F, Erden I. An unusual case of neurobrucellosis presenting with unilateral abducens nerve palsy: Clinical and MRI findings. Diagn Interv Radiol. 2009;15(4):236-8.

[6] Asadipooya K, Dehghanian A, Omrani GH, Abbasi F. Short-course treatment in neurobrucellosis: A study in Iran. Neurol India. 2011;59(1):101-3.

[7] Guenifi W, Rais M, Gasmi A, Ouyahia A, Boukhrissa H, Mechakra S, Houari M, Nouasria B, Lacheheb A. [Neurobrucellosis: Description of 5 cases in Setif Hospital, Algeria]. Med Trop (Mars). 2010;70(3):309-10.

[8] Baykal T, Baygutalp F, Senel K, Levent A, Erdal A, Ugur M, Ozgocmen S. Spastic paraparesis and sensorineural hearing loss in a patient with neurobrucellosis. J Back Musculoskelet Rehabil. 2012;25(3):157-9.

[9] Babamahmoodi F, Babamahmoodi A. Brucellosis, presenting with guillain-barré syndrome. J Glob Infect Dis. 2011;3(4):390-2.

[10] Demiroğlu YZ, Turunç T, Karaca S, Arlıer Z, Alışkan H, Colakoğlu S, Arslan H. Neurological involvement in brucellosis; clinical classification, treatment and results. Mikrobiyol Bul. 2011;45(3):401-10.

[11] Işıkay S, Yılmaz K, Ölmez A. Neurobrucellosis developing unilateral oculomotor nerve paralysis. Am J Emerg Med. 2012;30(9):2085.e5-7.

[12] Marques R, Martins C, Machado I, Monteiro JP, Campos N, Calhau P. Unilateral optic neuritis as a presentation of neurobrucellosis. Pediatr Rep. 2011;3(2):e11.

[13] Guneri EA, Kirkim G, Serbetcioglu BM, Erdag TK, Guneri A. Cochlear implantation in neurobrucellosis. Otol Neurotol. 2009;30(6):747-9.

[14] Guney F, Gumus H, Ogmegul A, Kandemir B, Emlik D, Arslan U, Tuncer I. First case report of neurobrucellosis associated with hydrocephalus. Clin Neurol Neurosurg. 2008;110(7):739-42.

[15] Erdem M, Namiduru M, Karaoglan I, Kecik VB, Aydin A, Tanriverdi M. Unusual presentation of neurobrucellosis: A solitary intracranial mass lesion mimicking a cerebral tumor: A case of encephalitis caused by Brucella melitensis. J Infect Chemother. 2012;18(5):767-70.

[16] Awada A, Korri H, Issa Z, Ali Y, Beaini M. Progressive paraparesis with sensorineural deafness and leukoencephalopathy revealing neurobrucellosis. Rev Neurol (Paris). 2011;167(2):181-4.

[17] Faraji F, Didgar F, Talaie-Zanjani A, Mohammadbeigi A. Uncontrolled seizures resulting from cerebral venous sinus thrombosis complicating neurobrucellosis. J Neurosci Rural Pract. 2013;4(3):313-6.

[18] Ceran N, Turkoglu R, Erdem I, Inan A, Engin D, Tireli H, Goktas P. Neurobrucellosis: Clinical, diagnostic, therapeutic features and outcome. Unusual clinical presentations in an endemic region. Braz J Infect Dis. 2011;15(1):52-9.

[19] Bektaş O, Ozdemir H, Yılmaz A, Fitöz S, Ciftçi E, Ince E, Aksoy E, Deda G. An unusual case of neurobrucellosis presenting as demyelination disorder. Turk J Pediatr. 2013; 55(2):210-3.

[20] Daglioglu E, Bayazit N, Okay O, Dalgic A, Hatipoglu HG, Ergungor F. Lumbar epidural abscess caused by brucella species: Report of two cases. Neurocirugia (Astur). 2009;20(2):159-62.

[21] Keihani-Douste Z, Daneshjou K, Ghasemi M. A quadriplegic child with multiple brain abscesses: Case report of neurobrucellosis. Med Sci Monit. 2006;12(12):CS119-122.

[22] Nas K, Tasdemir N, Cakmak E, Kemaloglu MS, Bukte Y, Geyik MF. Cervical intramedullary granuloma of Brucella: A case report and review of the literature. Eur Spine J. 2007;16 Suppl 3:255-9.

[23] Yetkin MA, Bulut C, Erdinc FS, Oral B, Tulek N. Evaluation of the clinical presentations in neurobrucellosis. Int J Infect Dis. 2006;10(6):446-52.

[24] Gul HC, Erdem H, Bek S. Overview of neurobrucellosis: A pooled analysis of 187 cases. Int J Infect Dis. 2009;13(6):e339-43.

[25] Guven T, Ugurlu K, Ergonul O, Celikbas AK, Gok SE, Comoglu S, Baykam N, Dokuzoguz B. Neurobrucellosis: Clinical and diagnostic features. Clin Infect Dis. 2013;56(10):1407-12.

[26] Karsen H, Tekin Koruk S, Duygu F, Yapici K, Kati M. Review of 17 cases of neurobrucellosis: Clinical manifestations, diagnosis, and management. Arch Iran Med. 2012;15(8):491-4.

[27] Shehata GA, Abdel-Baky L, Rashed H, Elamin H. Neuropsychiatric evaluation of patients with brucellosis. J Neurovirol. 2010;16(1):48-55.

[28] Al-Otaibi A, Almuneef M, Shaalan MA. Brucella melitensis infection of ventriculoperitoneal shunt: A form of neurobrucellosis manifested as gastrointestinal symptoms. J Infect Public Health. 2014 Feb;7(1):62-5.

[29] Baldi PC, Giambartolomei GH. Immunopathology of Brucella infection. Recent Pat Antiinfect Drug Discov. 2013;8(1):18-26.

[30] Miraglia MC, Scian R, Samartino CG, Barrionuevo P, Rodriguez AM, Ibañez AE, Coria LM, Velásquez LN, Baldi PC, Cassataro J, Delpino MV, Giambartolomei GH. Brucella abortus induces TNF-α-dependent astroglial MMP-9 secretion through mitogen-activated protein kinases. J Neuroinflammation. 2013;10:47.

[31] García Samartino C, Delpino MV, Pott Godoy C, Di Genaro MS, Pasquevich KA, Zwerdling A, Barrionuevo P, Mathieu P, Cassataro J, Pitossi F, Giambartolomei GH. Brucella abortus induces the secretion of proinflammatory mediators from glial cells leading to astrocyte apoptosis. Am J Pathol. 2010;176(3):1323-38.

[32] Altas M, Evirgen O, Arica V, Tutanc M. Pediatric neurobrucellosis associated with hydrocephalus. J Pediatr Neurosci. 2010;5(2):144-6.

[33] Ceran N, Turkoglu R, Erdem I, Inan A, Engin D, Tireli H, Goktas P. Neurobrucellosis: Clinical, diagnostic, therapeutic features and outcome. Unusual clinical presentations in an endemic region. Braz J Infect Dis. 2011;15(1):52-9.

[34] Budnik I, Fuchs I, Shelef I, Krymko H, Greenberg D. Unusual presentations of pediatric neurobrucellosis. Am J Trop Med Hyg. 2012;86(2):258-60.

[35] Erdem H, Kilic S, Sener B, Acikel C, Alp E, Karahocagil M, Yetkin F, Inan A, Kecik-I. Bosnak V, Gul HC, Tekin-Koruk S, Ceran N, Demirdal T, Yilmaz G, Ulu-Kilic A, Cey-

lan B, Dogan-Celik A, Nayman-Alpat S, Tekin R, Yalci A, Turhan V, Karaoglan I, Yilmaz H, Mete B, Batirel A, Ulcay A, Dayan S, Seza Inal A, Ahmed SS, Tufan ZK, Karakas A, Teker B, Namiduru M, Savasci U, Pappas G. Diagnosis of chronic brucellar meningitis and meningoencephalitis: the results of the Istanbul-2 study. Clin Microbiol Infect. 2013;19(2):E80-6.

[36] Karsen H, Koruk ST, Karahocagil MK, Calisir C, Baran FC. Comparative analysis of cerebrospinal fluid adenosine deaminase activity in meningitis. Swiss Med Wkly. 2011;141:w13214.

[37] Sinopidis X, Kaleyias J, Mitropoulou K, Triga M, Kothare SV, Mantagos S. An uncommon case of pediatric neurobrucellosis associated with intracranial hypertension. Case Rep Infect Dis. 2012;2012:492467.

[38] Kizilkilic O, Calli C. Neurobrucellosis. Neuroimaging Clin N Am. 2011;21(4):927-37.

[39] Tekin-Koruk S, Duygu F, Gursoy B, Karaagac L, Bayraktar M. A rare case of seronegative neurobrucellosis. Ann Saudi Med. 2010;30(5):412-4.

[40] Erdem H, Ulu-Kilic A, Kilic S, Karahocagil M, Shehata G, Eren-Tulek N, Yetkin F, Celen MK, Ceran N, Gul HC, Mert G, Tekin-Koruk S, Dizbay M, Inal AS, Nayman-Alpat S, Bosilkovski M, Inan D, Saltoglu N, Abdel-Baky L, Adeva-Bartolome MT, Ceylan B, Sacar S, Turhan V, Yilmaz E, Elaldi N, Kocak-Tufan Z, Ugurlu K, Dokuzoguz B, Yilmaz H, Gundes S, Guner R, Ozgunes N, Ulcay A, Unal S, Dayan S, Gorenek L, Karakas A, Tasova Y, Usluer G, Bayindir Y, Kurtaran B, Sipahi OR, Leblebicioglu H. Efficacy and tolerability of antibiotic combinations in neurobrucellosis: Results of the Istanbul study. Antimicrob Agents Chemother. 2012;56(3):1523-8.

[41] Gul HC, Erdem H, Gorenek L, Ozdag MF, Kalpakci Y, Avci IY, Besirbellioglu BA, Eyigun CP. Management of neurobrucellosis: An assessment of 11 cases. Intern Med. 2008;47(11):995-1001.

Chapter 7

Brucellosis – Granulomatous Spine Infection

Ana M. Cerván, Miguel Hirschfeld, Miguel Rodriguez and Enrique Guerado

Additional information is available at the end of the chapter

http://dx.doi.org/10.5772/61214

Abstract

Brucellosis mainly affects the musculoskeletal system, with the spine as the most common location. Diagnosis is based on clinical symptoms, but in some cases, they may be lacking. Laboratory diagnosis is mainly made on the combination of high erythrocyte sedimentation rate (ESR) together with high levels of C-reactive protein (CRP) and leukocytosis. Blood culture is a very cost-effective investigation; plain radiographs may be useful, but magnetic resonance images (MRI) with gadolinium enhancement is the choice for diagnosing osteoarticular and spinal complications of human brucellosis. MRI diffusion-weighted imaging fast sequence is the most sensitive for differentiating acute and chronic forms of spondylodiscitis. The basis for treatment is usually the medical management. The indications for surgical treatment (endoscopy or open) are when: no microorganism has been isolated, spinal cord or dural compression is seen in MRI, or there's spinal instability or severe deformity. Open surgery is the standard: the anterior approach allows for anterior disc and bone debridement. If there is an epidural abscess or posterior elements are involved it's indicated as a posterior approach. To prevent relapses and reduce the rate of sequelae, it's necessary to have an appropriate duration of antimicrobial therapy and a timely indication to perform surgery.

Keywords: Brucellosis, spine brucellosis, spondylodiscitis, granulomatous infection, surgical treatment

1. Introduction

Spondylodiscitis refers to an infection affecting the intervertebral disk, the vertebral body, or the posterior arch of the vertebra. Aetiologically, spinal infection can be classified as pyogenic, granulomatous (tuberculosis, brucellosis, or fungal infection), or parasitic. Brucellosis mainly affects the musculoskeletal system, with the spine as the most common location.

Epidemiology. Brucella, one of the world's major zoonotic pathogens, is responsible for huge economic losses, as well as significant human morbidity in endemic areas [1]. It is caused by an aerobic, Gram-negative rods of the genus Brucella, discovered by David Bruce in 1887 [2]. In humans, this disease is also called Maltese fever, Bang's disease, undulant fever, or Mediterranean fever [3]. Human brucellosis involves an important public health problem in most developing countries including those of the Mediterranean, Balkans, the Middle East, Central Asia, and Central and South America. New foci of human brucellosis have emerged, particularly in Central Asia [4].

Pathogenic. Brucellosis is a systemic disease and many organ systems (nervous system, heart, skeletal system, bone marrow, etc.) may become involved following hematogenous dissemination. However, osteoarticular involvement is the most common complication of brucellosis, being reported in 10%–85% in most series [5]. The sacroiliac joint and arthritis are generally affected in the acute form. However the spine is usually affected in the subacute and chronic forms of this disease. The sacroiliac joint involvement and arthritis occur in patients under 30 years old, whereas the spine affectation is characteristic of older patients [6]. In the musculoskeletal system the spine is the most often affected location [7, 8]. The incidence of spinal involvement can be quite different, from 2%–54%, it depends on the type of population you study [9]. The radiographic changes will appear between the third to the twelfth week of the start of clinical symptoms [10]. The L4-L5 and L5-S1 junctions are the most frequent locations affected [11].

Clinical syndrome. Brucellosis is an acute (25%–77%), subacute (12.5%–59%), or chronic (5%–27.5%) illness that presents with a spectrum of nonspecific signs and symptoms. The disease is severely disabling with fever, sweating, fatigue, weight loss, headache, and joint pain that can persist for weeks to months. Spinal manifestations tend to occur during chronic infections [12, 13]. Clinical presentation varies widely [14] and approximately one-third of the patients have a more fulminant illness with acute onset of systemic toxicity [15]. The earliest sign of spondylitis is localized spine pain [16], since some degree of neurologic compromise may occur between 10%–43% of those with spondylitis [17], and in 10%–20% a paraspinal abscess develops. In a multicenter prospective study of 593 patients with brucellosis [18], 9.7% had spondylitis; neurologic deficits occurred in five (71%) of the patients with cervical spondylitis, two (11%) of the patients presented thoracic involvement, and nine (21%) developed lumbar disease. Paraspinal and epidural abscesses were more frequent in patients with cervical and thoracic disease; the worst prognosis was for those having cervical spine involvement. Complications of spinal brucellosis, with affectation of neighboring vertebrae with paraspinal, psoas, or epidural abscesses, with or without neurological affectation is uncommon; however, several series have published cases of complicated spinal brucellosis [19–22], although possible multilevel involvement may occur [23].

Diagnosis. It is not always easy. Suspected diagnosis of spondylodiscitis is based on clinical symptoms (pain, fever, and deformity), although, in some cases, they may be lacking. Patients complaining of back pain, particularly in endemic areas, should be accurately investigated. Laboratory diagnosis is mainly made in the presence of combination of high erythrocyte sedimentation rate (ESR) together with high levels of C-reactive protein (CRP) and, less useful, leukocytosis. Blood cultures are positive in less than half the cases overall but indeed in 70% of patients with acute B. melitensis infection. An agglutination reaction with a Brucella antibody titer of 1 : 160 or greater is presumptive evidence of infection, but an increasing titer is a more helpful sign of active infection [16, 17].

The diagnostic confirmation of spinal spondylitic granulomatous can be done by the polymerase chain reaction (PCR). If we have a case of prior antibiotic used or the presence of fastidious microorganisms, the molecular diagnostic can be done using broad-range 16S rDNA PCR [24]. By amplification of the mec A gene, doing species-specific PCR, especially targeting the Staphylococcus aureus, the sensitivity can increase, providing methicillin susceptibility [25]. But these methods are not completely unerring by themselves; in fact, nowadays, they are considered as an important complementary to standard cultures particularly those harvested through image-guided surgery [25]. Blood culture is a very cost-effective investigation. Plain radiographs may be useful; however, even large destructive spondylodiscitis may go undetected on X-rays as changes take several months to appear. Furthermore, usually in more aged patients, it may be difficult to distinguish between infection destruction and degenerative changes. The first radiological sign that we will find is osteoporosis of the affected vertebral body and erosion of the anterior-superior endplate, so-called Pons' sign, also a vacuum phenomenon may be observed in the anterior part of the disc (accumulation of gas with the crevices of the intervertebral or adjacent discs). The appearance of destructive changes on plain radiographs appears from the third month of the disease.

Radionuclide tests are currently less used. If magnetic resonance images (MRI) cannot distinguish among degenerative changes and infection, the fluorine-18 fluorodeoxyglucose positron emission tomography (FDG-PET) can be useful [26].The most useful image test, with the higher sensitivity and specificity for the diagnosis of spondylodiscitis, is MRI with gadolinium enhancement, which also provides information on anatomy [27]. CT-scan is useful in assessing the bone destruction and also for surgical planning, as well as contributes greatly in the CT-guided needle percutaneous biopsy [28]. MRI is the method of choice for diagnosing osteoarticular and spinal human brucellosis and its complications, especially during the early phase [29, 30]. It has been published [31] that diffusion-weighted imaging fast sequence is the most sensitive diagnosis tool for differentiating between acute and chronic forms of spondylodiscitis.

Sometimes diagnosis of brucellar spondylodiscitis becomes a major task as clinical findings are usually nonspecific and radiological features may mimic those of other bacterial, fungical, inflammatory, and neoplastic diseases. Likewise, it is very common to confuse spinal brucellosis with tuberculosis.

Differential diagnosis must be performed with tuberculous spondylitis, salmonella spondylitis, pyogenic spondylitis, disc herniation, and metastatic lesions [32–34]. The radiologic findings for tuberculous and brucellar spondylodiscitis are similar, so serologic testing for brucellosis is necessary in such cases [11]; and also the MRI findings are different as tuberculosis produces more severe changes with more deformity and abscess formation [35]. There are also differences regarding the involvement of the intervertebral disc spaces, whereas in brucellar spondylodiscitis intervertebral discs are narrowed, in metastatic diseases or in tuberculous spondylitis intervertebral discs are rarely affected. However, in brucellar spondylodiscitis the affectation of the posterior elements is very uncommon, while it may be frequently encountered in metastatic disease and tuberculosis spondylodiscitis. Paravertebral and epidural abscess formation and spinal cord and root compression are considered very rare findings in brucellar spondylodiscitis and are generally considered to be findings for tuberculosis and pyogenic spondylodiscitis.

Findings characteristic of MRI for brucellar spondylitis [36] are: vertebral body signal changes without morphologic changes, marked signal increase in the intervertebral disc on T2-weighted and contrast-enhanced sequences, vertebral endplate defects mimicking Schmorl's nodules, obliteration of muscle fat borders, moderate amount of paraspinal granulation tissue, and gas accumulation in the disc space and facet joint involvement. Nevertheless, some of these signs, such as the presence of gas, can also be present in pyogenic infections. In any case, the most useful method for detecting the presence and extension of brucellar spondylitis is the MRI, particularly using the fat-suppression technique with contrast. Even in extensive cases, vertebral collapse and gibbus deformity are rare findings, and the vertebral body is usually morphologically intact (Figures 1, 2, 3).

Biopsy is necessary to confirm the diagnosis in only 5% of the cases, in contrast to pyogenic and tuberculosis spondylitis [37].

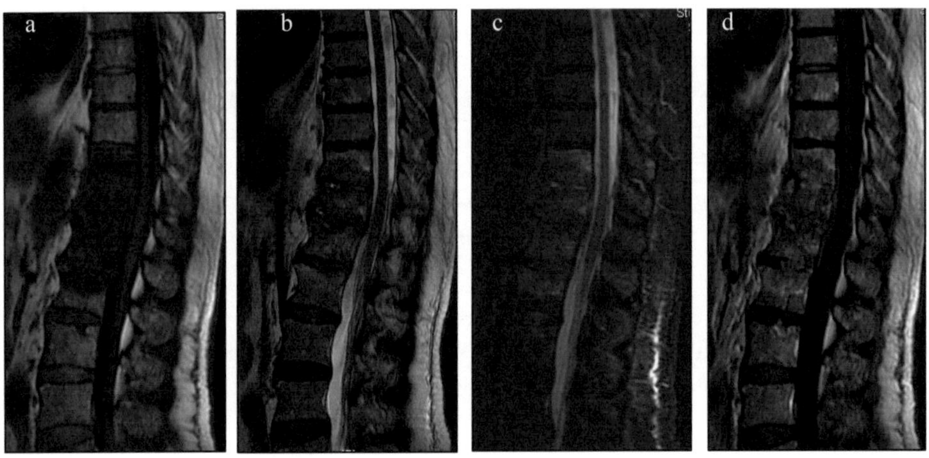

Figure 1. Sagittal magnetic resonance images from a 62-year-old man with brucellar spondylodiscitis. a. T1-weighted image showing irregularity and destruction of vertebral endplates and hypointensity at T11 to L2. b. T2-weighted image showing increase signal intensity of the disc and loss of intervertebral disc height. c. Sagittal STIR image showing hyperintense lesions vertebral contiguous. d. Contrast-enhanced, T1-weighted sagittal image shows involvement of intervertebral disc space between T11-L2 vertebral levels, vertebral bodies, and vertebral endplate.

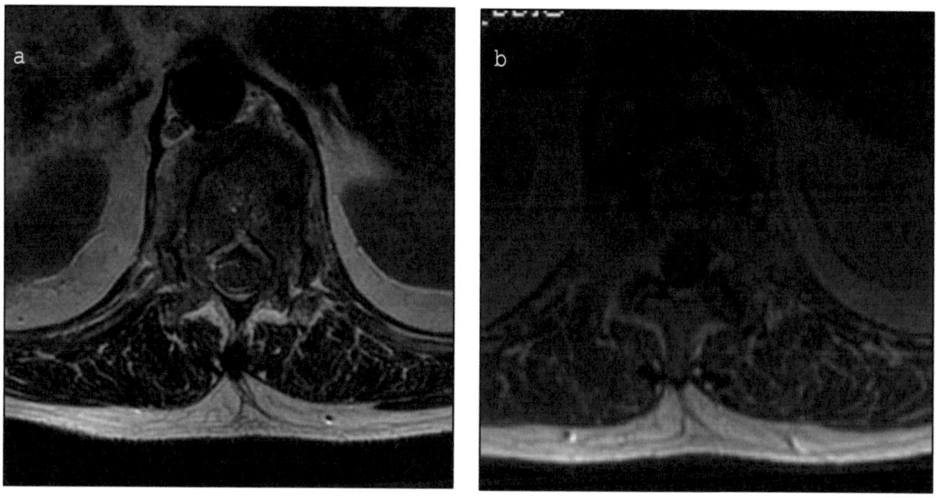

Figure 2. a. Axial T2-weighted image reveals a paravertebral abscess. b. Contrast enhanced T1-weighted axial image shows enhancement in affected vertebra and paravertebral soft tissue.

2. Treatment

The treatment of spinal brucellosis is mainly medical. The surgical intervention is reserved for biopsy, severe neurological impairment, and rarely for spinal stabilization.

The combination of tetracycline (tetracycline, 500 mg every 6 hours given orally or doxycycline, 100 mg every 12 hours) for 6 weeks together with an aminoglycoside (preferably, streptomycin, 1 g/day intramuscularly for 2–3 weeks or gentamicin 5 mg/kg/day intravenously or intramuscularly for 7–10 days) is the current first line therapy for brucellosis as recommended by the World Health Organization. The combination of rifampicine (600–900 mg/day orally administrated) and doxycycline (100 mg every 12 hours orally administrated) for 6 weeks is suggested as the principal alternative therapy. In spinal brucellosis, it is noted that the same regimens can be given, but the duration of therapy should be longer. A combination of doxycycline (200 mg/day, for at least 12 weeks) with streptomycin (1 g/day, for 2 or 3 weeks) is still the first-line antimicrobial regimen in spinal brucellosis. For a long time Doxycycline + rifampin or co-trimoxazole + rifampin or ciprofloxacin + rifampin or ciprofloxacin + streptomycin could be used as an alternative when adverse reactions or contraindications (ototoxicity, nephrotoxicity, pregnancy, lactation, etc.) are present [38]. The combination of doxycycline and streptomycin has been used for a long time for complications and severe disease [39]. However, therapeutic failure and relapse are still reported with this regimen [40]. Response to treatment is monitored with repeated agglutination tests. Lifeso and colleagues [17] recommend continuing antibiotic therapy until the agglutination test titer is equal or less than 1 : 160 and there is clinical and radiographic evidence of disease resolution. Relapses seldom

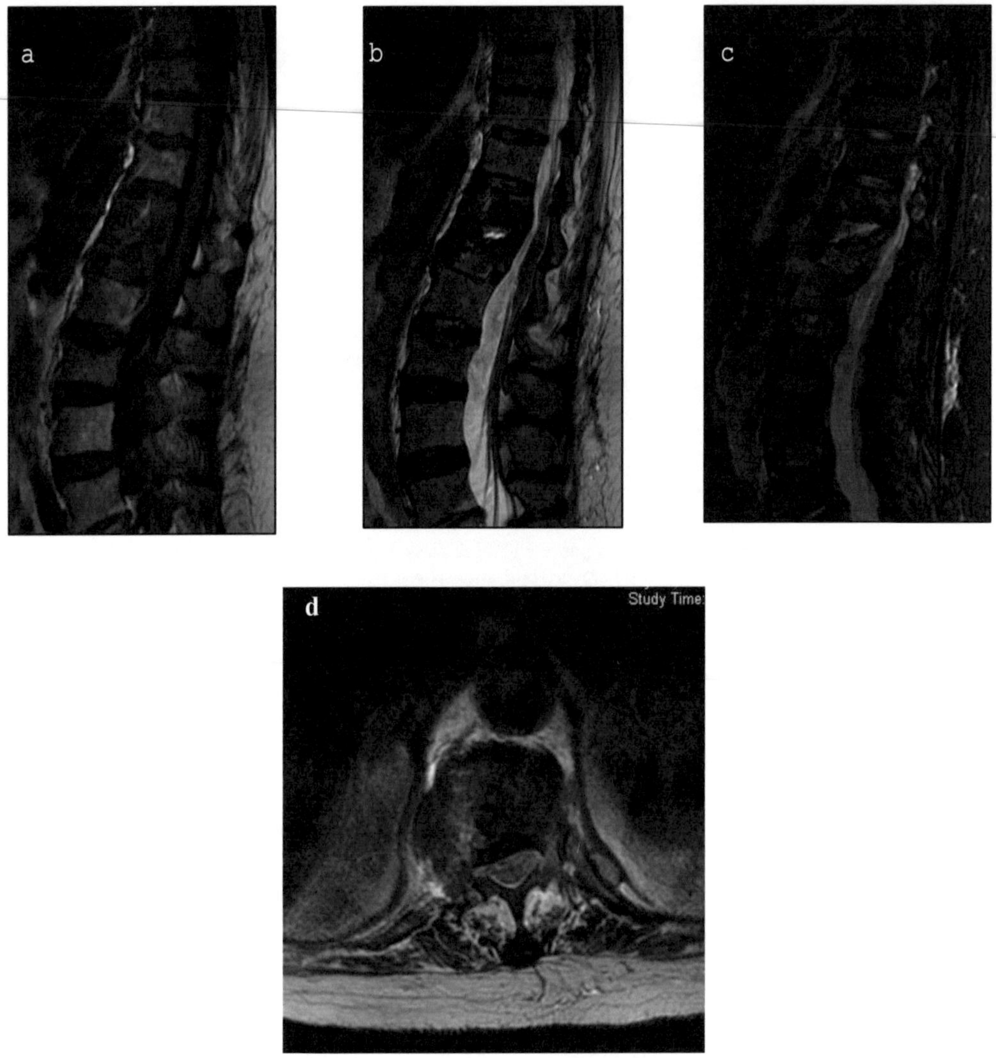

Figure 3. Sagittal magnetic resonance images from an 69-year-old woman with brucellar spondylodiscitis a. The T1-weighted image reveals complete signal loss at the T12 and L1 vertebrae bodies. b. The T2-weighted image reveals high signal intensity at T12-L1, medullar compression by the T12 pedicle. c. Sagittal STIR image shows hyperintense lesions at T12-L1. d. Axial T2-weighted image shows paravertebral and muscle abscesses. A medullar compression by T12 right pedicle is observed.

occur in patients who do not receive appropriate treatment and are often the result of focal suppurative complications such as spondylitis.

Conservative treatment is indicate in patients without spine instability or neurological deficits and with high surgical risk [41]. The doubt may arise in case of minor neurological deficits, for that some authors [42] prefer conservative treatment if there is no spinal instability as neurological symptoms will be improved with antibiotics. It is of paramount importance to achieve proper immobilization of the affected spinal segment; orthoses could be used for that purpose and in same instances, protected bed rest, although home confinement now is being abandoned [43].

If after 4 to 6 weeks of conservative treatment there are signs of spine instability, progressive deformity, or no clinical improvement, surgical treatment must be the choice.

On the other hand, early surgical treatment should be performed in the presence of sepsis or neurological deficits. Patients with spinal epidural abscess have high rates of morbidity and mortality, therefore, in these urgent surgical cases surgical treatment is essential [44].

Surgery is indicated in the presence of spinal instability, cord compression or radiculopathy [45]. Whenever a root, spinal cord, or dura mater compression is seen on MRI (epidural abscess with an anterior longitudinal ligament bulge), the patient must be taken to the theatre [46]. A clear indication for surgical treatment is spinal instability due to a great deformity or due to bone destruction. In case of an anterior abscess larger than 2.5 cm, a surgical evacuation must be carried out. Also, if there is concomitant vertebral body destruction, bone debridement with subsequent anterior body reconstruction must done, too. There are other indications for surgery such as: unsuccessful medical treatment, negative biopsy or lingering pain [47]. The main role for surgery is to perform a debridement and biopsy for culture, and also if there is biomechanical instability a stabilizing surgery will be performed at this moment or at another time [48].

Nowadays, there are two different surgical treatment options: less invasive or classic open surgery.

Less invasive techniques can facilitate debridement [49] (e.g., endoscopy, CT-scan percutaneous-guided surgery) and reconstruction (posterior percutaneous instrumentation is already regularly used in patients undergoing a double approach) [50] (Figure 4). Thoracoscopy has very much changed the philosophy of the current surgical treatment for the spondylodiscitic thoracic spine.

Open surgery can use any standard approach (anterior, posterior, or combined). The choice will depend on the location of the infection, the degree of bone destruction, and the presence of neurological deficits.

Thus, open surgery can be either anterior, posterior, or a combination of both, performed either in one or two stages. Usually, open surgery consists of an anterior approach and a secondary posterior approach. During the anterior approach, full disc and affected vertebral bone sequestra must be performed, followed by inserting a tricortical bone graft piece in between the above and below vertebral bodies for anterior vertebral bodies bridging. Ostheosynthesis through the combined posterior approach (in epidural abscess, important kyphosis and/or instability) with pedicular instrumentation is advisable to complement anterior debridement and fusion.

The anterior approach is the standard for anterior vertebral body debridement and stabilization. Most authors agree with the conclusion of the Medical Research Council that the Hong Kong procedure [51] of anterior radical debridement and reconstruction of the large anterior

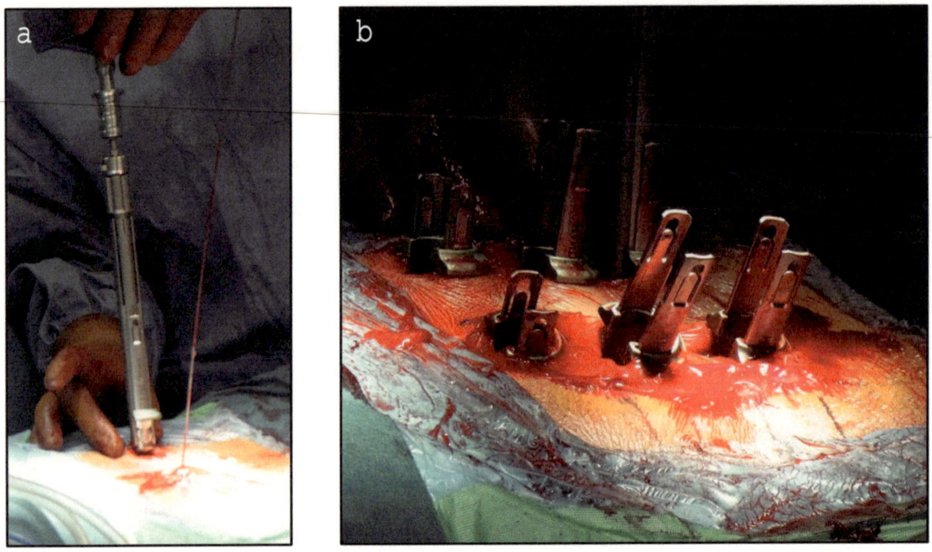

Figure 4. Pedicular instrumentation can be accomplished by percutaneous instrumentation where the surgeons use x-ray fluoroscopic imaging to guide the placement of special cannulated screws into the vertebrae. This is a minimally invasive procedure, it does not split and retract the muscle off the spine through a much larger incision and has more benefits that include less pain, less damage to the muscle, smaller scars, and prompt recovery.

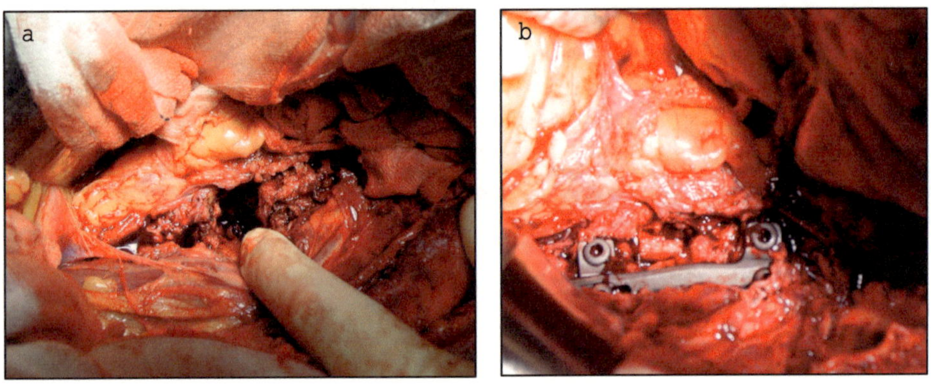

Figure 5. a. Large debridement (disc and vertebrae bodies) was performed by an anterior approach. b. Autologous graft insertion and a plate was carried out for anterior stabilization.

gap with strut graft is superior to any other procedure, and must be combined with posterior stabilization. Some authors prefer to start with a posterior approach for mechanical stabilization followed by radical anterior debridement; this has the advantage of having a very stable spine for radical anterior debridement [52, 53] (Figure 5).

In many series, radical debridement and anterior insertion is followed by the insertion of a titanium cage, filled with autogenous bone graft, together with a posterior less invasive approach for pedicle screw fixation in order to eliminate posterior soft tissue injury, preserve blood supply, and reduce surgical time, blood loss, and surgical complications [54]. Interbody cages have the function of providing an anterior support to compression forces, without the morbidity of tricortical harvesting [55]. Though, if we do a literature review, it seems that interbody cages have not completely resolved the complications and problems of interbody spinal fusions [56, 57].

The posterior approach is the first choice in cases of epidural abscess at the lumbar level in order to perform proper drainage, followed by pedicular instrumentation. If only one level is approached, instrumentation can be avoided. Large multilevel laminectomies without instrumentation are contraindicated, as it increases instability that already exists, provoked by the destruction of the anterior spine; it therefore, may result in paraplegia. Thus, in cases of substantial anterior destruction, collapse, spinal deformity, and when great debridement is recommended, an anterior approach must be the choice [58, 59]. A two-stage (posterior and anterior) surgical treatment for pyogenic or granulomatous spondylitis (first, the placement of posterior instrumentation and then anterior debridement and bone graft) provided satisfactory results; however, should kyphosis exists, changes in sagittal alignment may be difficult to be corrected [60].

In smaller defects, autograft is usually harvested from the iliac crest and ribs, and for larger bone deficits the choice is fibular graft [61]. In severe cases, only fibular grafts can allow a buttressing support, with a tension band principle if a concurrent pedicular instrumentation is also performed [62]. Louw [63] reported high fusion rates with vascularized rib grafts for stabilization and also good results with fibular graft for large defects used with stabilization by a posterior instrumentation. The use of BMPs combined with structural bone graft for spinal fusion has been claimed to provide good results and improve posterior fusion rates in pyogenic vertebral osteomyelitis after a 11–30 months follow up [64], though more studies are needed with longer follow-up.

According to the level of infection, surgical planning will be different. To the cervical spine, upper C1-C2 spine can be approached by a transpolar access; a posterior approach for occiput-C2 fusion may be necessary whenever a major instability is observed. The C3-C7 segment can be approached either anteriorly, posteriorly, or both, depending on abscess localization, instability, and fusion technique for this segment. Usually an anterior approach is recommended for debridement, decompression (eventual corpectomy), and fusion with bone graft associated with anterior plate stabilization (Figure 6). If it is a multilevel intervention, this must be complemented with pedicular instrumentation [65].

The thoracic spine can be approached either through an anterior transthoracic, posterior costotransversectomy, or an extra pleural anterolateral approach. Transthoracic approach give better results than lateral costotrasversectomy, for debridement, fusion rates, and mortality. At this spine level, it is recommended to use autograft and pedicular instrumentation.

The lumbar spine retroperitoneal approach is very useful, but opening the peritoneum must be avoided as intraperitoneal complications can occur. Debridement, abscesses drainage, and anterior instrumentation are easily performed by this approach.

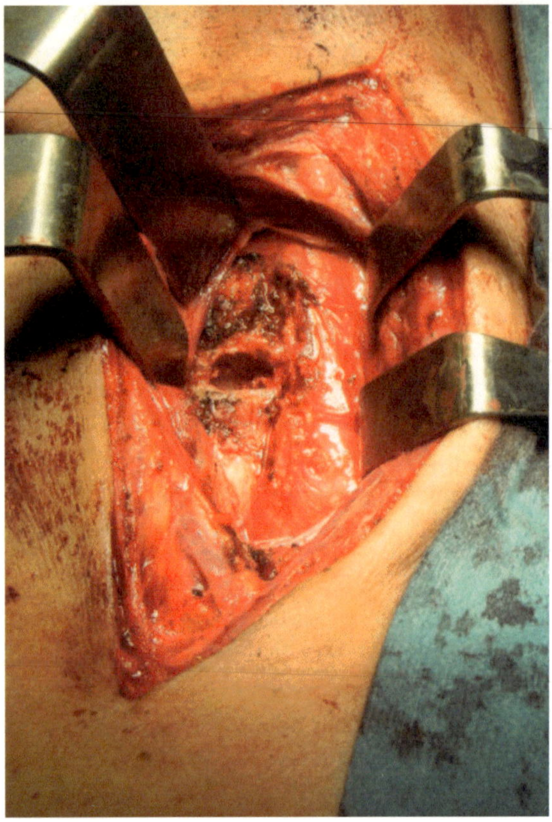

Figure 6. An anterior approach is the technique of choice for disc and vertebrae debridement at the C3-C7 segment.

Despite a properly treatment, sequelae, such as back pain or residual neurological symptoms, will persist due to degenerative changes secondary to destruction and instability caused by the infectious process.

In order to prevent relapses and reduce the rate of sequelae, it is necessary that an appropriate duration of antimicrobial therapy (antimicrobial treatment should be prolonged in complicated spinal forms of brucellosis [65]) and a timely indication to perform surgery, if necessary.

Author details

Ana M. Cerván*, Miguel Hirschfeld, Miguel Rodriguez and Enrique Guerado

*Address all correspondence to: anacervan@me.com

Department of Orthopedic Surgery and Traumatology, Hospital Costa del Sol, University of Málaga, Marbella, Spain

http://dx.doi.org/10.5772/61214

References

[1] Boschiroli ML, Foulongue V, O'Callaghan D. Brucellosis: A worldwide zoonosis. Curr Opin Microbiol. 2001;4:58-64.

[2] Bruce D. Note on the discovery of a microorganism in Malta fever. Practitioner. 1887;39:161-70.

[3] Galinska EM, Zagórski J. Brucellosis in humans—etiology, diagnostics, clinical forms. Ann Agric Environ Med. 2013;20:233-8.

[4] Pappas G, Papadimitriou P, Akritidis N, et al. The new global map of human brucellosis. Lancet Infect Dis. 2006;6:91-9.

[5] Doganay M, Aygen B. Human brucellosis: An overview. Int J Infect Dis. 2003;7:173-82.

[6] Chelli Bouaziz M, Ladeb MF, Chakroun M, Chaabane S. Spinal brucellosis: A review. Skeletal Radiol. 2008;37:785-90.

[7] Franco MP, Mulder M, Gilman RH, Smits HL. Human brucellosis. Lancet Infect Dis. 2007;7:775-86.

[8] Franco MP, Mulder M, Smits HL. Persistence and relapse in brucellosis and need for improved treatment. Trans R Soc Trop Med Hyg. 2007;101:854-55.

[9] Mousa AR, Muhtaseb SA, Almudallal DS, Khodeir SM, Marafie AA. Osteoarthicular complications of brucellosis: A study of 169 cases. Rev Infect Dis. 1987;9:531-43.

[10] Geyik MF, Gu°r A, Nas K, Cevik R, Sarac J, Dikici B, et al. Musculoskeletal involvement in brucellosis in different age groups: A study of 195 cases. Swiss Med Wkly. 2002;132:98-105.

[11] Pourbagher A, Pourbagher MA, Savas L, Turunc T, Demiroglu YZ, Erol I, et al. Epidemiologic, clinical, and imaging findings in brucellosis patients with osteoarticular involvement. AJR Am J Roentgenol. 2006;187:873-80.

[12] Pappas G, Akritidis N, Bosilkovski M, Tsianos E. Brucellosis. N Engl J Med. 2005;352:2325-36.

[13] Pappas G, Akritidis N, Tsianos E. Effective treatments in the management of brucellosis. Expert Opin Pharmacother. 2005;6:201-9.

[14] Zribi MA, Ammari L, Masmoudi A, Tiouiri H, Fendri C. Clinical manifestations, complications and treatment of brucellosis: 45-patient study. Pathol Biol (Paris). 2009;57:349-52.

[15] Young EJ: Brucella specia. 1995 Churchill Livingstone New York 2053-2060.

[16] Keenan JD, Metz CW Jr. Brucella spondylitis. A brief review and case report. Clin Orthop Relat Res. 1972;82:87-91.

[17] Lifeso RM, Harder E, McCorkell SJ. Spinal brucellosis. J Bone Joint Surg Br. 1985;67:345-51.

[18] Colmenero JD, Cisneros JM, Orjuela DL, et al. Clinical course and prognosis of Brucella spondylitis. Infection. 1992;20:38-42.

[19] Ulu-Kilic A, Sayar MS, Tütüncü E, Sezen F, Sencan I. Complicated brucellar spondylodiscitis: Experience from an endemic area. Rheumatol Int. 2013;33:2909-12.

[20] Colmenero JD, Ruiz-Mesa JD, Plata A, et al. Clinical findings, therapeutic approach, and outcome of brucellar vertebral osteomyelitis. Clin Infect Dis. 2008;46:426-33.

[21] Buzgan T, Karahocagil MK, Irmak H, et al. Clinical manifestations and complications in 1028 cases of brucellosis: A retrospective evaluation and review of the literature. Int J Infect Dis. 2010;14: e469-78.

[22] Ates O, Cayli SR, Kocak A, Kutlu R, Onal RE, Tekiner A. Spinal epidural abscess caused by brucellosis two case reports. Neurol Med Chir (Tokyo). 2005;45:66-70.

[23] Bouaziz MC, Bougamra I, Kaffel D, Hamdi W, Ghannouchi M, Kchir MM. Noncontiguous multifocal spondylitis: An exceptional presentation of spinal brucellosis. Tunis Med. 2010;88:280-84.

[24] Sontakke S, Cadenas MB, Maggi RG, Diniz PP, Breitschwerdt EB. Use of broad range16S rDNA PCR in clinical microbiology. J Microbiol Methods. 2009;76(3): 217-25.

[25] Gouliouris T, Aliyu SN, Brown MN. Spondylodiscitis: Update on diagnosis and management. J Antimicrob Chemother. 2010;65(Suppl 3):11-24.

[26] Stumpe KD, Zanetti M, Weishaupt D, Hodler J, Boos N, Von Schulthess GK. FDG positron emission tomography for differentiation of degenerative and infectious endplate abnormalities in the lumbar spine detected on MR imaging. AJR Am J Roentgenol. 2002;179:115-7.

[27] Modic MT, Feiglin DH, Piraino DW, Boumphrey F, Weinstein MA, Duchesneau PM, Rehm S. Vertebral osteomyelitis: Assessment using MR. Radiology. 1985;157:157-66.

[28] Michel SC, Pfirrmann CW, Boos N, Hodler J. CT-guided core biopsy of subchondral bone and intervertebral space in suspected spondylodiskitis. AJR Am J Roentgenol. 2006;186:977-80.

[29] Yang X, Zhang Q, Guo X. Value of magnetic resonance imaging in brucellar spondylodiscitis. Radiol Med. 2014 Dec;119:928-33.

[30] Bozgeyik Z, Aglamis S, Bozdag PG, Denk A. Magnetic resonance imaging findings of musculoskeletal brucellosis. Clin Imaging. 2014;38:719-23.

[31] Oztekin O, Calli C, Adibelli Z, Kitis O, Eren C, Altinok T. Brucellar spondylodiscitis: Magnetic resonance imaging features with conventional sequences and diffusion-weighted imaging. Radiol Med. 2010;115:794-803.

[32] Tali ET. Spinal infections. Eur J Radiol. 2004;50:120-33.

[33] Turunc T, Demiroglu YZ, Uncu H, Colakoglu S, Arslan H. A comparative analysis of tuberculous, brucellar and pyogenic spontaneous spondylodiscitis patients. J Infect. 2007;55:158-63.

[34] Ozaksoy D, Yucesoy K, Yucesoy M, Kovanlıkaya I, Yuce A, Naderi S. Brucellar spondylitis: MRI findings. Eur Spine J. 2001;10:529-33.

[35] Sharif HS, Aideyan OA, Clark DC, et al. Brucellar and tuberculous spondylitis: Comparative imaging features. Radiology. 1989;171:419-425.

[36] Alp E, Doganay M. Current therapeutic strategy in spinal brucellosis. Int J Infect Dis. 2008;12:573-7.

[37] Colmenero JD, Jimenez-Mejias ME, Sanchez-Lora FJ, et al. Pyogenic, tuberculous, and brucellar vertebral osteomyelitis: A descriptive and comparative study of 219 cases. Ann Rheum Dis. 1997;56:709-15.

[38] Corbel MJ. Brucellosis in humans and animals. Geneva, Switzerland: World Health Organization Publications, 2006.

[39] Alavi SM, Alavi L. Treatment of brucellosis: A systematic review of studies in recent twenty years. Caspian J Intern Med. 2013;4:636-41.

[40] Aygen B, Doganay M, Sumerkan B, Yildiz O, Kayabas U. Clinical manifestations, complications and treatment of brucellosis: A retrospective evaluation of 480 patients. Med Mal Infect. 2002;32:485-93.

[41] Sobottke R, Seifert H, Fätkenheuer G, Schmidt M, et al. Current diagnosis and treatment of spondylodiscitis. Dtsch Arztebl Int. 2008;105:181-87.

[42] Duarte RM, Vaccaro AR. Spinal infection: State of the art and management algorithm. Eur Spine J. 2013;22:2787-99.

[43] Cramer J, Haase N, Behre I, Ostermann PAW. Spondylitis und Spondylodiszitis. Trauma und Berufskrankheit. 2003;5:336-341.

[44] Lu CH, Chang WN, Lui CC, Lee PY, Chang HW. Adult spinal epidural abscess: Clinical features and prognostic factors. Clin Neurol Neurosurg. 2002;104:306-10.

[45] Nas K, Gur A, Kemaloglu MS, et al. Management of spinal brucellosis and outcome of rehabilitation. Spinal Cord. 2001;39:223-7.

[46] Darouiche RO. Spinal epidural abscess. N Engl J Med. 2006;355:2012-20.

[47] Chen WH, Jiang LS, Dai LY. Surgical treatment of pyogenic vertebral osteomyelitis with spinal instrumentation. Eur Spine J. 2007;16:1307-16.

[48] Guerado E, Cerván AM. Surgical treatment of spondylodiscitis. An update. Int Orthop. 2012;36:413-20.

[49] Yang SC, Fu TS, Chen LH, Chen WJ, Tu YK. Identifying pathogens of spondylodiscitis: Percutaneous endoscopy or CT-guided biopsy. Clin Orthop Relat Res. 2008;466:3086-92.

[50] Mückley T, Schütz T, Schmidt MH, Potulski M, Bühren V, Beisse R. The role of thoracoscopic spinal surgery in the management of pyogenic vertebral osteomyelitis. Spine. 2004;29:E227-33.

[51] Five-year assessments of controlled trials of ambulatory treatment, debridement and anterior spinal fusion in the management of the tuberculosis of the spine. Studies in Vulawayo (Rhodesia) and in Hong Kong. Sixth report of the Medical Research Council Working Party on Tuberculosis of the spine. J Bone Joint Surg Br. 1978;60:163-77.

[52] Moon MS, Woo YK, Lee KS, Ha KY, Kim SS, Sun DH. Posterior instrumentation and anterior interbody fusion for tuberculous kyphosis of dorsal and lumbar spine. Spine. 1995;20:1910-68.

[53] Turgut M. Spinal tuberculosis (Potts disease): Its clinical presentation, surgical management and outcome: A survey study on 694 patients. Neurosurg Rev. 2001;24:8-13.

[54] Korovessis P, Petsinis G, Koureas G, Iliopoulos P, Zacharatos S. Anterior surgery with insertion of titanium mesh cage and posterior instrumented fusion performed sequentially on the same day under one anesthesia for septic spondylitis of thoracolumbar spine: Is the use of titanium mesh cages safe? Spine. 2006;31:1014-9.

[55] Hee HT, Majd ME, Holt RT, Pienkowski D. Better treatment of vertebral osteomyelitis using posterior stabilization and titanium mesh cages. J Spinal Disord Tech. 2002;15:149-56;discussion 156.

[56] Smith AJ, Arginteanu M, Moore F, Steinberger A, Camins M. Increased incidence of cage migration and nonunion in instrumented transforaminal lumbar interbody fusion with bioabsorbable cages. J Neurosurg Spine. 2010;13:388-93.

[57] Reinhold M, Knop C, Beisse R, Audigé L, Kandziora F, Pizanis A, et al. Operative treatment of 733 patients with acute thoracolumbar spinal injuries: comprehensive results from the second, prospective, Internet-based multicenter study of the Spine Study Group of the German Association of Trauma Surgery. Eur Spine J. 2010; 19:1657-76

[58] Zarghooni K, et al. Treatment of spondylodiscitis. Int Orthop. 2012;36:405-11

[59] Linhardt O, Matussek J, Refior HJ, Krödel A. Long-term results of ventro-dorsal versus ventral instrumentation fusion in the treatment of spondylitis. Int Orthop. 2007;31:113-9

[60] Fukuta S1, Miyamoto K, Masuda T, Hosoe H, Kodama H, Nishimoto H, Sakaeda H, Shimizu K. Two-stage (posterior and anterior) surgical treatment using posterior spinal instrumentation for pyogenic and tuberculotic spondylitis. Spine (Phila Pa 1976). 2003 Aug 1;28:E302-8.

[61] Hirakawa A, Miyamoto K, Masuda T, Fukuta S, Hosoe H, Iinuma N, et al. Surgical outcome of 2-stage (posterior and anterior) surgical treatment using spinal instrumentation for tuberculous spondylitis. Spinal Disord Tech. 2010 Apr;23:133-8.

[62] Guerado E, Fuerstenberg CH. What bone graft substitutes should we use in post-traumatic spinal fusion? Injury Suppl. 2011;2:S64–S71.

[63] Louw JA. Spinal tuberculosis with neurologic deficit: Treatment with vascularized rib grafts, posterior osteotomies and fusion. J Bone Joint Surg Br. 1986;72:686-93.

[64] Allen RT, Lee YP, Stimson E, Garfin SR. Bone morphogenetic protein-2 (BMP-2) in the treatment of pyogenic vertebral osteomyelitis. Spine. 2007;32:2996-3006.

[65] Pola E, Rossi B, Nasto LA, Colangelo D, Logroscino CA. Surgical treatment of tuberculous spondylodiscitis. Eur Rev Med Pharmacol Sci. 2012;16 Suppl 2:79-85.

[66] Ulu-Kilic A, Karakas A, Erdem H, Turker T, Inal AS, Ak O, et al. Update on treatment options for spinal brucellosis. Clin Microbiol Infect. 2014;20:O75-82.

Chapter 8

Blood Cultures for the Diagnosis of Human Brucellosis

Pablo Yagupsky

Additional information is available at the end of the chapter

http://dx.doi.org/10.5772/61143

Abstract

Brucellosis represents a serious health threat to human populations living in areas endemic for the disease. The clinical manifestations of brucellosis are protean and non-specific, and laboratory confirmation of the diagnosis is crucial for an adequate management of the patient and implementation of infection control measures aimed to control the disease in affected herds. Although brucellosis can be confirmed by serologic tests and nucleic acid amplification assays, culture detection of circulating *Brucella* organisms remains a diagnostic cornerstone. Traditionally, prolonged incubation of media and performance of blind subcultures of negative blood culture vials have been recommended to maximize isolation of the organism. In recent years, modern automated blood culture systems have revolutionized the diagnosis of human brucellosis by improving sensitivity and enabling detection of brucellae within the routine one-week incubation protocol followed in most Clinical Microbiology laboratories. Development of molecular techniques and mass-spectrometry technology have also shortened the time needed to identify members of the genus, whereas use of biological safety cabinets considerably reduce the risks of contagion to laboratory personnel.

Keywords: Human brucellosis, blood cultures, diagnosis, identification, safety

1. Introduction

Because of the non-specific clinical manifestations of human brucellosis and the need for prolonged combination therapy with antibiotics that are not routinely prescribed for other infectious diseases, laboratory confirmation of the diagnosis is of paramount importance for the adequate patient management. In addition, evidence of brucellosis has serious public health implications because it discloses exposure to a contaminated source (infected animals or their products, unsafe laboratory practices, or a potential biological warfare attack).

The current laboratory diagnosis of human brucellosis is based on culture, serology, and nucleic acid amplification assays. Although the culture strategy is hampered by the slow growing features of *Brucella* species, safety problems, and the reduced sensitivity of the method for detecting chronic cases, isolation of the organism remains a diagnostic cornerstone. Recovery of the brucellae is an irrefutable evidence of the disease; it permits speciation and typing of the recovered strain for epidemiological studies [1] and enables determination of antibiotic susceptibility, when indicated. Blood cultures may also allow diagnosis of brucellosis in the acute period of the disease, when serological test results may still be negative or exhibit borderline antibody titers [2]. An additional advantage of the culture approach is the fact that it enables the diagnosis in cases in which brucellosis is not suspected. This is an important consideration because the clinical presentation of human brucellosis is frequently not specific, and patients may present with symptoms and signs suggestive of other diagnoses, including a variety of infections, rheumatic, hematologic, or neurologic conditions, hepatitis, etc. If the possibility of brucellosis is not considered, specific serologic tests or nucleic acid amplification assays will not be ordered and, under these circumstances, the diagnosis of the disease can be missed altogether, unless a positive blood culture was obtained. Isolation of *Brucella* organisms can be, then, the first and only proof of the disease. For instance, in a study conducted in a highly endemic area for *B. melitensis* in southern Israel, 27 blood cultures obtained from 21 patients with suspected brucellosis grew the organism, as did 42 cultures drawn from 27 patients in whom possibility of the disease was not entertained [3].

The current prevalence of brucellosis in most Western countries is low and, therefore, microbiology laboratories are frequently unfamiliar with the tools available for isolating the organism. The purpose of this review is to summarize published information on the performance of the different blood culture techniques for the detection of brucellae. Because anaerobic conditions do not support growth of the strictly aerobic members of the genus, only data on the performance of aerobic media will be included in the chapter.

1.1. Role of blood cultures in the diagnosis of human brucellosis

Brucellosis is a systemic infection in which the bacterium initially localizes in the regional lymph nodes and then disseminates by the hematogenous route to macrophages-rich tissues where it adopts an intracellular lifestyle [4]. In the early stages of the disease, patients experience continuous brucellemia, facilitating the culture diagnosis of the disease. As the infection progresses, bacteremia tends to wane, making the recovery of the organism increasingly difficult [5]. However, *Brucella* organisms may reappear in the bloodstream intermittently [5], and their isolation is associated with an increased risk of relapse, probably because a demonstrable bacteremia implies a high bacterial burden [6, 7]. Even in localized infections, the pathogenesis of brucellosis in the human host always implies a bacteremic phase and, therefore, blood cultures may represent an adequate tool for establishing the diagnosis, although their sensitivity varies widely (between 10% and 90%) in different series [5].

http://dx.doi.org/10.5772/61143

2. Blood culture methods

The sensitivity of blood cultures for detecting circulating brucellae may be negatively influenced by a variety of factors such as patient's age [8], prolonged or chronic clinical course [9–12], or previous exposure to antibiotics [12, 13], as well as technical aspects including blood sample volume, incubation time, frequency of growth monitoring, or the performance of blood culture media and detection systems. Despite these drawbacks, blood culture techniques have also been adopted for the isolation of *Brucella* spp. from normally sterile specimens other than blood [14], such as bone marrow [12, 15, 16], synovial fluid aspirates [17], pancreatic exudate [18], or cerebrospinal fluid [19], and have been shown to be comparable or more sensitive than conventional culture methods on solid media.

2.1. Manual monophasic methods

Although *Brucella* organisms may be recovered by routine bacteriological culture methods, detection of the organism in clinical specimens is frequently hindered by its slow growth. Because seemingly negative blood culture vials are routinely discarded after a one-week incubation period, unless physicians and laboratory personnel are aware of the possibility of brucellosis, the diagnosis may be missed altogether. To maximize the detection of fastidious members of the genus, incubation of blood cultures for 30 days and performance of blind subcultures have been advised [20, 21]. This approach has obvious drawbacks: it is labor intensive, prolonged incubation of blood culture vials requires large laboratory space and costly equipment, and diagnosis of the disease is substantially delayed.

2.2. Biphasic methods

To circumvent the necessity of making repeat subcultures, an ingenious biphasic flask, containing solid agar and a liquid phase, was developed by Ruiz-Castañeda in the late 1940s [11, 14, 21, 22]. After inoculation, the flask is supplemented with 10% CO_2 and tilted so that the liquid covers the solid medium and incubated in the upright position. Flasks are examined every 3 days for the presence of colonies [14, 21, 22]. If no growth is observed, flasks are tilted again and re-incubated, and the cycle is repeated for at least 35 days [14, 21, 22].

Gotuzzo *et al.* reported their experience with the Castañeda method in Peru and observed that brucellae colonies developed within one week, with a mean time-to-detection of 4.3 days when seeded with bone marrow specimens, and 6.7 days when inoculated with peripheral blood, and all positive results were obtained within 15 days of incubation [10]. In a Spanish study, however, the time-to-detection was more prolonged, and the majority of flasks required between one and three weeks of incubation [23]. Differences in the patients' population, the biological characteristics of the *Brucella* strains, or the composition and quality of homemade media may explain the observed discrepancies in the performance of the method.

The capability of a commercial biphasic blood culture flask (Hémoline biphasic medium, bioMérieux, Marcy l'Etoile, France) to recover *Brucella melitensis* was prospectively assessed by Ruiz et al. [24]. Flasks were inoculated with 10 ml of blood obtained from patients with suspected brucellosis, incubated for three weeks, and subjected to blind subcultures on day 21. Although the median time-to-positivity was 5 days only, four out of 19 (21.1%) positive cultures were detected after 7 to 9 incubation days [24].

2.3. Lysis centrifugation: In-house and commercial methods

Braun and Kelsh developed a membrane filter technique for isolating *Brucella* spp. and evaluated its performance in a rabbit animal model [25]. A heparinized blood specimen obtained from animals experimentally inoculated with *Brucella* organisms was subjected to osmotic lysis and filtered through a sterile Millipore filter under negative pressure. Filters were placed on the surface of solid media and incubated, and organisms trapped in the membrane developed as colonies on the agar. The technique was abandoned because it was too cumbersome, time and labor intensive, and filters became easily plugged with cellular components of the blood.

A new and original method was subsequently developed in which blood cells were osmotically lysed, and this step was followed by centrifugation and spread of the lysate on the surface of solid culture media [26, 27]. In 1984, Etemadi et al. evaluated this lysis centrifugation procedure —also known as lysis concentration—and compared its performance with that of the Castañeda flask for the detection of *B. melitensis* from blood and other normally sterile body fluids [26]. All cultures, including 14 peripheral blood samples, two bone marrow, and two cerebrospinal fluid specimens, were positive by the lysis centrifugation method within 48 hours, whereas all 18 Castañeda flasks remained negative after 21 days of incubation [26].

A similar lysis centrifugation method was used by Mantur and Mangalgi who compared it with the biphasic Castañeda vial in patients with acute and chronic brucellosis confirmed by a standard agglutination test (SAT) titer ≥160 [28]. Of 121 patients with acute brucellosis, the Castañeda method identified 87 (71.8%), whereas the lysis centrifugation was positive in 110 (90.9%) patients (*P=0.001*), and the time-to-detection was 6.7±2.2 and 2.4±0.9 days, respectively (*P<0.001*). Of the 27 patients with chronic disease, the detection rates were 3.3% (n=9) for the Castañeda flask and 74.1% (n=20) for the lysis centrifugation method (*P=0.087*), and the time-to-detection was 7.2±2.6 and 2.7±1.4 days, respectively (*P=0.001*). In a more recent study, the lysis centrifugation recovered *B. melitensis* in 73 (43.1%) of 169 serologically-confirmed human cases, compared to 42 (24.8%) detected by the blood clot culture and 59 (34.9%) by the Castañeda technique, and the detection time was significantly shorter [29].

Encouraging results were also obtained in Peru by Espinosa et al. who compared the performance of the traditional Castañeda method with that of Etemadi's lysis centrifugation technique in 88 patients in which the disease was suspected on the bases of compatible clinical symptoms and a SAT titer ≥1:25 [9]. The two methods were similar in terms of sensitivity: the lysis centrifugation procedure detected *Brucella* organisms in 38 (43.2%) patients while the Castañeda flask succeeded in 31 (35.2%) patients (*P>0.05*). However, the detection times differed significantly and were 3.8±0.8 days for the lysis centrifugation and 13.6±6.5 days for the Castañeda method (*P<0.001*). In a prospective study, Kolman et al. obtained blood cultures from Israeli patients with serologically proven brucellosis [27]. Blood sample aliquots were subjected to an in-house lysis centrifugation procedure and inoculated into an aerobic radiometric BACTEC system (Becton Dickinson Diagnostic Instrument Systems, Towson, Md., USA) vial [27]. The lysis centrifugation detected *B. melitensis* in only 15 (27.8%) out of 54 patients, whereas the comparator succeeded in 19 (35.2%) patients. The lysis centrifugation method, however, detected brucellae after an average of 3.5 days (range 2–4 days) vs.14 days (range 7–30 days) by the automated system.

The traditional in-house lysis concentration methods have been replaced in recent decades by a commercial blood culture system (the Isolator Microbial Tube, Wampole Laboratories, Cranbury, NJ, USA). Collected blood samples are inoculated into a vial containing a mixture of the anticoagulant sodium polyethol sulfonate (SPS) and detergent. The detergent lyses the blood cells releasing already phagocytized but still viable organisms, and the lysate is then seeded onto appropriate solid media and incubated. The system has two versions: a small tube for use in pediatric patients that accommodate up to 1.5 ml of blood and, therefore, is plated directly; and a larger 10 ml-containing tube for use in adult patients that require a preliminary centrifugation step to concentrate the lysate before plating.

In a prospective study, Navas et al. inoculated 10 ml of blood obtained from patients with presumptive brucellosis into an Isolator Microbial Tube, and two 5 ml-aliquots were inoculated into one aerobic (NR6A) and one anaerobic (NR7A) BACTEC NR660 vials [30]. The two methods were comparable in terms of sensitivity, the Isolator Microbial Tube detected 7 positive cultures system vs. 6 identified by the automated system. [30]. The lysis concentration technique reduced the time-to-detection to 2–5 days vs.17 to 29 days with a mean of 20.6 days for the BACTEC blood culture system. It should be noted, however, that because anaerobic bottles do not support the growth of strictly aerobic *Brucella* organisms, the effective blood volume inoculated into the BACTEC system was, in fact, only half of that seeded onto the Isolator Microbial Tube plates [30].

A study conducted in a region endemic for *B. melitensis* in Israel confirmed the capability of the Isolator Microbial Tube system to accelerate the detection of the organism as compared to traditional methods, and 15 out of 22 (68.2%) blood cultures were already positive after 72 hours [31]. When compared with the automated BACTEC 9240 system, however, the Isolator Microbial Tube was inferior in terms of both time-to-detection and sensitivity (see "Comparative studies involving fully automated blood culture systems" section).

2.4. Automated blood culture systems

In the past, detection of positive blood culture vials relied on periodic examination of inoculated vials for the presence of turbidity as an indication that microorganisms have multiplied in the broth and reached a high concentration. Over the last few decades, the diagnosis of bacteremic infections has been revolutionized by the development of automated blood culture systems. The novel technologies are based on detections of increasing concentrations of CO_2 released by the metabolic activity of a growing mass of organisms, or consumption of the available oxygen. Significant changes in the gas content of the blood culture vials can be detected before cloudiness becomes visible, resulting in the gain of precious time and allowing early diagnosis of bacteremia. The detecting technology evolved over the years; the pioneer semi-automated BACTEC 460 detected release of radioactive CO_2 generated by the metabolism of ^{14}C-containing substrates by penetrating the vial top and aspirating the headspace above the fluid level. The subsequent generations consisted of fully-automated instruments that employed either detection of CO_2 levels by invasive infrared reading (BACTEC NR), non-invasive measurement of increasing fluorescence as the concentration of CO_2 increases or the O_2 content decreases (the BACTEC 9000 and FX series of instruments), colorimetric CO_2 measurement (BacT/ALERT, bioMérieux, Marcy l'Etoile, France), or quenching of fluorescence by CO_2 production and acidification or reduction of the culture broth (VITAL, bioMérieux, Marcy l'Etoile, France). Overall, published studies indicate that technical advances in the detection technologies and improvements in the composition of broth culture media have resulted in gradual increase in sensitivity, shortened time-to-detection of *Brucella* organisms, enabling labor saving by continuous hands-off monitoring of a large number of blood culture vials and decrease in culture contamination rates.

Experience with the isolation of *Brucella* spp. by automated blood culture systems has been accumulating at a slow pace. Although the disease is still prevalent in many developing countries, use of modern bacteriologic techniques in endemic areas is limited because of their high cost, whereas in the more affluent Western world, where use of modern automated systems is widespread, brucellosis has been successfully controlled or eradicated altogether.

2.5. Factors influencing detection of brucellae by automated systems

In general terms, detection of CO_2 production in blood culture broths depends on the initial number of bacteria inoculated (which reflects the concentration of circulating organisms and the volume of the blood sample drawn), duplication time of the species, its intrinsic metabolic activity, composition of the media, presence of growth promoters or inhibitory factors, frequency of readings, sensitivity of the sensor, and threshold levels.

Obviously, obtaining a large blood specimen should improve the sensitivity of the blood culture tool for detecting bacteremia. In practice, the volume of blood inoculated in the bottle varies little (usually between 1 to 3 ml per bottle in children and 3 to 5 ml in adults) because of the requirement to keep at least a 1:5 to 1:10 blood-to-broth ratio to reduce the concentration of detrimental factors such as complement, antibodies, or antibiotics contained in the clinical specimen.

The magnitude of *Brucella* bacteremia is frequently low with a median of 88 CFU/ml [31, 32] and a range of 1.3 CFU/ml to >1,000 CFU/ml in children [31]. As it should be expected, the time-to-positivity of automated blood culture systems correlates inversely with the concentration of circulating organisms, validating the results of experimental studies with simulated blood cultures [33, 34]. In addition, *Brucella* organisms have a relatively long (2.5 to 3.5 hours) doubling time compared to other pathogenic bacteria [32]. This feature, coupled with the low CO_2 production by members of the genus, results in delayed detection of brucellae by some automated blood culture systems. In a series of in vitro studies using the BacT/ALERT system, a slow release of CO_2 by *B. melitensis* compared with other human pathogens was observed, and the peak concentrations of the gas were inferior [33]. In a series of experiments with BACTEC NR730 vials inoculated with brucellae, Gamazo et al. reported that noticeable

http://dx.doi.org/10.5772/61143

turbidity was noted in the vial on average 24 hours earlier than detection by the automated instrument [32].

With the purpose of improving CO_2 production by *Brucella* organisms, the effect of adding a variety of supplements (pyruvate, alanine, glutarate, urea, glucose, and erythritol), as well as changing the pH of the culture broth was investigated [32]. Only alanine and pyruvate resulted in a mild increase in the CO_2 production, while lowering the pH of the medium from 7.2 to 6.2 coupled with pyruvate supplementation, induced a more pronounced increment. Although these experimental results suggest that modifications in the formulation of blood culture media may reduce the time-to-detection of *Brucella* bacteremia, changes in the broth composition may not necessarily sustain growth of other bacterial species. In the same study, a harmful effect of the anticoagulant SPS contained in the blood culture vials was demonstrated. Unfortunately, blood culture systems cannot dispense with the use of SPS because there are no good alternatives to the antiphagocytic, anticomplementary, and aminoglycoside-neutralizing effects of this compound. In the vials of the 9000 series of BACTEC instruments, the concentration of SPS has been reduced to 0.025% compared with 0.035% in the NR660 and BacT/ALERT media and the total volume of broth has been increased from 30 ml in the NR660 system to 40 ml in the BACTEC 9000 instruments vials, improvements that may explain the better performance of the latter systems for detecting fastidious *Brucella* organisms [35].

2.6. Radiometric detection of brucellae

The BACTEC 460, developed in the early 1970s was the first in a series of modern blood culture systems. Published experience with the use of this method for the recovery of brucellae from blood is limited and obtained results were suboptimal [27, 36–38]. In 1984, Arnow et al. investigated a cluster of foodborne *B. melitensis* infections among travelers to endemic Spain [36]. Overall, 15 out of 19 (78.9%) blood cultures derived from 6 patients were detected by the automated instrument between 4 and 8 days of incubation. In another report, brucellae were only recovered from a blind subculture performed in a three-day-old vial that remained radiometrically negative despite having been incubated for 6 additional days [37].

In a comparative study, Serrano et al. obtained 83 blood culture sets from 42 patients with positive *Brucella* agglutinin titers [38]. Five ml of blood were inoculated into an aerobic BACTEC 460 vial and an identical volume was inoculated into a Castañeda flask, incubated for 10 days, and subjected to blind subcultures on days 5 and 10. By day 5, 14 cultures were positive. The Castañeda method detected 12 positive cultures (85.7%) and the BACTEC bottle 10 (71.4%), of which only 2 were detected radiometrically and the remaining by subculture only. On day 10, 49 cultures were already positive by the biphasic flask and 56 by the radiometric medium ($P>0.05$), of which only 27 reached the radiometric positivity threshold [38].

2.7. Infrared detection system

Data on the use of infrared detection technology (BACTEC NR instruments) for the detection of *Brucella* spp. are also scarce [3, 27, 30, 34, 39, 40]. Zimmerman et al. recovered *B. abortus* by subculture of two five-day-old blood cultures and from a seven-day-old bone marrow culture inoculated into aerobic BACTEC NR vials [34]. Once the diagnosis was made, additional blood cultures were obtained and 15 vials, including aerobic, osmotically stabilized (aerobic hypertonic), and anaerobic media were inoculated and monitored by the automated instrument. All five aerobic and four osmotically stabilized vials became positive between 7 and 20 days, whereas, as expected, all five anaerobic bottles remained negative.

In a Spanish study, inoculated BACTEC NR vials and biphasic Hémoline flasks were monitored for three weeks, and negative media were blindly subcultured on day 21. The biphasic system detected 28 positive cultures, obtained from 18 patients, after an average of 7 days. The BACTEC NR system detected only 12 positive bottles, missed 10 patients, and the mean time-to-positivity was substantially longer (19.6 days) [39]. Furthermore, 11 of these 12 BACTEC NR positive vials gave negative infrared readings during the three-week incubation period, and the organism was detected by subculture only [39].

In the aforementioned study by Navas et al., the BACTEC NR instrument detected only 12 out of 16 (75.0%) blood culture sets obtained from 7 patients and missed the diagnosis in 1 patient, whereas the Isolator Microbial Tube detected all 7 patients, and the time-to-positivity was significantly shorter [30]. Employing the BACTEC NR system, Gedikoglu isolated brucellae in 22 patients with a median detection time of 72 hours [40]. Because vials were only kept for 7 days and no blind subcultures of negative bottles were performed, the study does not allow assessment of the sensitivity of the system for detecting brucellae within the routine one-week incubation protocol.

To assess the capability of the BACTEC NR blood culture system to detect *B. melitensis* within the conventional one-week incubation schedule, we conducted a prospective study in southern Israel [3]. Blood culture vials were monitored by the automated instrument and subcultured once a week for four weeks, and the proportion of positive cultures detected by the instrument within the first week was determined. During the two-year study period, 27 of 373 (7.2%) blood cultures, drawn from 21 patients, were positive for brucellae. Twenty-one (78.8%) of these cultures were detected by the BACTEC NR instrument within 7 days, and 6 positive cultures (22.2%) were detected by subculture after two or three weeks, corroborating that prolonged incubation and periodic performance of subcultures of negative bottles were still required to optimize the detection of *B. melitensis* by the non-radiometric BACTEC technology.

2.8. Continuous monitoring systems

BacT/ALERT system. The published experience with the use of the BacT/ALERT system for the recovery of circulating brucellae remains limited [18, 33, 41]. In 1992, Solomon and Jackson isolated *B. melitensis* in a traveler to the Middle East after only 2.8 days [33]. Two years later, Casas et al. drew blood cultures from 6 patients with serologically-confirmed infection [41]. Inoculated bottles were monitored by the BacT/ALERT instrument for 10 consecutive days and were then transferred to a regular incubator for 10 additional days, and blind subcultures on solid media were performed on days 10 and 20. Only 1 of 9 positive bottles was detected by the automated instrument after 2.9 days, while the remaining bottles were detected by subculture only: 7 on day 10, and 1 on day 20 [41]. A different experience was reported by Roiz et al. who found that all 9 blood cultures, obtained from 5 patients, yielded the organism within

3.7 days, and a blood culture vial, inoculated with pancreatic fluid, was detected positive after 13.3 hours only [18].

BACTEC 9000 instruments. In 1996, Gedikoglu et al. summarized the experience accumulated in a Turkish hospital with the use of the BACTEC 9120 system with a one-week monitoring protocol [40]. Thirty blood cultures, drawn from 15 patients grew *B. melitensis* within 84 hours of incubation. Akcam et al. compared the BACTEC 9120 blood culture system and conventional cultures for culturing normally-sterile body fluids other than blood employing the aerobic pediatric vial and a 7-day incubation protocol, and reported that the five clinical specimens containing *B. melitensis* were only detected by the automated instrument [14].

Kurtoglu et al. summarized the experience accumulated with the BACTEC small 9050 instrument and the medium-size 9120 model for culturing blood in an endemic area for brucellosis in Turkey. The study employed a routine 5-day protocol but extended the incubation period to 14 days when brucellosis was suspected [42]. All brucellae were recovered within 10 days but no precise information on the time-to-positivity was reported, and the fraction of organisms detected within the routine protocol's timetable was not stated. Using the BACTEC 9240, a larger version of the system, and a similar incubation protocol, we detected 59 of 77 (76.6%) positive *Brucella* cultures within 4 days (unpublished data).

Despite these encouraging results, limiting incubation of blood culture vials to the traditional one-week period instituted in most clinical laboratories cannot be adopted in regions endemic for brucellosis, unless it is convincingly demonstrated that no significant number of positive cultures are missed by a short incubation schedule. Adequate assessment of the capability of any blood culture system to detect brucellae within the routine one-week incubation protocol requires keeping of inoculated vials for a longer period and performance of blind subculture of negative vials to assure that no positive cultures are overlooked.

The capability of the BACTEC blood culture system to detect brucellae within 7 days was prospectively investigated among febrile children in southern Israel [43]. Following the traditional recommendations by the World Health Organization [20] and the American Society for Microbiology [21], inoculated aerobic pediatric blood culture vials were monitored by the BACTEC 9240 instrument for four consecutive weeks, and blind subcultures of negative vials were performed once a week [43]. Of a total of 2,579 blood cultures drawn, 42 (1.6%) were positive for *B. melitensis*, of which 41 (97.6%) were detected by the automated instrument within 2 to 6 days, and the remaining positive vial was missed by the instrument and detected by blind subculture performed on day 7. Cumulative positivity rates by the automated detection were 0.0%, 23.6%, 78.9%, 86.8%, 92.1%, 97.6%, and 97.6% for days 1 through 7, respectively.

Similar results were obtained in a study conducted in Saudi Arabia in a mixed population of children and adult patients [35]. BACTEC 9240 aerobic/F (for adults) and Peds Plus vials (used for pediatric patients) were kept for up to 21 days, but no blind subcultures of negative vials were performed, precluding an adequate assessment of the sensitivity of the method. Overall, the BACTEC instrument detected 90 out of 97 (92.7%) positive cultures, of which 85 yielded *B. melitensis* and 12 *B. abortus* isolates within 5 days of incubation, and only 3 cultures (3.1%) became positive after the seventh day (2 on day 8 and 1 on day 9) [35].

Durmaz et al. reviewed their five-year experience with the BACTEC 9120 system in a Turkish hospital [44]. Vials were monitored by the automated instrument for 7 days and vials negative at the end of period were Gram-stained and subcultured. Overall, 20 vials yielded *B. melitensis* after a median 69.9 hours (mean: 30.0 hours, range: 31.2–117.5 hours), and no false negative automated readings were recorded.

However, in another Turkish study, 8 of 136 cultures obtained from 60 patients, remained undetected by the instrument and were recovered on blind subcultures performed after 30 days of incubation [45]. A similar experience was recorded in the investigation of an outbreak of *B. melitensis* infections involving 16 adult Spanish patients [46]. The researchers employed the BACTEC 9050 that differs from the other instruments of the BACTEC 9000 series in that agitation of the bottles is continuous, a factor that may accelerate bacterial growth, whereas in the other models is intermittent. Inoculated bottles were incubated for 21 days, and negative vials were subcultured blindly at the end of the study period [46]. Overall, 13 patients had demonstrable *Brucella* bacteremia. Growth of the organism was detected by the instrument within one week in only 9 (69.2%) bacteremic individuals, in 2 additional patients on the 8th and 11th day, and in the remaining 2 patients, brucellae were entirely missed by the instrument and detected by the final subculture.

Although the reasons for these discrepancies are not obvious, the superior performance of the automated BACTEC system in the aforementioned communication by Yagupsky et al. [43] could be explained by the fact that their study population consisted entirely of children presenting to the Pediatric Emergency Department with an acute febrile disease, probably characterized by continuous high-magnitude bacteremia, whereas other investigations enrolled mostly adult patients with a more prolonged disease and, therefore, a lower bacterial load.

The BACTEC MYCO/F LYTIC medium has been recently developed to improve the recovery of intracellular pathogens such as fungi and mycobacteria by lysing leucocytes with saponin [47]. Because brucellae are facultative intracellular bacteria, it was assumed that use of the automated blood culture system coupled with this novel medium would improve both sensitivity and time-to-detection of circulating organisms. However, in a prospective study in which the performance of the traditional pediatric (Peds Plus /F) and adult (PlusAerobic/F) aerobic vials were compared with that of the MYCO/F LYTIC vial, the sensitivity was comparable but the time-to-positivity was significantly longer in the latter (101.4±46.7 hours) vs. 65.5±18.9 hours for the traditional media combined (*P=0.004*), and after 72 hours of incubation, only 5 out of the 16 (31.2%) MYCO/F LYTIC vials were already positive, compared to 16 out of 19 (84.2%) aerobic adult and pediatric vials (*P=0.005*).

2.9. Comparative studies involving fully automated blood culture systems

In a prospective study in which blood aliquots drawn from children with suspected brucellosis were inoculated into a BACTEC 9240 aerobic vial and into an Isolator Microbial Tube, the sensitivity and time-to-positivity of the two methods were compared [31]. Overall, 122 pairs of blood cultures were obtained and 28 (22.8%) were positive by at least one method. The BACTEC system detected all 28 positive cultures and the Isolator Microbial Tube detected 22 positive cultures (sensitivity: 78.6%, $P<0.023$). Among those 22 cultures positive by both methods, 21 (95.5%) and 15 (68.2%) were found to be positive within 3 days by the BACTEC and by the lysis centrifugation systems, respectively. Eight cultures (36.4%) were detected at least 1 day earlier by the BACTEC instrument, and the remaining 14 were detected by the two systems on the same day ($P<0.05$). In summary, the automated BACTEC system was significantly superior than the compactor in terms of sensitivity and also reduced the time-to-positivity.

The performance of the two most popular automated blood culture systems for the detection of brucellae was compared in a single study [48]. BacT/ALERT and BACTEC 9,240 vials were inoculated with 10 ml of adult patients' blood and monitored for 7 days. Overall, the BACTEC system detected 9 out of 17 (52.9%) positive cultures whereas the BacT/ALERT detected 14 (82.3%) ($P=0.067$), and the time-to-detection of the positive vials were similar (2.8 vs. 2.5 days, respectively). Apparently, no blind subcultures of negative vials were performed, and it is unknown whether a more prolonged incubation would have improved the recovery rate.

The performance of three blood culture systems [the automated BACTEC 9120 and VITAL (bioMérieux) systems, and the Hémoline biphasic flask] was compared in a prospective study involving 19 positive blood cultures drawn from Spanish patients with brucellosis [24]. The Hémoline medium detected all 19 positive cultures, whereas the BACTEC and the VITAL systems missed one positive culture each (sensitivity: 94.7%). By using a 5-day incubation protocol, 47.4%, 78.9%, and 10.5% cultures were detected by the three blood culture systems, respectively. When the incubation was extended to 7 days, the results were 73.7%, 94.7%, and 47.4%, respectively, indicating that the BACTEC system was significantly faster than the comparators ($P<0.05$). The delayed detection of brucellae by the VITAL system was confirmed in two later studies in which the time-to-positivity for members of the genus was 119.7 and 211.7 hours [49, 50].

2.10. Bone marrow vs. blood cultures

Because of the suboptimal recovery rate of brucellae from blood, it has been suggested that cultures of bone marrow [14, 10, 11, 51, 52], liver tissue [53, 54], or lymph nodes [55] may improve the recovery of the organism. The rationale for these alternative approaches is that *Brucella* organisms survive the intracellular killing by phagocytes and polymorphonuclear leukocytes and localize in the reticuloendothelial system [10, 52].

Ganado and Bannister demonstrated that in one-fifth of patients in whom bone marrow cultures were positive for brucellae, the organism could not be isolated from the blood [39]. Gotuzzo et al. reported that among 50 patients with proven brucellosis detected by cultures of blood, bone marrow, or both, bone marrow cultures were positive in 46 (92.0%) patients whereas blood cultures were positive in only 35 (70.0%) [10]. Despite the small volume of bone marrow cultured (usually less than 1 ml) compared to the much larger blood volumes (between 5 and 10 ml), brucellae grew more rapidly from bone marrow samples, suggesting that higher bacterial concentrations may be present in this macrophages-rich specimen type. In a prospective study by Mantur et al., blood samples and bone marrow aspirates obtained from 103 Indian patients with serologically confirmed brucellosis were inoculated into Castañeda flasks

[15]. The sensitivity of bone marrow cultures was significantly superior and recovered *Brucella* organisms in 85 (82.5%) patients vs. 47 (45.6%) detected by blood cultures *($P<0.001$)*, and the time-to-recovery was significantly shorter (2.8±0.7 and 7.2±2.4 days, respectively, *$P=0.001$*) [15]. It is noticeable that the superior performance of the bone marrow culture was observed in acute, as well as in chronic cases.

Özkurt et al. obtained blood and bone marrow samples from 50 Turkish patients with suspected brucellosis, of which 48 exhibited SAT titers ≥1:160 [12]. Specimens were inoculated into BacT/ALERT vials and into a homemade *Brucella* broth medium. Seeded BacT/ALERT vials were incubated for 7 days. Negative vials at day 7 were incubated for two additional weeks and subcultured on solid media every 2 days. The non-commercial *Brucella* broth media were incubated for four weeks and subcultured blindly every 2 days. The bone marrow specimens proved to be more sensitive for the detection of *B. melitensis* and, overall, 35 of 50 (70.0%) bone marrow cultures, but only 24 of 50 (48.0%) blood cultures grew the organism (*$P<0.05$*).

On the other hand, Magill and Killough found that in their experience, blood cultures were more reliable (sensitivity: 90%) than bone marrow cultures (sensitivity: 40%) [56]. Similarly, Shehabi et al. reported a sensitivity of 44.4% for blood cultures compared to 27.7% for bone marrow cultures [57]; and Iseri et al., employing the BACTEC 9050 instrument, also found peripheral blood cultures to be more sensitive than bone marrow aspirates [detection rates 39 out of 102 (48.0%) and 35 out of 102 (34.3%), respectively (*$P<0.05$*)] [16].

Although current evidence regarding the relative merits of bone marrow vs. peripheral blood cultures remains controversial, most experts considered the former as the gold standard specimen for diagnosis [4]. However, it should be pointed out that blood cultures have the clear advantage of being easy to obtain and repeat, and the fact that they can serendipitously identify cases in which the diagnosis was not entertained; whereas aspiration of bone marrow samples for detecting brucellae requires, *a priori,* a high index of suspicion.

2.11. Blood clot cultures

Because the serum of patients with brucellosis may have antibacterial activity, culture of the blood clot, where organisms phagocytized by leukocytes may be trapped, appears as a rational strategy. The method consists of collecting a blood sample in a sterile tube and allowing it to cloth. The tube is then centrifuged and the serum is separated aseptically and used for serological assays, whereas the clot is disrupted by shaking the tube and seeded into appropriate media [29]. Available data on the advantages of this technique, however, are limited and contentious. Escamilla et al. employed two types of clot cultures, one with added taurocholate-streptokinase and the other with bile, and compared their yield with that of conventional cultures of whole blood in an area endemic for brucellosis in Peru and found the clot cultures were far less sensitive and more labor-intensive than the comparator method [58]. Whereas the conventional cultures detected 28 of 30 (93.3%) positive cultures, the taurocholate-streptokinase was positive in 21 (70.0%) and the bile-clot recovered the organism in a single culture (3.3%). It is unclear whether culturing of the clot without the additives could have provided better results.

http://dx.doi.org/10.5772/61143

In a comparative study of 169 serologically confirmed patients, Mangalgi and Sajjan reported a detection rate of 34.9% for the clot culture, 24.8% for the Castañeda flask, and 43.1% for the lysis concentration method; the mean±SD recovery times were 5.8±1.4, 9.6±1.7, and 4.1±0.9 days, respectively [29]. In a second study by the same research group, blood clot cultures were clearly superior to conventional broth cultures of whole blood for isolating brucellae, increasing the yield by >20% and shortening the time-to-positivity from an average of 8.2 days to 3.1 days [59]. If these favorable results are confirmed by additional research, this simple and inexpensive method could represent a real contribution to the diagnosis of brucellosis in developing countries where more advanced and expensive laboratory technologies are not available.

3. From detection to identification

3.1. Conventional identification of blood culture isolates

Once bacterial growth is detected in a blood culture vial, prompt and precise identification of the isolate is of paramount importance for adequate patient management and avoidance of exposure of laboratory technicians to infective *Brucella* organisms. Traditionally, a Gram stain of the positive broth is performed and, unless the biphasic Castañeda method is employed, it is subcultured onto solid media. Identification of members of the genus *Brucella* is based of the presence of typical small Gram-negative coccobacilli (see Figure 1); positive oxidase, catalase, and urease tests; no fermentation of sugars; CO_2 requirement; lack of motility; and confirmed by a positive agglutination reaction with specific antiserum [14] or, alternatively, the isolate'sbiochemical profile is determined by a commercial system. The main drawbacks of this traditional approach is the slow turnaround time (2 to 3 days) and the possible misidentification of brucellae as *Ochrobactrum anthropi* [60], *Ochrobactrum intermedium* [61], *Bergeyella zoohelcum* [62], or *Moraxella phenylpyruvica* by commercial kits; a serious mistake that has already lead to an outbreak of laboratory-acquired infection [63].

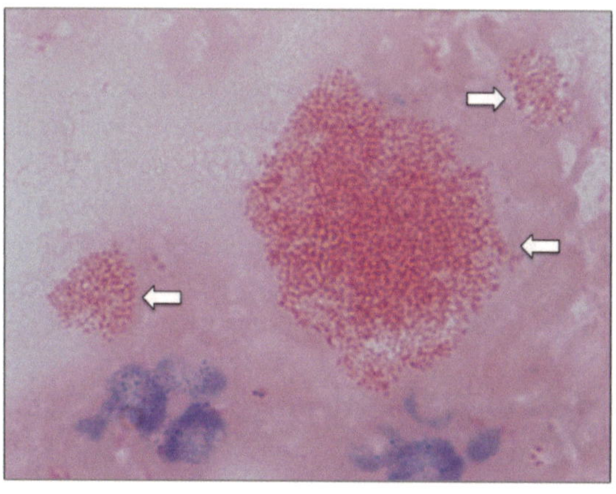

Figure 1. Gram stain of a positive aerobic BACTEC blood culture vial showing *Brucella melitensis* microcolonies (white arrows).

3.2. Rapid phenotypic identification methods

A simple and rapid method was proposed by Rich and co-investigators in Saudi Arabia for the presumptive identification of brucellae from signal-positive BACTEC 9240 blood culture vials [64]. Thirty-three positive BACTEC broths containing Gram-negative coccobacilli and 32 with no visible organisms were subcultured on urea slants and incubated in a CO_2-enriched atmosphere. Of the 44 *Brucella* isolates eventually recovered, 37 gave a positive urease reaction within 4 hours and the remaining were positive after overnight incubation. The urease test showed good specificity and only 2 isolates other than brucellae (both *Haemophilus influenzae*) gave a delayed positive urease reaction. Favorable results were also reported by Maleknejad et al. in an endemic area of Iran using a slight modification of the procedure [65]. The investigators combined the routine Gram staining procedure of positive vials with the high sensitivity of the acridine orange staining, and inoculated positive media onto urea slants. The procedure correctly identified the 41 blood cultures positive for brucellae within 4 hours and was negative in 61 slants seeded with blood culture broths that grew other bacterial species.

In recent years, introduction of matrix-assisted laser desorption ionization-time of flight mass spectrometry (MALDI-TOF) technology in the Clinical Microbiology laboratory has revolutionized the field of bacterial speciation, enabling precise, reproducible, and cost-effective identification of isolates within minutes. The method obviates the need for biochemical testing and, thus, is suitable for high-throughput by less skilled laboratory personnel [66, 67]. This novel approach can be employed on bacterial colonies growing on agar plates, as well as from positive culture broths and, therefore, it enables direct identification of organisms from blood culture vials [68]. Available data with type strains and simulated blood cultures indicate that the MALDI-TOF procedure reliably identifies isolates as members of the genus *Brucella*. It should be pointed out that because of the high transmissibility of *Brucella* organisms, an initial bacterial inactivation step with absolute ethanol was added as a measure of caution, to be followed by extraction with formic acid and acetonitrile [69, 70]. Although in some studies, the method also enabled discrimination at the species level and even at the biovar level for *B. suis* [66, 67], other investigators reported unreliable discrimination between the different *Brucella* species [68].

In summary, major advancements in spectrometry technology over the last decade have opened the possibility of accurate and rapid identification of brucellae directly from blood culture vials. Data on the use of MALDI-TOF method for this purpose, however, are still limited because, although the cost for specimen processing is low, MALDI-TOF instruments are expensive and, thus, unavailable in most resources-poor rural areas endemic for brucellosis. Although experimental results are promising, this encouraging experience awaits confirmation with real cultures derived from actual patients.

3.3. Identification of brucellae by DNA technology

A variety of molecular approaches have also been proposed to shorten the identification process and enable correct identification of *Brucella* isolates. A fluorescence *in-situ* hybridization (FISH) assay targeting a part of the *16S* rRNA gene and containing an unlabeled competitor differing from the probe at one base with the purpose of preventing cross-binding, has been

http://dx.doi.org/10.5772/61143

developed and evaluated with actual blood cultures [71]. The test was employed directly in positive blood culture broths and enabled rapid and correct identification of *B. melitensis* at a low cost, and was negative in cultures that grew a variety of other bacterial species.

Sequencing of the *16S* rRNA gene, which is in widespread use for bacterial identification, can be misleading and *Brucella* organisms cannot be accurately distinguished from the closely related α-protobacterial *Ochrobacterium* species [72]. A novel *recA* gene-based, multi-primer, single-target PCR assay has been recently developed and succeeded in differentiating between brucellae and *Ochrobacterium anthropi* and *O. intermedium* [73], although the test has a more prolonged turnaround time and is more expensive than the FISH test.

4. Blood cultures for brucellae and laboratory safety

Brucellosis remains among the most commonly recognized causes of laboratory-transmitted infections, and 2% of all brucellosis cases are laboratory-acquired [74]. Several biological characteristics make brucellae easily transmissible within the close confinement of the Clinical Microbiology laboratory: the infecting dose for humans is very low (10 to 100 bacteria); the organism may enter the body in many ways relevant to laboratory practices, including through the respiratory mucosa, conjunctivae, gastrointestinal tract, or abraded skin [74]; and the long-term persistence of viable microorganisms on inanimate surfaces [13, 75].

Because of the protean manifestations of brucellosis in humans, a wide array of clinical samples submitted to the Clinical Microbiology laboratory for culture, including normally sterile body fluids, exudates, and tissues, may contain viable bacteria, although blood cultures represent the largest number of specimens. The concentration of circulating brucellae in the patients' blood is frequently low [31], and unless a serious breach of safety practices has occurred, blood specimens do not pose a tangible threat of contagion to laboratory personnel. In addition, current automated blood culture instruments monitor CO_2 production without penetrating the blood culture vial and, thus, avoid creation of risky aerosols. However, the danger of significant exposure increases exponentially after incubation, and routine bacteriologic procedures such as preparing, centrifuging, and vortexing of bacterial suspensions, performing subcultures and biochemical testing, particularly the catalase test, entail a substantial potential for nebulization of bacteria, accidental spillage, and contamination of the laboratory environment [76].

In regions endemic for brucellosis, the number of positive cultures for the organism and, consequently, the risk for transmission to laboratory personnel can be extremely high. In a Clinical Microbiology laboratory in Ankara, Turkey, an annual average of 400 cultures were positive for *Brucella* spp. and the disease was diagnosed in 10 (18%) of 55 laboratory workers, representing a calculated hazard of 8% per employee-year [77]. In a study conducted in 1997 at the Soroka University Medical Center (SUMC) that serves an endemic area for the disease in southern Israel, 127 of 3,974 (3.2%) aerobic blood culture vials detected as positive by the automated BACTEC instrument, as well as 11 of 126 (8.7%) Isolator Microbial Tube cultures, grew *B. melitensis* [78]. From 2002–2009, the organism was isolated from 514 of 20,620 (2.5%)

positive blood culture vials and, as expected, the detection rate showed a significant seasonal pattern and was higher between April and September (3.3%) compared with the October-March period (0.9%, *P<0.001*) [79].

To increase laboratory safety, the Centers for Disease Control (CDC) has strongly recommended that all manipulations with live *Brucella* cultures should be confined to a Class II biologic safety cabinet [80]. However, by the time bacterial isolates are identified as brucellae, extensive manipulation of culture media has usually been performed and inadvertent exposure of laboratory personnel may have already occurred. Following a large outbreak of laboratory-acquired brucellosis at the SUMC in 1997 [78], all positive blood cultures are initially processed in safety cabinets until the presence of the organism is ruled-out, and performance of unnecessary antibiotic susceptibility testing of *Brucella* isolates and aerosol-generating procedures has been discontinued, and no further cases of the disease have been detected ever since. It seems, then, prudent to recommend that all positive blood culture vials in endemic areas should be processed in a safety cabinet, when available, pending final identification of the isolate.

5. Conclusions

Although the diagnosis of human brucellosis can be established by serologic and nucleic acid amplification assays, culture confirmation of the disease has not lost its traditional clinical and epidemiological importance. In the past, isolation of brucellae was hindered by the slow growth of the organism and the lack of a suitable commercial blood culture system. To improve recovery of this fastidious bacterium, use of biphasic media, prolonged incubation of vials, and periodic performance of blind subcultures have been traditionally recommended. Development of automated blood culture systems in recent decades has resulted in the gradual increase in sensitivity and shortening of detection time of *Brucella* species. Nowadays, use of modern blood culture systems makes possible the diagnosis of more than 95% of positive cultures within the routine 7-day incubation protocol, and performance of subcultures of negative media is no longer necessary. Additional advances, especially the development of MALDI-TOF technology and nucleic acid amplification and hybridization assays, in recent years, enable a rapid and precise identification of the genus.

Author details

Pablo Yagupsky*

Address all correspondence to: yagupsky@bgu.ac.il

Director of the Clinical Microbiology Laboratory, Soroka University Medical Center, Ben-Gurion University of the Negev, Beer-Sheva, Israel

References

[1] Lee S, Hwang KJ, Park MY, Hwang SD, Chai HY, Chu H, Park SH. Evaluation and selection of multilocus variable-number tandem-repeat analysis primers for genotyping *Brucella abortus* biovar 1 isolated from human patients. Osong Public Health Res Perspect 2013; 4:265-270.

[2] Shemesh AA, Yagupsky P. Limitations of the standard agglutination test for detecting patients with *Brucella melitensis* bacteremia. Vector Borne Zoonotic Dis 2011; 11:1599-1601.

[3] Yagupsky P. Detection of *Brucella melitensis* by BACTEC NR660 blood culture system. J Clin Microbiol 1994; 32:1889-1901.

[4] Pappas G, Akritidis, Bosilkovski M, Tsianos E. Brucellosis. N Eng J Med 2005; 352:2325-2336.

[5] Pappas G, Papadimitriou P. Challenges in *Brucella* bacteremia. Int J Antimicrob Agents 2007; 30; Supp. l1:S29-S31.

[6] Ariza J, Corredoira J, Pallares R, Viladrich PF, Rufi G, Pujol M, Gudiol F. Characteristics of and risk factors for relapse of brucellosis in humans. Clin Infect Dis 1995; 20: 1241-1249.

[7] Solera J, Martinez-Alfaro E, Espinosa A, Castillejos ML, Geijo P, Rodriguez-Zapata M. Multivariate model for predicting relapse in human brucellosis. J Infect 1998; 36:85-88.

[8] Apa H, Devrim I, Memur S, Günay I, Gülfidan G, Çelegen M, Bayram N, Karaarslan U, Bag O, Isgüder R, Özturk A, Inan S, Ünal N. Factors affecting *Brucella* spp. blood culture positivity in children. Vector Borne Zoonotic Dis 2013; 13:176-180.

[9] Espinosa BJ, Chacaltana J, Mulder M, Franco MP, Blazes DL, Gilman RH, Smits HL, Hall ER. Comparison of culture techniques at different stages of brucellosis. Am J Trop Med Hyg 2009; 80:625-627.

[10] Gotuzzo E, Carrillo C, Guerra J, Llosa L. An evaluation of diagnostic methods for brucellosis-the value of bone marrow culture. J Infect Dis 1986; 153:122-125.

[11] Ruiz Castañeda, M. Laboratory diagnosis of brucellosis in man. Bull World Health Org 1961; 24:73-84.

[12] Özkurt Z, Erol S, Tasyaran MA, Kaya A. Detection of *Brucella melitensis* by the BacT/ALERT automated system and *Brucella* broth culture. Clin Microbiol Infect 2002; 8:749-752.

[13] Doganay M, Aygen B. Human brucellosis: An overview. Int J Infect Dis 2003; 7:173-182.

[14] Akcam FZ, Yayli G, Uskun E, Kaya O, Demir C. Evaluation of the Bactec microbial detection system for culturing miscellaneous sterile body fluids. Res Microbiol 2006; 157:433-436.

[15] Mantur BG, Mulimani MS, Bidari LH, Akki AS, Tikare NV. Bacteremia is as unpredictable as clinical manifestations in human brucellosis. Int J Infect Dis 2008; 12:303-307.

[16] Iseri S, Bulut C, Kinikli S, Demiröz AP, Tülek N. Comparison of the diagnostic value of blood and bone marrow cultures in brucellosis. Microbiyol Bul 2006; 40:201-206.

[17] Yagupsky P, Peled N. Use of the Isolator 1.5 Microbial Tube for detection of *Brucella melitensis* in synovial fluid. J Clin Microbiol 2002; 40:3878.

[18] Roiz MP, Peralta FG, Valle R, Arjona R. Microbiological diagnosis of brucellosis. J Clin Microbiol 1998; 36:1819.

[19] Raj A, Gautam V, Gupta PK, Sethi S, Rana S, Ray P. Rapid detection of *Brucella* by an automated blood culture system at a tertiary care hospital of north India. Indian J Med Res 2014; 139:776-778.

[20] Alton GG, Jones LM. Bacteriological methods, 1967; pp. 13-17. *In* Laboratory techniques in brucellosis, World Health Organization, Geneva.

[21] Moyer NP, Holcomb LA. *Brucella*, 1995; pp. 549-555. *In* Murray PR, E J Baron, Pfaller MA, Tenover FC, Yolken RH (ed.), Manual of clinical microbiology, 6th ed. American Society for Microbiology, Washington, D.C.

[22] Ruiz Castañeda M. A practical method for routine blood cultures in brucellosis. Proc Soc Exp Biol Med 1947; 64:114-115.

[23] Rodríguez-Torres A, Fermoso J, Landinez R. Brucelosis. Medicine (Spanish Ed.) 1983; 48:3126-3136.

[24] Ruiz J, Lorente I, Perez J, Simarro E, Martínez-Campos L. Diagnosis of brucellosis by using blood cultures. J Clin Microbiol 1997; 35:2417-2418.

[25] Braun W, Kelsh J. Improved method for cultivation of *Brucella* from the blood. Proc Soc Exp Biol Med 1954; 85:154-155.

[26] Etemadi H, Raissadat A, Pickett MJ, Zafari Y, Vahedifar P. Isolation of *Brucella* spp. from clinical specimens. J Clin Microbiol 1984; 64:115.

[27] Kolman S, Maayan MC, Gotesman G, Rozenszajn LA, Wolach B, Lang R. Comparison of the BACTEC and lysis concentration methods for recovery of *Brucella* species from clinical specimens. Eur J Clin. Microbiol Infect Dis 1991; 10:647-648.

[28] Mantur BG, Mangalgi SS. Evaluation of conventional Castañeda and lysis centrifugation blood culture techniques for diagnosis of human brucellosis. J Clin Microbiol 2004; 42:4327-4328.

[29] Mangalgi S, Sajjan A. Comparison of three blood culture techniques in the diagnosis of human brucellosis. J Lab Physicians 2014; 6:14-17.

[30] Navas E, Guerrero A, Cobo J, Loza E. Faster isolation of *Brucella* spp. from blood by Isolator compared with BACTEC NR. Diagn Microbiol Infect Dis 1993; 16:79-81.

[31] Yagupsky P, Peled N, Press J, Abramson O, Abu-Rashid M. Comparison of BACTEC 9240 Peds Plus medium and Isolator 1.5 Microbial Tube for detection of *Brucella melitensis* from blood cultures. J Clin Microbiol 1997; 35:1382-1384.

[32] Gamazo C, Vitas AI, Lopez-Goñi I, Diaz R, Moriyon I. Factors affecting detection of *Brucella melitensis* by BACTEC NR730, a nonradiometric system for hemocultures. J Clin Microbiol 1993; 31:3200-3203.

[33] Solomon HM, Jackson D. Rapid diagnosis of *Brucella melitensis* in blood: some operational characteristics of the BACT/ALERT. J Clin Microbiol 1992; 30:222-224.

[34] Zimmerman SJ, Gillikin S, Sofat N, Bartholomew WR, Amsterdam D. Case report and seeded blood culture study of *Brucella* bacteremia. J Clin Microbiol 1990; 28:2139-2141.

[35] Bannatyne RM, Jackson MC, Memish Z. Rapid diagnosis of *Brucella bacteremia* by using the BACTEC 9240 system. J Clin Microbiol 1997; 35:2673-2674.

[36] Arnow PM, Smaron M, Ormiste V. Brucellosis in a group of travelers to Spain. J Am Med Assoc 1984; 251:505-507.

[37] Menard RR, Choudhury SP, Naini MG, Wilk JT. A case of brucellosis: The importance of physician/laboratory communication. Clin Microbiol Newsl 1989; 11:157-158.

[38] Serrano ML, Llosa J, Castells C, Mendoza J, Navarro JM, de la Rosa M. Detección radiométrica de bacteriemias por *Brucella*. Enferm Infec Microbiol Clin (Spain) 1987; 5:139-142.

[39] García Rodríguez JA, García Sánchez JE, Muñoz Bellido JL, Canut-Blasco A. 1988. Comparison of a biphasic system and non-radiometric system for blood culture. Eur J Clin Microbiol Infect Dis 1988; 7:666-668.

[40] Gedikoglu S, Helvaci S, Ozakin C, Gokirmak F, Kilicturgay K. Detection of *Brucella melitensis* by BACTEC NR 730 and BACTEC 9120 systems. Eur J Epidemiol 1996; 12:649-650.

[41] Casas J, Partal Y, Llosa J, Leiva J, Navarro JM, de la Rosa M. Detección de *Brucella* por un sistema automático de hemocultivos: Bact/ALERT. Enferm Infec Microbiol Clin 1994; 12:497-500.

[42] Kurtoglu MG, Bozkurt H, Tuncer O, Kesli R, Berktas M. Distribution, optimum detection time and antibiotic susceptibility rates of the microorganisms isolated from blood cultures over a 4-year time period in a Turkish university hospital and a review of the international literature. J Intern Med Res 2008; 36:3-13.

[43] Yagupsky P, Peled N, Press J, Abu-Rashid M, Abramson O. Rapid detection of *Brucella melitensis* from blood cultures by a commercial system. Eur J Clin Microbiol Infect Dis 1997; 16:605-607.

[44] Durmaz G, Us T, Aydinli A, Kiremitci A, Kiraz N, Akgun Y. Optimum detection times for bacteria and yeast species with the BACTEC 9120 aerobic blood culture system: evaluation for a 5-year period in a Turkish university hospital. J Clin Microbiol 2003; 41:819-821.

[45] Ayaslioglu E, Kiliç D, Kaygusuz S, Kücük S, Ceken S, Erol O, Alpay Y. The detection of *Brucella* spp. by BACTEC 9050 blood culture system. Microbiyol Bul 2004; 38:415-419.

[46] Lepe JA, Guerrero FJ, Garrido A, Perea R. Deteccion de *Brucella melitensis* por el sistema BACTEC 9050. Enferm Infecc Microbiol Clin 2001; 19:267-269.

[47] Yagupsky P. Use of the MYCO/F LYTIC medium for detection of *Brucella melitensis* bacteremia. J Clin MIcrobiol 2004; 42:2207-2208.

[48] Baysallar M, Aydogan H, Kilic A, Kucukkaraaslan A, Doganci L. Evaluation of the BacT/ALERT and BACTEC 9240 automated blood culture systems for growth time of *Brucella* species in a Turkish tertiary hospital. Med Sci Monitor 2006; 12:235-238.

[49] Giménez M, Prat C, Vallés X, Matas L, Arnal J, Ausina V. Evaluation of the VITAL (bioMérieux) automated blood culture system using blind subculture. Clin Microbiol Infect 2002; 8:222-228.

[50] Melo-Cristino J, Salgado MJ. Detection of *Brucella* bacteremia by using the VITAL automated system and trypticase broth culture. Clin Microbiol Infect 1999; 5:706-709.

[51] Ganado W, Bannister W. Bacteremia in human brucellosis. Br Med J 1960; 1:601-603.

[52] Young EJ. An overview of human brucellosis. Clin Infect Dis 1995; 21:283-290.

[53] Cohen FB, Robins B, Lipstein W. Isolation of *Brucella abortus* by percutaneous liver biopsy. New Eng J Med 1957; 257:228-230.

[54] Fogel R, Lewis S. Diagnosis of *Brucella melitensis* by percutaneous needle biopsy of the liver. Ann Intern Med 1960; 53:204-206.

[55] Poston MA, Parsons PB. Isolation of *Brucella* from lymph nodes. J Infect Dis 1940; 66:86-90.

[56] Magill GB, Killough JH. Cortisone and combined antibiotic therapy of acute brucellosis melitensis. Am J Med 1954; 16:810-817.

[57] Shehabi A, Shakir K, El-Khateeb M, Qubain H, Fararjeh N, Abu Shamat AR. 1990. Diagnosis and treatment of 106 cases of human brucellosis. J Infect 1990; 20:5-10.

[58] Escamilla J, Florez-Ugarte H, Kilpatrick ME. Evaluation of blood clot cultures for isolation of *Salmonella typhi, Salmonella paratyphi*-A, and *Brucella melitensis*. J Clin Microbiol 1986; 24:388-390.

[59] Mantur BG, Bidari LH, Akki AS, Mulimani MS, Tikare NV. Diagnostic yield of blood clot culture in the accurate diagnosis of enteric fever and human brucellosis. Clin Lab 2007; 53:57-61.

[60] Elsaghir AA, James EA. Misidentification of *Brucella melitensis* as *Ochrobactrum anthropi* by API 20NE. J Med Microbiol 2003; 52:441-442.

[61] Hubálek Z, Sholz HC, Sedláceck I, Melzer F, Sanogo Y, Nesbadbová JJ. Brucellosis of the common vole (*Microtus arvalis*). Vector Borne Zoonotic Dis 2007; 7:679-687.

[62] Dash N, Al-Zarouni M, Rattan A, Panigrahi D. Misidentification of *Brucella melitensis* as *Bergeylla zoohelcum* by Microscan WalkAway: A case report. Med Princ Pract 2012; 21:495-497.

[63] Batchelor BI, Brindlr RJ, Gilks GF, Stelton JB. Biochemical mis-identification of *Brucella melitensis* and subsequent laboratory acquired infections. J Hosp Infect 1992; 22:159-162.

[64] Rich M, Bannatyne RA, Memish ZA. Direct urease test on BACTEC blood cultures. Early presumptive diagnosis of brucellosis in an area of endemicity. J Clin Microbiol 2000; 38:1706.

[65] Maleknejad P, Hashemi FB, Fatollahzadeh B, Jafari S, Peeri Dogaheh H. Direct urease test and acridine orange staining on BACTEC blood culture for rapid presumptive diagnosis of brucellosis. Iranian J Public Health 2005; 34:52-55.

[66] Lista F, Reubsaet FAG, De Santis R, Parchen RR, de Jong AL, Kieboom J, van der Laaken AL, Voskamp-Visser IA, Fillo S, Jansen HJ, Van der Plas J, Paauw A. Reliable identification at the species level of *Brucella* isolated with MALDI-TOF. BMC Microbiol 2011; 11:267. doi: 10.1186/1471-2180-11-267.

[67] Karger A, Melzer F, Timke M, Bettin B, Kostrzewa M, Nöcler K, Hohman A, Tomasoo H, Neubauer H, Al Dahouk S. Interlaboratory comparison of intact-cell matrix-assisted laser desorption ionization-time of flight mass spectrometry results for identification and differentiation of *Brucella* spp. J Clin Microbiol 2013; 51:3123-3126.

[68] Ferreira L, Vega Castaño S, Sánchez-Juanes F, González-Cabrero S, Menegotto F, Orduña-Domingo A, González-Buitrago JM, Muñoz-Bellido JL. Identification of *Brucella* by MALDI-TOF mass spectrometry. Fast and reliable identification from agar plates and blood cultures. PloS ONE 2010; 5:e14235. doi:m10.1371/journal.pone.0014235.

[69] Drevinek M, Dresler J, Klimentova J, Pisa L, Hubalek M. Evaluation of sample preparation methods for MALSI-TOF MS identification of highly dangerous bacteria. Lett Appl Microbiol 2012; 55:40-46.

[70] Marklein G, Josten M, Klanke U, Müller E, Horré R, Maier T, Wenzel T, Kostrzewa M, Bierbaum G, Hoerauf A, Sahl HG. Matrix-assisted laser desorption ionization-time of flight mass spectrometry for fast and reliable identification of clinical yeast isolates. J Clin Microbiol 2009; 47:2912-2917.

[71] Wellinghousen N, Nöckler K, Sigge A, Bartel M, Essig A, Poppert S. Rapid detection of *Brucella* spp. in blood cultures by fluorescence in situ hybridization. J Clin Microbiol 2006; 44:1828-1830.

[72] Horvat RT, El Atrouni W, Hammoud K, Hawkinson D, Cowden S. Ribosomal RNA sequence analysis of *Brucella* infection misidentified as *Ochrobactrum anthropi.* J Clin Microbiol 2011; 49:1165-1168.

[73] Scholz HC, Pfeffer M, Witte A, Neubauer H, Al Dahouk S, Wernery U, Tomaso H. Specific detection and differentiation of *Ochrobactrum anthropi* and *Ochrobactrum intermedium* and *Brucella* spp. by a multi-primer PCR that targets the *recA* gene. J Med Microbiol 2008; 57:64-71.

[74] Yagupsky P, Baron EJ. Laboratory-exposures to brucellae and implications for bioterrorism. Emerg Infect Dis 2005; 11:1180-1185.

[75] Calfee MW, Wendling M. The effects of environmental conditions on persistence and inactivation of *Brucella suis* on building material surfaces. Lett Appl Microbiol 2012; 54:504-510.

[76] Noviello S, Gallo R, Kelly M, Linberger RJ, DeAngelis K, Cain L, Wallace B, Duma N. Laboratory-acquired bucellosis. Emerg Infect Dis 2004; 10:1848-1850.

[77] Ergonul O, Celikbas A, Tezeren D, Guvener E, Dokuzoguz B. Analysis of risk factors for laboratory-acquired *Brucella* infections. J Hosp Infect 2004; 56:223-227.

[78] Yagupsky P, Peled N, Riesenberg K, Banai M. Exposure of hospital personnel to *Brucella melitensis* and occurrence of laboratory-acquired disease in an endemic area. Scand J Infect Dis 2000; 32:31-35.

[79] Shemesh AA, Yagupsky P. Isolation rates of *Brucella melitensis* in an endemic area and implications for laboratory safety. Eur J Clin Microbiol Infect Dis 2012; 31:441-443.

[80] Centers for Disease Control and National Institutes of Health Biosafety in Microbiological and Biomedical Laboratories, Publication no. 17-40-508-3. 1988. U.S. Government Printing Office, Washington, DC.

Chapter 9

Antibiotic Susceptibility Testing of *Brucella* Species - Old and New Drugs

Max Maurin

Additional information is available at the end of the chapter

http://dx.doi.org/10.5772/61706

Abstract

Brucella species cause brucellosis in humans and animals, a zoonosis that can manifest not only as acute or chronic diseases but also as silent infections persisting throughout life with recurrences potentially occurring after several decades. *In vitro* and *in vivo* methods have been developed to evaluate the bacteriostatic and bactericidal activity of antibiotics against *Brucella* sp. Especially eukaryotic cells and animal models have been used to evaluate the ability of antibiotics, alone or in combination, to eradicate these bacteria from their intracellular reservoir. Although treatment recommendations have been established for common clinical forms of brucellosis, optimized therapeutic alternatives are still needed for severe forms of the disease, and for infections occurring in young children and pregnant women. Moreover, acquired resistance to first-line treatments of brucellosis is a current concern. This chapter will summarize current knowledge on *in vitro* and *in vivo* interactions between *Brucella* species and antibiotics and new therapeutic strategies that have been evaluated.

Keywords: *Brucella*, brucellosis, antibiotic susceptibility testing, antibiotic resistance, treatment

1. Introduction

Most *Brucella* species are highly infectious in humans and thus are considered class 3 biological agents [1–3] and potential biological threat agents by the CDC (class B) [4,5]. Because of a high risk of human infections, especially through inhalation of infectious aerosols, the *Brucella* cultures should be handled in a biosafety level 3 laboratory. Also, in many countries, detention of these pathogens is now subject to strict regulations. The clinical symptoms of brucellosis are often unspecific. Therefore, the diagnosis may be delayed, especially in geographic areas where the disease is rare and thus often not evoked by physicians in febrile patients. A definite diagnosis of brucellosis relies on isolation of *Brucella* sp. from infected patients, mainly from blood samples during the first few weeks following the onset of symptoms. Serological methods lack specificity, and only represent a stopgap for brucellosis diagnosis. PCR-based techniques are useful to detect *Brucella* DNA in clinical samples, especially in patients with suppurated secondary locations. A specific antibiotic therapy should be started as soon as possible to avoid severe complications (including neurological and cardiac involvement), and evolution to a chronic debilitating disease. However, current treatment alternatives are still scarce in adult patients, and even more limited in young children and pregnant women. Although rarely fatal, brucellosis remains a major public health problem worldwide, and a significant economic burden in livestock because of its abortive nature. This chapter will summarize current knowledge on antibiotic susceptibilities of *Brucella* species and treatment alternatives for human brucellosis. In the first part of this chapter, experimental models currently used for the evaluation of the activity of antibiotics against *Brucella* species will be presented, including *in vitro* models with or without eukaryotic cells, and animal models. The results obtained in these experimental models will be summarized and tentatively correlated with each other and with current knowledge on the clinical efficacy of antibiotics in brucellosis patients. The available data on antibiotic resistances in *Brucella* species will be presented, with their potential impact in clinical situations. The second part of this chapter will present current strategies for the development of new therapeutic alternatives for human brucellosis. These may include the development of new drugs inhibiting the intracellular growth of *Brucella* sp., reducing the virulence of this pathogen or enhancing the host response to *Brucella* infection.

2. Experimental models for evaluation of the activity of antibiotics against *Brucella* spp.

Routine antibiotic susceptibility testing (AST) of *Brucella* sp. is not currently advocated because of lack of acquired resistances to clinically useful antibiotics and a high risk of laboratory-acquired brucellosis [6,7]. Three types of experimental models have been used to assess the activities of antibiotics against *Brucella* sp.: AST in cell-free liquid or solid media (minimum inhibitory concentration (MICs)), AST in *Brucella*-infected eukaryotic cell models, and *Brucella*-infected animal models. We will summarize data obtained in these three models and their respective predictive value of the clinical efficacy of antibiotics in brucellosis patients.

2.1. AST in axenic media

2.1.1. Bacteriostatic activity by class of antibiotics

Current reference methods for the *in vitro* determination of the minimum inhibitory concentration (MIC) of antibiotics against bacteria in axenic media do not apply to the fastidious and slow growth of *Brucella* species. The method recommended by the Clinical and Laboratory Standards Institute (CLSI) includes the use of *Brucella* medium (pH 7.1), inoculated with a 0.5 McFarland standard inoculum, and an incubation at 35 ± 2°C in aerobic atmosphere for 48 h before reading MICs [8]. An incubation in 5% CO_2-enriched atmosphere may be required for some *Brucella* strains, but this usually increases MIC levels [9–11]. Using this method, susceptibility breakpoints for *Brucella* are ≤ 8 mg/L for streptomycin; ≤ 4 mg/L for gentamicin; ≤ 1 mg/L for tetracycline, doxycycline, and rifampicin; and ≤ 2/38 mg/L for the combination of trimethoprim (TMP) plus sulfamethoxazole (SMX) (i.e., cotrimoxazole).

In the literature, however, the multiplicity of methods used for MIC determination for *Brucella* strains shows a lack of standardization (Tables 1 and 2). MICs were determined using either the Kirby–Bauer agar disk diffusion method, the E-test strip method, a broth dilution or microdilution method, or the agar dilution method. Culture media have included Brucella broth, Mueller Hinton agar with or without 5% sheep blood, Mueller Hinton broth supplemented with 1% polyvitex with or without 1% hemoglobin, Trypticase soy broth, and Iso-Sensitest® Agar (Oxoid, CM47L). The tested bacterial inoculum was expressed in McFarland standard, cfu/mL, or cfu per spot, often without any correspondence between units, and it varied between studies (e.g., 10^5–10^6 cfu/mL, 0.5–1 McFarland). The incubation atmosphere varied from 35°C to 37°C, with 0%–10% CO_2. The incubation time before reading MICs varied from 24 h to 48 h. Obviously, all these parameters may change MIC levels. Several studies have shown that a high bacterial load and a low pH of the culture medium increase MICs by two to four times or even more [9,11–15].

A first interesting finding is the variability in susceptibility to beta-lactams among *Brucella* strains (Table 2). In cell-free media, MICs to ampicillin varied from 0.02 mg/L to 8 mg/L, with MIC90 of 2–4 mg/L [9,16–19]. For ceftriaxone, a third-generation cephalosporin, MICs varied from 0.064 mg/L to 4 mg/L, with MIC90 of 0.5–1 mg/L [20–23]. For thienamycin, a carbapenem compound, MICs varied from 0.1 mg/L to 2 mg/L, with an MIC90 of 2 mg/L [24]. These variations were also observed for other beta-lactams tested, although *Brucella* species were less susceptible to aztreonam [20]. Because heterogeneity in MICs was observed whatever the methodology used, they may represent true variations in genetic backgrounds among *Brucella* strains. However, beta-lactamases have never been characterized in these species, neither variations in penicillin-binding proteins (PBP).

The tetracyclines display the lowest MICs against *Brucella* spp. in cell-free media (Table 1). However, these MICs greatly vary according to the methodology used. Doxycycline, which is currently recommended as first-line treatment of brucellosis, displayed MICs ranging from 0.6 to 0.25 mg/L (MIC90 of 0.12–0.25 mg/L), when using the agar dilution method with either the CM47L medium or Mueller Hinton agar, supplemented with hemoglobin and polyvitex (1% each) [23,25]. The broth microdilution method gave MICs ranging from 0.01 to 0.5 mg/L (MIC90 of 0.06–0.3 mg/L), using various media and incubation conditions [9,10,19]. However, MICs up to 8 mg/L were reported in a Turkish study of 43 human strains of *B. melitensis* [11]. The only significant difference in the methodology might have been the use of a high bacterial inoculum (i.e., 10^5–10^6 cfu per well). The E-test method, using sheep blood-supplemented Mueller Hinton agar and a 0.5 McFarland standard inoculum, gave MICs ranging from 0.023 to 0.5 mg/L (MIC90 of 0.064–0.38 mg/L) [21,22,26–28]. Using the E-test method, much higher MICs ranging from 8 to 32 mg/L were recently reported for 19 Chinese strains of *B. melitensis*, although the incubation time before the MIC reading was only 24 h [17]. Tigecycline was no more effective than doxycycline, with MICs ranging from 0.019 to 0.5 mg/L using the E-test method [26,27,29].

Antibiotics	Country /host	Collected isolates: species, n, period[£]	Method[$] (medium, inoculum, %$CO_2$ temperature and hours of incubation)	MIC_{90} (mg/L)	MIC ranges (mg/L)	Reference
Aminoglycosides						
Streptomycin	US/HA	Bru, 27, (1970)	Broth microdilution (BB, NA, 10%, 37°C, 48 h)	2.5	0.15->100	[9]
	Israel/H	Bru, 31, 1978–82	Agar dilution (CM47L, 10^4/mL, 10%, 37°C, 48 h)	2	0.125-4	[12]
		Bru, 31, 1978–82	Agar dilution (CM47L, 10^5/mL, 10%, 37°C, 48 h)	8	0.06-8	[12]
		Bru, 31, 1978–82	Agar dilution (CM47L, 10^6/mL, 10%, 37°C, 48 h)	8	0.25-8	[12]
	Spain/H	Bm, 95, 1980–84	Agar dilution (CM47L, 10^5cfu/ spot, 0%, 37°C, 48 h)	0.5	0.12-1	[23]
	US-Mexico/HA	Bru, 15, (1986)	Broth microdilution (TSB,5 × 10^5cfu/mL,6%,35°C,48 h)	4	1-4	[18]
	Saudi Arabia	Bm, 47, (1989)	Broth dilution (BB,5 × 10^5cfu/mL, 0%, 35°C, 48 h)	2.5	0.15-5	[13]
	Israel/H	Bm, 86, (1991)	Broth microdilution (BB, 5 × 10^5cfu/mL,5%,37°C,48 h)	3.1	NA	[33]
	Turkey/H	Bm, 43, 1991–94	Broth microdilution (MH-P/ 7,$10^{5\text{-}6}$cfu,0%,35°C,48 h)	2	0.25-8	[11]
	Turkey/H	Bm, 43, 1991–94	Broth microdilution (MH-P/ 5,$10^{5\text{-}6}$cfu,0%,35°C,48 h)	128	8-256	[11]
	Spain/HA	Bru, 62, (1993)	Agar dilution (MH-HP,10^4cfu/ spot,10%,35°C,48 h)	4	0.1-4	[30]
	Spain/H	Bm, 160, 1997	Agar dilution (MH-HP,10^4cfu/ spot,10%,35°C,48 h)	8	4-16	[25]
	Korea/C	Bab, 85, 1998–2006	Broth microdilution (TSB, 0.5 McFd, 5%, 37°C, 48 h)	2	0.5-2	[19]
	Greece/HA	Bru, 74, 1999–2005	E-test (SB-MH, 0.5 McFd, 5%, 35°C, 48 h)	2	0.125-4	[16]
	Egypt/H	Bm, 355, 1999–2007	E-test (SB-MH, 0.5 McFd, 5%, NA, 48 h)	2	0.125-3	[22]

Antibiotics	Country /host	Collected isolates: species, n, period[£]	Method[$] (medium, inoculum, %$CO_2$ temperature and hours of incubation)	MIC_{90} (mg/L)	MIC ranges (mg/L)	Reference
	Syria	Bm, 100, 2004–07	Broth microdilution (BB/7, 5 × 10^6 cfu/mL,37°C, 48 h)	>128	64->128	[15]
	Syria	Bm, 100, 2004–07	Broth microdilution (BB/5, 5 × 10^6 cfu/mL,37°C, 48 h)	>128	>128	[15]
	Turkey/H	Bru, 56, 2008–09	E-test (SB-MH, 0.5 McFd, 0%, 35°C, 48 h)	1	0.064-1.5	[27]
	Turkey/H	Bm, 73, 2009–11	E-test (SB-MH, 0.5 McFd, NA, 37°C, 48 h)	1	0.5-1.5	[26]
	Turkey/H	Bm, 76, 2001–06	E-test (SB-MH, 1 McFd, 0%, 35°C,48 h)	1	0.064-1.5	[29]
	US/H	Bru, 39, (2010)	Broth microdilution (BB, NA, 0%, 35°C, 48 h)	2	1-8	[10]
		Bru, 39, (2010)	Broth microdilution (BB, NA, 5%, 35°C, 48 h)	4	2-16	[10]
Gentamicin	US/HA	Bru, 27, (1970)	Broth microdilution (BB, NA, 10%, 37°C, 48 h)	0.3	0.02-2.5	[9]
	Israel/H	Bru, 31, 1978–82	Agar dilution (CM47L, 10^4/mL, 10%, 37°C, 48 h)	0.25	0.03-0.25	[12]
		Bru, 31, 1978–82	Agar dilution (CM47L, 10^5/mL, 10%, 37°C, 48 h)	1	0.03-1	[12]
		Bru, 31, 1978–82	Agar dilution (CM47L, 10^6/mL, 10%, 37°C, 48 h)	2	0.03-2	[12]
	US-Mexico/HA	Bru, 15, (1986)	Broth microdilution (TSB,5 × 10^5cfu/mL,6%,35°C,48 h)	1	0.25-2	[18]
	Saudi Arabia	Bm, 116, (1995)	Broth dilution (MH,10^{5-6}cfu/mL, 5%, 35°C, 48 h)	0.5	<0.25-0.5	[31]
	Korea/C	Bab, 85, 1998–2006	Broth microdilution (TSB, 0.5 McFd, 5%, 37°C, 48 h)	1	0.5-2	[19]
	Greece/HA	Bru, 74, 1999–2005	E-test (SB-MH, 0.5 McFd, 5%, 35°C, 48 h)	2	0.03-1.5	[16]
	Egypt/H	Bm, 355, 1999–2007	E-test (SB-MH, 0.5 McFd, 5%, NA, 48 h)	1	0.094-3	[22]
	Peru/H	Bm, 48, 2000–06	E-test (SB-MH, 0.5 McFd, NA, NA, 48 h)	0.25	0.032-0.25	[28]

Antibiotics	Country /host	Collected isolates: species, n, period£	Method$ (medium, inoculum, %CO_2 temperature and hours of incubation)	MIC_{90} (mg/L)	MIC ranges (mg/L)	Reference
	Turkey/H	Bm, 76, 2001–06	E-test (SB-MH, 1 McFd, 0%, 35°C,48 h)	0.5	0.064-0.75	[29]
	US/H	Bru, 39, (2010)	Broth microdilution (BB, ND, 0%, 35°C, 48 h)	2	0.5-2	[10]
		Bru, 39, (2010)	Broth microdilution (BB, ND, 5%, 35°C, 48 h)	4	0.5-8	[10]
	China/H	Bm, 19, 2010–12	E-test (BA-MH, 0.5 McFd, 5%, 35°C, 24 h)	0.75	0.5-0.75	[17]
Tobramycin	US-Mexico/HA	Bru, 15, (1986)	Broth microdilution (TSB,5 × 10^5cfu/mL,6%,35°C,48 h)	2	0.5-4	[18]
Kanamycin	US/HA	Bru, 27, (1970)	Broth microdilution (BB, NA, 10%, 37°C, 48 h)	2.5	0.02-5	[9]
Amikacin	US-Mexico/HA	Bru, 15, (1986)	Broth microdilution (TSB,5 × 10^5cfu/mL,6%,35°C,48 h)	4	1-4	[18]
	China/H	Bm, 19, 2010–12	E-test (BA-MH, 0.5 McFd, 5%, 35°C, 24 h)	12	4-12	[17]
Tetracyclines						
Tetracycline	US/HA	Bru, 27, (1970)	Broth microdilution (BB, NA, 10%, 37°C, 48 h)	0.04	0.001-0.15	[9]
	Israel/H	Bru, 31, 1978–82	Agar dilution (CM47L, 10^4/mL, 10%, 37°C, 48 h)	0.25	≤0.06-0.5	[12]
		Bru, 31, 1978–82	Agar dilution (CM47L, 10^5/mL, 10%, 37°C, 48 h)	0.5	≤0.06-0.5	[12]
		Bru, 31, 1978–82	Agar dilution (CM47L, 10^6/mL, 10%, 37°C, 48 h)	1	≤0.06-2	[12]
	Spain/H	Bm, 95, 1980–84	Agar dilution (CM47L, 10^5cfu/ spot, 0%, 37°C, 48 h)	0.25	0.6-0.25	[23]
	Spain/H	Bm, 98, (1982)	Agar dilution (CM47L, 10^5cfu/ spot, 0%, 37°C, 48 h)	0.39	0.1-0.5	[24]
	US-Mexico/HA	Bru, 15, (1986)	Broth microdilution (TSB,5 × 10^5cfu/mL,6%,35°C,48 h)	0.25	≤0.13-0.25	[18]
	Spain/H	Bm, 358, 1987–89	Agar dilution (CM471, 10^5cfu/ spot, 0%, 37°C, 48 h)	0.25	0.06-0.5	[32]

Antibiotics	Country /host	Collected isolates: species, n, period[£]	Method[$] (medium, inoculum, %$CO_2$ temperature and hours of incubation)	MIC_{90} (mg/L)	MIC ranges (mg/L)	Reference
	Saudi Arabia	Bm, 47, (1989)	Broth dilution (BB,5 × 10^5cfu/mL, 0%, 35°C, 48 h)	0.04	0.001-0.6	[13]
	Spain/HA	Bru, 62, (1993)	Agar dilution (MH-HP, 10^4cfu/ spot, 10%, 35°C, 48 h)	0.2	0.01-0.2	[30]
	Saudi Arabia	Bm, 116, (1995)	Broth dilution (MH, $10^{5\text{-}6}$cfu/mL, 5%, 35°C, 48 h)	0.5	<0.25-0.5	[31]
	Greece/HA	Bru, 74, 1999–2005	E-test (SB-MH, 0.5 McFd, 5%, 35°C, 48 h)	0.5	0.03-1.5	[16]
	Korea/C	Bab, 85, 1998–2006	Broth microdilution (TSB, 0.5 McFd, 5%, 37°C, 48 h)	0.25	0.125-0.5	[19]
	Egypt/H	Bm, 355, 1999–2007	E-test (SB-MH, 0.5 McFd, 5%, NA, 48 h)	0.19	0.023-0.75	[22]
	Syria	Bm, 100, 2004–07	Broth microdilution (BB/7, 5 × 10^6 cfu/mL, 37°C, 48 h)	16	0.25-16	[15]
	Syria	Bm, 100, 2004–07	Broth microdilution (BB/5, 5 × 10^6 cfu/mL, 37°C, 48 h)	16	0.25-16	[15]
	US/H	Bru, 39, (2010)	Broth microdilution (BB, ND, 0%, 35°C, 48 h)	0.25	0.06-0.5	[10]
		Bru, 39, (2010)	Broth microdilution (BB, ND, 5%, 35°C, 48 h)	0.25	0.03-0.5	[10]
Doxycycline	US/HA	Bru, 27, (1970)	Broth microdilution (BB, NA, 10%, 37°C, 48 h)	0.3	0.01-0.3	[9]
	Spain/H	Bm, 95, 1980–84	Agar dilution (CM47L, 10^5cfu/ spot, 0%, 37°C, 48 h)	0.12	0.6-0.25	[23]
	Turkey/H	Bm, 43, 1991–94	Broth microdilution (MH-P/ 7,$10^{5\text{-}6}$cfu,0%, 35°C,48 h)	<0.125	<0.125-8	[11]
	Turkey/H	Bm, 43, 1991–94	Broth microdilution (MH-P/ 5,$10^{5\text{-}6}$cfu,0%, 35°C,48 h)	2	<0.125-8	[11]
	Spain/H	Bm, 160, 1997	Agar dilution (MH-HP, 10^4cfu/ spot, 10%, 35°C,48 h)	0.25	0.12-0.25	[25]
	Korea/C	Bab, 85, 1998–2006	Broth microdilution (TSB, 0.5 McFd, 5%, 37°C, 48 h)	0.25	0.063-0.5	[19]
	Egypt/H	Bm, 355, 1999–2007	E-test (SB-MH, 0.5 McFd, 5%, NA, 48 h)	0.25	0.016-0.5	[22]

Antibiotics	Country /host	Collected isolates: species, n, period£	Method$ (medium, inoculum, %CO_2 temperature and hours of incubation)	MIC_{90} (mg/L)	MIC ranges (mg/L)	Reference
	Peru/H	Bm, 48, 2000–06	E-test (SB-MH, 0.5 McFd, NA, NA, 48 h)	0.38	0.032-0.5	[28]
	Turkey/H	Bm, 76, 2001–06	E-test (SB-MH, 1 McFd, 0%, 35°C,48 h)	0.125	0.016-0.19	[29]
	Syria	Bm, 100, 2004–07	Broth microdilution (BB/7, 5 × 10^6 cfu/mL, 37°C, 48 h)	16	0.5-16	[15]
	Syria	Bm, 100, 2004–07	Broth microdilution (BB/5, 5 × 10^6 cfu/mL, 37°C, 48 h)	8	0.5-8	[15]
	Italy/H	Bru, 20, 2005–06	E-test (SB-MH, 0.5 McFd, 5%, 37°C, 48 h)	ND	0.06-0.125	[21]
	Turkey/H	Bru, 56, 2008–09	E-test (SB-MH, 0.5 McFd, 0%, 35°C, 48 h)	0.064	0.023-0.125	[27]
	Turkey/H	Bm, 73, 2009–11	E-test (SB-MH, 0.5 McFd, NA, 37°C, 48 h)	0.094	0.023-0.19	[26]
	US/H	Bru, 39, (2010)	Broth microdilution (BB, ND, 0%, 35°C, 48 h)	0.25	0.06-0.5	[10]
		Bru, 39, (2010)	Broth microdilution (BB, ND, 5%, 35°C, 48 h)	0.5	0.03-1	[10]
	China/H	Bm, 19, 2010–12	E-test (BA-MH, 0.5 McFd, 5%, 35°C, 24 h)	32	8-32	[17]
Minocycline	US/HA	Bru, 27, (1970)	Broth microdilution (BB, NA, 10%, 37°C, 48 h)	0.3	0.01-1.25	[9]
	Israel/H	Bm, 86, (1991)	Broth microdilution (BB, 5 × 10^5cfu/mL, 5%, 37°C, 48 h)	0.4	NA	[33]
	Korea/C	Bab, 85, 1998–2006	Broth microdilution (TSB, 0.5 McFd, 5%, 37°C, 48 h)	0.125	0.063-0.25	[19]
Tigecycline	Turkey/H	Bru, 56, 2008–09	E-test (SB-MH, 0.5 McFd, 0%, 35°C, 48 h)	0.094	0.019-0.25	[27]
	Turkey/H	Bm, 73, 2009–11	E-test (SB-MH, 0.5 McFd, NA, 37°C, 48 h)	0.125	0.047-0.19	[26]
	Turkey/H	Bm, 76, 2001–06	E-test (SB-MH, 1 McFd, 0%, 35°C, 48 h)	0.094	0.023-0.5	[29]
	Turkey/H	Bm, 38, (2010)	E-test (SB, NA, NA, 35°C, 48 h)	0.5	0.032-0.5	[76]

Antibiotics	Country /host	Collected isolates: species, n, period[£]	Method[$] (medium, inoculum, %$CO_2$ temperature and hours of incubation)	MIC_{90} (mg/L)	MIC ranges (mg/L)	Reference
	Turkey/H	Bm, 38, (2010)	E-test (BA, NA, NA, 35°C, 48 h)	1	0.0125-1	[76]
Rifampin	US/HA	Bru, 27, (1970)	Broth microdilution (BB, NA, 10%, 37°C, 48 h)	1.25	0.02-12.5	[9]
	Spain/H	Bm, 98, (1982)	Agar dilution (CM47L, 10^5cfu/spot, 0%, 37°C, 48 h)	0.5	0.06-1	[24]
	Spain/H	Bm, 95, 1980–84	Agar dilution (CM47L, 10^5cfu/spot, 0%, 37°C, 48 h)	2	0.12-4	[23]
	US-Mexico/HA	Bru, 15, (1986)	Broth microdilution (TSB, 5 × 10^5cfu/mL, 6%, 35°C, 48 h)	1	0.06-1	[18]
	Saudi Arabia	Bm, 47, (1989)	Broth dilution (BB, 5 × 10^5cfu/mL, 0%, 35°C, 48 h)	1.25	0.02-2.5	[13]
	Israel/H	Bm, 86, (1991)	Broth microdilution (BB, 5 × 10^5cfu/mL, 5%, 37°C, 48 h)	4	NA	[33]
	Turkey/H	Bm, 43, 1991–94	Broth microdilution (MH-P/7,$10^{5\text{-}6}$cfu, 0%, 35°C, 48 h)	2	1-32	[11]
	Turkey/H	Bm, 43, 1991–94	Broth microdilution (MH-P/5,$10^{5\text{-}6}$cfu, 0%, 35°C, 48 h)	1	<0.125-1	[11]
	Spain/HA	Bru, 62, (1993)	Agar dilution (MH-HP, 10^4cfu/spot, 10%, 35°C, 48 h)	1	0.1-4	[30]
	Saudi Arabia	Bm, 116, (1995)	Broth dilution (MH, $10^{5\text{-}6}$cfu/mL, 5%, 35°C, 48 h)	1	0.25-1	[31]
	Spain/H	Bm, 160, 1997	Agar dilution (MH-HP, 10^4cfu/spot, 10%, 35°C, 48 h)	1	0.5-1	[25]
	Korea/C	Bab, 85, 1998–2006	Broth microdilution (TSB, 0.5 McFd, 5%, 37°C, 48 h)	2	0.5-4	[19]
	Greece/HA	Bru, 74, 1999–2005	E-test (SB-MH, 0.5 McFd, 5%, 35°C, 48 h)	1	0.09-1.5	[16]
	Egypt/H	Bm, 355, 1999–2007	E-test (SB-MH, 0.5 McFd, 5%, NA, 48 h)	4	0.25-6	[22]
	Peru/H	Bm, 48, 2000–06	E-test (SB-MH, 0.5 McFd, NA, NA, 48 h)	0.75	0.19-1	[28]
	Turkey/H	Bm, 76, 2001–06	E-test (SB-MH, 1 McFd, 0%, 35°C,48 h)	1.5	0.064-3	[29]

Antibiotics	Country /host	Collected isolates: species, n, period[£]	Method[$] (medium, inoculum, %$CO_2$ temperature and hours of incubation)	MIC_{90} (mg/L)	MIC ranges (mg/L)	Reference
	Syria	Bm, 100, 2004–07	Broth microdilution (BB/7, 5 × 10^6 cfu/mL,37°C, 48 h)	64	2-64	[15]
	Syria	Bm, 100, 2004–07	Broth microdilution (BB/5, 5 × 10^6 cfu/mL,37°C, 48 h)	64	2-64	[15]
	Italy/H	Bru, 20, 2005–06	E-test (SB-MH, 0.5 McFd, 5%, 37°C, 48 h)	ND	0.75-2	[21]
	Turkey/H	Bru, 56, 2008–09	E-test (SB-MH, 0.5 McFd, 0%, 35°C, 48 h)	2	0.5-2	[27]
	Turkey/H	Bm, 73, 2009–11	E-test (SB-MH, 0.5 McFd, NA, 37°C, 48 h)	2	0.38-3	[26]
	US/H	Bru, 39, (2010)	Broth microdilution (BB, ND, 0%, 35°C, 48 h)	2	0.25-2	[10]
		Bru, 39, (2010)	Broth microdilution (BB, ND, 5%, 35°C, 48 h)	2	0.25->8	[10]
	China/H	Bm, 19, 2010–12	E-test (BA-MH, 0.5 McFd, 5%, 35°C, 24 h)	2	0.06-2	[17]
Rifapentine	Spain/HA	Bru, 62, (1993)	Agar dilution (MH-HP, 10^4cfu/ spot, 10%, 35°C, 48 h)	1	0.2-4	[30]

NA, data not available; Bm, *B. melitensis*; Bab, *B. abortus*; Bru, *Brucella* sp.

[£]Studies have been classified according to the period of isolation of the studied *Brucella* strains (e.g., 2010–12) and the date of the corresponding publication (e.g., (1993)) when the latter was unavailable.

[$]Method: Kirby–Bauer disk diffusion method (Kirby–Bauer); E-test strip method (E-test);

Medium: Mueller Hinton agar with 5% sheep blood (SB-MH) or unspecified percentage and type of blood (BA-MH); 5% sheep blood agar (SB); Brucella broth (BB); Brucella agar (BA); Trypticase soy broth (TSB); Iso-Sensitest® Agar CM47L (CM47L); Mueller Hinton broth supplemented with 1% polyvitex with (HP) or without (P) 1% hemoglobin, at pH 7 (/7) or pH 5 (/5); The bacterial inoculum used for antibiotic susceptibility testing is specified in cfu/mL or according to McFarland standards (McFd). Host: human (H), cattle (C), unspecified or various animals (A).

Table 1. Antibiotic susceptibilities of *Brucella* sp. to aminoglycosides, tetracyclines, and rifampin, as determined in cell-free media.

Rifampicin is the second most active compound against *Brucella* sp. in cell-free medium (Table 1). MICs ranged from 0.06 to 4 mg/L with the agar dilution method [23–25,30], 0.06 to 4 mg/L with the broth dilution method [10,11,13,18,19,31], and 0.06 to 6 mg/L with the E-test method [16,17,21,22,26–29]. Higher MICs (up to 12.5 mg/L) were reported in one study using *Brucella* broth and a 10% CO_2 atmosphere incubation [9]. Rifampicin MICs were lower at acidic pH [11], but higher at increasing concentrations of CO_2 [10,11].

The aminoglycosides are also highly active *in vitro* against *Brucella* sp. (Table 1). Streptomycin has long been used as first-line treatment of brucellosis, whereas gentamicin is now used in most countries because the former antibiotic is no longer available. MICs to streptomycin varied from 0.12 to 4 mg/L with the agar dilution method [23,30], although a more recent study from Spain reported higher MIC levels (4–16 mg/L) for 160 human strains of *B. melitensis* [25]. MICs varied from 0.1 to 16 mg/L with the broth dilution method [10,11,13,18,19,25]. An acidic pH of the broth medium and/or an incubation in 5%–10% CO_2-enriched atmosphere were associated with higher MICs [9–11]. Higher MIC levels (≥256 mg/L) were, however, occasionally reported with this technique [9,11]. MICs ranged from 0.06 to 4 mg/L with the E-test method [16,22,27,29]. Gentamicin displayed lower MICs, ranging from 0.02 to 2.5 mg/L [9,10,18,31] with the broth dilution method, and 0.03 to 3 mg/L with the E-test method [16,17,22,28,29].

The combination of trimethoprim (TMP) and sulfamethoxazole (SMX) was usually tested at a ratio of 1:19, and only TMP MICs were reported (Table 2). These varied from 0.06 to 4 mg/L with the agar dilution method [23,30], 0.006 to 4 mg/L with the broth microdilution method [10,18,31], and 0.06 to 1.5 mg/L with the E-test method [16,21,22,26–29]. Similar MIC ranges (0.8–3.2 mg/L) were obtained when using TMP/SMX at a ratio of 1:5 [17]. In contrast, higher MICs (5–25 mg/L of TMP) were reported in a study from Saudi Arabia [13], using a broth dilution method with high-volume (5 mL) medium culture and a high bacterial inoculum (2.5 × 10^6 cfu per test).

Antibiotics	Country /host	Collected isolates: species, n, period[£]	Method[$] (medium, inoculum, %$CO_2$ temperature and hours of incubation)	MIC_{90} (mg/L)	MIC ranges (mg/L)	Reference
β-lactams						
Penicillin G	US/HA	Bru, 27, (1970)	Broth microdilution (BB, NA, 10%, 37°C, 48 h)	25	0.3->100	[9]
	US-Mexico/HA	Bru, 15, (1986)	Broth microdilution (TSB,5 × 10^5cfu/mL,6%,35°C,48 h)	4	0.25-8	[18]
Ampicillin	US/HA	Bru, 27, (1970)	Broth microdilution (BB, NA, 10%, 37°C, 48 h)	2.5	0.02-5	[9]
	US-Mexico/HA	Bru, 15, (1986)	Broth microdilution (TSB,5 × 10^5cfu/mL,6%,35°C,48 h)	4	0.25-8	[18]
	Greece/HA	Bru, 74, 1999–2005	E-test (SB-MH, 0.5 McFd, 5%, 35°C, 48 h)	2	0.09-3	[16]
	Korea/C	Bab, 85, 1998–2006	Broth microdilution (TSB, 0.5 McFd, 5%, 37°C, 48 h)	4	0.125-4	[19]
	China/H	Bm, 19, 2010–12	E-test (BA-MH, 0.5 McFd, 5%, 35°C, 24 h)	2	1.5-2	[17]

Antibiotics	Country /host	Collected isolates: species, n, period£	Method$ (medium, inoculum, $\%CO_2$ temperature and hours of incubation)	MIC_{90} (mg/L)	MIC ranges (mg/L)	Reference
Carbenicillin	US/HA	Bru, 27, (1970)	Broth microdilution (BB, NA, 10%, 37°C, 48 h)	50	0.6->100	[9]
Cephalothin	US/HA	Bru, 27, (1970)	Broth microdilution (BB, NA, 10%, 37°C, 48 h)	100	0.3->100	[9]
	US-Mexico/HA	Bru, 15, (1986)	Broth microdilution (TSB,5 × 10^5cfu/mL,6%,35°C,48 h)	32	1-64	[18]
Cefoxitine	Spain/H	Bm, 98, (1982)	Agar dilution (CM47L, 10^5 cfu/spot, 0%, 37°C, 48 h)	64	8-128	[24]
	US-Mexico/HA	Bru, 15, (1986)	Broth microdilution (TSB,5 × 10^5cfu/mL,6%,35°C,48 h)	16	2-16	[18]
Cefuroxime	Spain/H	Bm, 83, (1986)	Agar dilution (CM47L, 10^5 cfu/spot, 0%, 37°C, 48 h)	32	8-64	[20]
Ceftizoxime	Spain/H	Bm, 83, (1986)	Agar dilution (CM47L, 10^5 cfu/spot, 0%, 37°C, 48 h)	1	0.5-1	[20]
Cefoperazone	US-Mexico/HA	Bru, 15, (1986)	Broth microdilution (TSB,5 × 10^5cfu/mL,6%,35°C,48 h)	16	≤1-16	[18]
	Spain/H	Bm, 83, (1986)	Agar dilution (CM47L, 10^5 cfu/spot, 0%, 37°C, 48 h)	32	4-64	[20]
Cefotaxime	US-Mexico/HA	Bru, 15, (1986)	Broth microdilution (TSB,5 × 10^5cfu/mL, 6%,35°C,48 h)	2	≤0.5-4	[18]
	Spain/H	Bm, 83, (1986)	Agar dilution (CM47L, 10^5 cfu/spot, 0%, 37°C, 48 h)	2	≤0.5-2	[20]
Ceftriaxone	Spain/H	Bm, 95, 1980–84	Agar dilution (CM47L, 10^5cfu/spot, 0%, 37°C, 48 h)	0.5	0.12-1	[23]
	Spain/H	Bm, 83, (1986)	Agar dilution (CM47L, 10^5 cfu/spot, 0%, 37°C, 48 h)	1	≤0.25-1	[20]
	Egypt/H	Bm, 355, 1999–2007	E-test (SB-MH, 0.5 McFd, 5%, NA, 48 h)	1	0.064-4	[22]
	Italy/H	Bru, 20, 2005–06	E-test (SB-MH, 0.5 McFd, 5%, 37°C, 48 h)	NA	0.064-0.38	[21]
Ceftazidime	China/H	Bm, 19, 2010–12	E-test (BA-MH, 0.5 McFd, 5%, 35°C, 24 h)	8	2-8	[17]
Moxalactam	US-Mexico/HA	Bru, 15, (1986)	Broth microdilution (TSB,5 × 10^5cfu/mL, 6%,35°C,48 h)	16	1-16	[18]

Antibiotics	Country /host	Collected isolates: species, n, period£	Method$ (medium, inoculum, %CO_2 temperature and hours of incubation)	MIC_{90} (mg/L)	MIC ranges (mg/L)	Reference
	Spain/H	Bm, 83, (1986)	Agar dilution (CM47L, 10^5cfu/spot, 0%, 37°C, 48 h)	16	4-16	[20]
Aztreonam	Spain/H	Bm, 83, (1986)	Agar dilution (CM47L, 10^5cfu/spot, 0%, 37°C, 48 h)	>256	64->256	[20]
Thienamycin	Spain/H	Bm, 98, (1982)	Agar dilution (CM47L, 10^5cfu/spot, 0%, 37°C, 48 h)	2	0.1-2	[24]
TMP/SMX*	Spain/H	Bm, 98, (1982)	Agar dilution (CM47L, 10^5cfu/spot, 0%, 37°C, 48 h)	6.25	0.39-6.25	[24]*
	Spain/H	Bm, 95, 1980–84	Agar dilution (CM47L, 10^5cfu/spot, 0%, 37°C, 48 h)	0.25	0.06-0.5	[23]
	US-Mexico/HA	Bru, 15, (1986)	Broth microdilution (TSB,5 × 10^5cfu/mL,6%,35°C,48 h)	1	≤0.25-1	[18]
	Saudi Arabia	Bm, 47, (1989)	Broth dilution (BB,5 × 10^5cfu/mL, 0%, 35°C, 48 h)	5	5-25	[13]
	Spain/HA	Bru, 62, (1993)	Agar dilution (MH-HP,10^4cfu/spot,10%,35°C,48 h)	4	0.1-4	[30]
	Saudi Arabia	Bm, 116, (1995)	Broth dilution (MH, 10^{5-6}cfu/mL, 5%, 35°C, 48 h)	1	<0.25-1	[31]
	Greece/HA	Bru, 74, 1999–2005	E-test (SB-MH, 0.5 McFd, 5%, 35°C, 48 h)	0.75	0.032-1.5	[16]
	Egypt/H	Bm, 355, 1999–2007	E-test (SB-MH, 0.5 McFd, 5%, NA, 48 h)	0.19	0.006-0.75	[22]
	Peru/H	Bm, 48, 2000–06	E-test (SB-MH, 0.5 McFd, NA, NA, 48 h)	0.15	0.012-0.64	[28]
	Turkey/H	Bm, 76, 2001–06	E-test (SB-MH, 1 McFd, 0%, 35°C,48 h)	0.094	0.016-0.125	[29]
	Italy/H	Bru, 20, 2005–06	E-test (SB-MH, 0.5 McFd, 5%, 37°C, 48 h)	ND	0.012/0.064	[21]
	Turkey/H	Bru, 56, 2008–09	E-test (SB-MH, 0.5 McFd, 0%, 35°C, 48 h)	0.125	0.064-0.25	[27]
	Turkey/H	Bm, 73, 2009–11	E-test (SB-MH, 0.5 McFd, NA, 37°C, 48 h)	0.19	0.016-0.5	[26]
	China/H	Bm, 19, 2010–12	E-test (BA-MH, 0.5 McFd, 5%, 35°C, 24 h)	3.2	0.8-3.2	[17]*

Antibiotics	Country /host	Collected isolates: species, n, period£	Method$ (medium, inoculum, %CO_2 temperature and hours of incubation)	MIC_{90} (mg/L)	MIC ranges (mg/L)	Reference
	US/H	Bru, 39, (2010)	Broth microdilution (BB, ND, 0%, 35°C, 48 h)	2	0.25-2	[10]
		Bru, 39, (2010)	Broth microdilution (BB, ND, 5%, 35°C, 48 h)	2	0.25-4	[10]
Chloramphenicol	US/HA	Bru, 27, (1970)	Broth microdilution (BB, NA, 10%, 37°C, 48 h)		0.3->100	[9]
	Israel/H	Bru, 31, 1978–82	Agar dilution (CM47L, 10^4/mL, 10%, 37°C, 48 h)	2	0.125-4	[12]
		Bru, 31, 1978–82	Agar dilution (CM47L, 10^5/mL, 10%, 37°C, 48 h)	4	0.06-4	[12]
		Bru, 31, 1978–82	Agar dilution (CM47L, 10^6/mL, 10%, 37°C, 48 h)	8	0.06-8	[12]
	US-Mexico/HA	Bru, 15, (1986)	Broth microdilution (TSB,5 × 10^5cfu/mL,6%,35°C,48 h)	2	0.25-4	[18]
	Korea/C	Bab, 85, 1998–2006	Broth microdilution (TSB, 0.5 McFd, 5%, 37°C, 48 h)	5	0.15-12.5	[19]
Macrolides and azalides						
Erythromycin	US/HA	Bru, 27, (1970)	Broth microdilution (BB, NA, 10%, 37°C, 48 h)	0.6	0.02-2.5	[9]
	US-Mexico/HA	Bru, 15, (1986)	Broth microdilution (TSB,5 × 10^5cfu/mL,6%,35°C,48 h)	8	0.5-8	[18]
	Turkey/H	Bm, 43, 1991–94	Broth microdilution (MH-P/7,10^{5-6}cfu,0%,35°C,48 h)	128	0.5-256	[11]
	Turkey/H	Bm, 43, 1991–94	Broth microdilution (MH-P/5,10^{5-6}cfu,0%,35°C,48 h)	>256	32->256	[11]
	Spain/HA	Bru, 62, (1993)	Agar dilution (MH-HP,10^4cfu/spot,10%,35°C,48 h)	16	0.2-16	[30]
	Greece/HA	Bru, 74, 1999–2005	E-test (SB-MH, 0.5 McFd, 5%, 35°C, 48 h)	4	0.5-8	[16]
	Korea/C	Bab, 85, 1998–2006	Broth microdilution (TSB, 0.5 McFd, 5%, 37°C, 48 h)	2	1-4	[19]
Roxithromycin	Spain/HA	Bru, 62, (1993)	Agar dilution (MH-HP,10^4cfu/spot,10%,35°C,48 h)	16	0.1-32	[30]

Antibiotics	Country /host	Collected isolates: species, n, period[£]	Method[$] (medium, inoculum, %$CO_2$ temperature and hours of incubation)	MIC_{90} (mg/L)	MIC ranges (mg/L)	Reference
Dirithromycin	Spain/HA	Bru, 62, (1993)	Agar dilution (MH-HP,10^4cfu/ spot,10%,35°C,48 h)	16	0.5-16	[30]
Clarithromycin	Spain/HA	Bru, 62, (1993)	Agar dilution (MH-HP,10^4cfu/ spot,10%,35°C,48 h)	8	0.06-8	[30]
Azithromycin	Spain/H	Bm, 358, 1987–89	Agar dilution (CM471, 10^5cfu/ spot, 0%, 37°C, 48 h)	1	0.03-2	[32]
	Turkey/H	Bm, 43, 1991–94	Broth microdilution (MH-P/ 7,10^{5-6}cfu,0%,35°C,48 h)	1	<0.125-4	[11]
	Turkey/H	Bm, 43, 1991–94	Broth microdilution (MH-P/ 5,10^{5-6}cfu,0%,35°C,48 h)	>256	16->256	[11]
	Spain/HA	Bru, 62, (1993)	Agar dilution (MH-HP, 10^4cfu/ spot, 10%,35°C, 48 h)	2	0.1-4	[30]
	Saudi Arabia	Bm, 116, (1995)	Broth dilution (MH,10^{5-6}cfu/mL, 5%, 35°C, 48 h)	0.5	<0.25-2	[31]
	Peru/H	Bm, 48, 2000–06	E-test (SB-MH, 0.5 McFd, NA, NA, 48 h)	0.5	0.064-0.5	[28]
	Turkey/H	Bm, 73, 2009–11	E-test (SB-MH, 0.5 McFd, NA, 37°C, 48 h)	8	0.75-16	[26]
Fluoroquinolones						
Norfloxacin	Greece/HA	Bru, 74, 1999–2005	E-test (SB-MH, 0.5 McFd, 5%, 35°C, 48 h)	3	0.125-4	[16]
	Korea/C	Bab, 85, 1998–2006	Broth microdilution (TSB, 0.5 McFd, 5%, 37°C, 48 h)	8	4-16	[19]
Ofloxacin	Saudi Arabia	Bm, 47, (1989)	Broth dilution (BB,5 × 10^5cfu/mL, 0%, 35°C, 48 h)	0.02	0.02-0.3	[13]
	Israel/H	Bm, 86, (1991)	Broth microdilution (BB, 5 × 10^5cfu/mL,5%,37°C,48 h)	2.5	ND	[33]
	Turkey/H	Bm, 43, 1991–94	Broth microdilution (MH-P/ 7,10^{5-6}cfu,0%,35°C,48 h)	1	<0.125-4	[11]
	Turkey/H	Bm, 43, 1991–94	Broth microdilution (MH-P/ 5,10^{5-6}cfu,0%,35°C,48 h)	>16	4->16	[11]
	Spain/H	Bm, 160, 1997	Agar dilution (MH-HP,10^4cfu/ spot,10%,35°C,48 h)	2	1-2	[25]

Antibiotics	Country /host	Collected isolates: species, n, period£	Method$ (medium, inoculum, %CO_2 temperature and hours of incubation)	MIC_{90} (mg/L)	MIC ranges (mg/L)	Reference
	Korea/C	Bab, 85, 1998–2006	Broth microdilution (TSB, 0.5 McFd, 5%, 37°C, 48 h)	2	0.5-2	[19]
Levofloxacin	Spain/H	Bm, 160, 1997	Agar dilution (MH-HP,10^4cfu/ spot,10%,35°C,48 h)	0.5	0.5	[25]
	Greece/HA	Bru, 74, 1999–2005	E-test (SB-MH, 0.5 McFd, 5%, 35°C, 48 h)	0.5	0.06-0.75	[16]
	China/H	Bm, 19, 2010–12	E-test (BA-MH, 0.5 McFd, 5%, 35°C, 24 h)	8	2-8	[17]
Ciprofloxacin	Spain/H	Bm, 95, 1980–84	Agar dilution (CM47L, 10^5cfu/ spot, 0%, 37°C, 48 h)	0.5	0.12-0.5	[23]
	Saudi Arabia	Bm, 47, (1989)	Broth dilution (BB,5 × 10^5cfu/mL, 0%, 35°C, 48 h)	1.25	1.25-2.5	[13]
	Israel/H	Bm, 86, (1991)	Broth microdilution (BB,5 × 10^5cfu/mL,5%,37°C,48 h)	0.8	NA	[33]
	Spain/H	Bm, 34, (1991)	Agar dilution (MH-HP/7,10^3cfu/ spot,10%,35°C,48 h)	0.5	0.25-0.5	[14]
	Spain/H	Bm, 34, (1991)	Agar dilution (MH-HP/5,10^3cfu/ spot,10%,35°C,48 h)	1	0.5-1	[14]
	Spain/H	Bm, 34, (1991)	Agar dilution (MH-HP/7,10^4cfu/ spot,10%,35°C,48 h)	0.5	0.25-0.5	[14]
	Spain/H	Bm, 34, (1991)	Agar dilution (MH-HP/5,10^4cfu/ spot,10%,35°C,48 h)	1	0.5-1	[14]
	Spain/H	Bm, 34, (1991)	Agar dilution (MH-HP/7,10^6cfu/ spot,10%,35°C,48 h)	1	0.5-1	[14]
	Spain/H	Bm, 34, (1991)	Agar dilution (MH-HP/5,10^6cfu/ spot,10%,35°C,48 h)	2	1-2	[14]
	Turkey/H	Bm, 43, 1991–94	Broth microdilution (MH-P/ 7,10^{5-6}cfu,0%,35°C,48 h)	2	<0.125-8	[11]
	Turkey/H	Bm, 43, 1991–94	Broth microdilution (MH-P/ 5,10^{5-6}cfu,0%,35°C,48 h)	>16	2->16	[11]
	Spain/H	Bm, 160, 1997	Agar dilution (MH-HP,10^4cfu/ spot,10%,35°C,48 h)	1	0.25-1	[25]
	Korea/C	Bab, 85, 1998–2006	Broth microdilution (TSB, 0.5 McFd, 5%, 37°C, 48 h)	1	0.25-4	[19]

Antibiotics	Country /host	Collected isolates: species, n, period£	Method$ (medium, inoculum, %CO_2 temperature and hours of incubation)	MIC_{90} (mg/L)	MIC ranges (mg/L)	Reference
	Greece/HA	Bru, 74, 1999–2005	E-test (SB-MH, 0.5 McFd, 5%, 35°C, 48 h)	0.5	0.016-0.75	[16]
	Egypt/H	Bm, 355, 1999–2007	E-test (SB-MH, 0.5 McFd, 5%, NA, 48 h)	0.38	0.125-0.75	[22]
	Peru/H	Bm, 48, 2000–06	E-test (SB-MH, 0.5 McFd, NA, NA, 48 h)	0.25	0.064-0.25	[28]
	Turkey/H	Bm, 76, 2001–06	E-test (SB-MH, 1 McFd, 0%, 35°C,48 h)	0.38	0.064-0.5	[29]
	Syria	Bm, 100, 2004–07	Broth microdilution (BB/7, 5 × 10^6 cfu/mL,37°C, 48 h)	4	0.125-8	[15]
	Syria	Bm, 100, 2004–07	Broth microdilution (BB/5, 5 × 10^6 cfu/mL,37°C, 48 h)	8	0.125-8	[15]
	Italy/H	Bru, 20, 2005–06	E-test (SB-MH, 0.5 McFd, 5%, 37°C, 48 h)	ND	0.094-0.5	[21]
	Turkey/H	Bm, 73, 2009–11	E-test (SB-MH, 0.5 McFd, NA, 37°C, 48 h)	0.19	0.125-1	[26]
Sparfloxacin	Israel/H	Bm, 86, (1991)	Broth microdilution (BB, 5 × 10^5cfu/mL,5%,37°C,48 h)	1.5	NA	[33]
Moxifloxacin	Spain/H	Bm, 160, 1997	Agar dilution (MH-HP,10^4cfu/ spot,10%,35°C,48 h)	1	1	[25]
	Turkey/H	Bm, 76, 2001–06	E-test (SB-MH, 1 McFd, 0%, 35°C,48 h)	0.25	0.032-0.25	[29]

NA, data not available; Bm, *B. melitensis*; Bab, *B. abortus*; Bru, *Brucella* sp.

£Studies have been classified according to the period of isolation of the studied *Brucella* strains (e.g., 2010–12) and the date of the corresponding publication (e.g., 1993) when the latter was unavailable.

*TMP/SMX: cotrimoxazole, trimethoprim plus sulfamethoxazole combination at 1/19 ratio, or 1/20 for reference [19] and 1/5 for reference [17].

$Method: Kirby–Bauer disk diffusion method (Kirby-Bauer); E-test strip method (E-test);

Medium: Mueller Hinton agar with 5% sheep blood (SB-MH) or unspecified percentage and type of blood (BA-MH); 5% sheep blood agar (SB); Brucella broth (BB); Brucella agar (BA); Trypticase soy broth (TSB); Iso-Sensitest® Agar CM47L (CM47L); Mueller Hinton broth supplemented with 1% polyvitex with (HP) or without (P) 1% hemoglobin, at pH 7 (/7) or pH 5 (/5); The bacterial inoculum used for antibiotic susceptibility testing is specified in cfu/mL or according to McFarland standards (McFd). Host: human (H), cattle (C), unspecified or various animals (A).

Table 2. Antibiotic susceptibilities of *Brucella* sp. to β-lactams, cotrimoxazole, chloramphenicol, macrolides, and fluoroquinolones, as determined in cell-free media.

MICs determined for chloramphenicol were not consistent from one study to the other (Table 2): MICs ranged from 0.3 to higher than 100 [9], 0.25 to 4 mg/L [18], and 0.15 to 12.5 mg/L [19]. However, this antibiotic was globally considered poorly effective *in vitro* against *Brucella* spp.

The macrolides also display poor *in vitro* activity against these bacteria (Table 2). MICs to erythromycin ranged from 0.2 to 16 mg/L using the agar dilution method [30], 0.5 to 8 mg/L using the E-test method [16], and 0.02 to 256 mg/L using various broth microdilution methods [9,11,18,19]. However, the very high MICs found in some studies could be related to the use of a high bacterial inoculum, especially at acidic pH [11]. Azithromycin displayed similar MIC ranges: 0.03–4 mg/L with the agar dilution method [30,32], 0.06–16 mg/L with the E-test method [26,28], and <0.12–4 mg/L with the broth microdilution method [11,31], with a deleterious effect of acidic pH [11].

In recent years, the fluoroquinolones proved to be very active against *Brucella* spp. *in vitro* (Table 2). Ciprofloxacin remains the most effective compound. MICs ranged from 0.12 to 1 mg/L using the agar dilution method [23,25], 0.016 to 1 mg/L with the E-test method [16,21,22,26,28,29], and <0.12 to 8 mg/L with the broth dilution method [11,13,19,33]. However, Garcia-Rodriguez et al. [14] demonstrated that MICs of several fluoroquinolone compounds (including ciprofloxacin), against *B. melitensis* and *B. abortus* strains, could be increased up to fourfold at acidic pH and/or in the presence of high bacterial loads. These authors also showed higher susceptibility to fluoroquinolones of *B. melitensis* compared to *B. abortus* [14].

2.1.2. Bactericidal activity by class of antibiotics

The bactericidal activity of antibiotics against *Brucella* species has been evaluated by determination of the minimal bactericidal concentrations (MBCs) and by kill-time experiments (Table 3). However, various methodologies and definitions for bactericidal activity were used in different studies. Results greatly varied according to experimental conditions, including the tested bacterial inoculum and pH of the culture medium [14]. De Rycke et al. [34] reported higher bactericidal activity of rifampicin compared to tetracycline against *B. suis*. Assuming that a bactericidal effect is at least 3-log reduction of the initial bacterial inoculum within 24–48 h incubation for *Brucella* sp., a bactericidal activity was reported by Mateu-de-Antonio et al. [35] at concentrations ranging from two to four times the MIC for the aminoglycosides (streptomycin and gentamicin), rifampicin, and the fluoroquinolone (enrofloxacin), but not for the tetracyclines (doxycycline) and the macrolides (erythromycin, clarithromycin, and roxithromycin). Only the aminoglycosides displayed early bactericidal activity (i.e., within 24 h of incubation) against *Brucella* sp. [33]. Garcia-Rodriguez et al. [14] reported lack of bactericidal activity of fluoroquinolones against 21 strains of *B. melitensis*, with ciprofloxacin MBCs ranging from 2 to ≥ 8 mg/L at neutral pH, but higher than 8 mg/L at pH 5.

2.1.3. Antibiotic combinations

The checkerboard method is considered the most accurate technique for *in vitro* evaluation of the activity of antibiotic combinations against bacteria. Results are usually expressed as the sum of fractional inhibitory concentrations (ΣFIC), which is the sum of the ratio of MIC of each

Antibiotic	Species	Number of strains	MBC ranges (mg/L)	Reference
Doxycycline	*B. melitensis, B. canis*	6	4–>16	[35]
Minocycline	*B. melitensis, B. canis*	6	1–>16	[35]
Gentamicin	*B. melitensis, B. canis*	6	0.25–1	[35]
Streptomycin	*B. melitensis, B. canis*	6	0.25–8	[35]
Ciprofloxacin	*B. melitensis, B. canis*	6	0.5–2	[35]
	B. melitensis	21	2–≥8	[14]
Ofloxacin	*B. melitensis*	21	≥8	[14]
Sparfloxacin	*B. melitensis*	21	2–≥8	[14]
Temafloxacin	*B. melitensis*	21	2–≥8	[14]
Lomefloxacin	*B. melitensis*	21	≥8	[14]
Fleroxacin	*B. melitensis*	21	≥8	[14]
Enrofloxacin	*B. melitensis, B. canis*	6	0.25–2	[35]
Rifampin	*B. melitensis, B. canis*	6	0.25–16	[35]
Erythromycin	*B. melitensis, B. canis*	6	2–>16	[35]
Spiramycin	*B. melitensis, B. canis*	6	4–>16	[35]
Clarithromycin	*B. melitensis, B. canis*	6	8–>16	[35]
Roxithromycin	*B. melitensis, B. canis*	6	16–>16	[35]

Table 3. Minimal bactericidal concentrations (MBCs) of several antibiotics against *Brucella* strains, as determined in broth culture, at pH 7.

antibiotic used in combination (MIC^{Acomb} or MIC^{Bcomb}) divided by MIC of each antibiotic (MIC^{A} or MIC^{B}, for antibiotics A and B, respectively): $\Sigma FIC = MIC^{Acomb}/MIC^{A} + MIC^{Bcomb}/MIC^{B}$. The antibiotic interactions are considered either synergistic ($\Sigma FIC \leq 0.5$, or $\Sigma FIC \leq 0.75$), additive ($\Sigma FIC > 0.5$ but ≤ 1, or $\Sigma FIC > 0.75$ but ≤ 1), indifferent ($\Sigma FIC > 1$ but ≤ 2), or antagonistic ($\Sigma FIC > 2$).

Using this method, Mortensen et al. [18] reported a synergistic effect of the combination of tetracycline with rifampicin, but indifference or antagonism with the combinations of tetracycline plus either streptomycin or gentamicin. Doxycycline plus rifampicin was reported to be synergistic in several studies [11,15,35,36]. A synergistic effect was also found for most *Brucella* strains tested for the combinations of doxycycline with either streptomycin or gentamicin [11,35,36]. The rifampicin and streptomycin combination was mainly indifferent [15]. The combinations of a fluoroquinolone (ofloxacin, ciprofloxacin, or sparfloxacin) with tetracycline, doxycycline, rifampicin, or streptomycin were mainly indifferent [11,15]. The rifampicin–azithromycin combination was also mainly indifferent [11], while ciprofloxacin plus azithromycin combination displayed variable activity (synergistic to antagonistic) according to the strains tested [36]. Interestingly, only the combination of doxycycline with rifampicin retained its synergistic activity at pH 5 [11,15]. It is to be noted also that Rubinstein et al. [33] did not find any synergistic effect of either of the previously mentioned antibiotic combinations.

The E-test method has also been used for the evaluation of the activity of antibiotic combinations [29,37]. Mueller Hinton agar plates supplemented with 5% sheep blood were inoculated with a 0.5–1 McFarland turbidity standard suspension of *Brucella* sp. The E-test strips were then successively applied to the inoculated surface so as MICs overlap at the same position. The first strip was removed after 1-h incubation, while the second was left on the agar for the 48-h incubation at 35°C. The ΣFIC index was used to interpret results: synergism ($\Sigma FIC \leq 0.5$), additive ($\Sigma FIC > 0.5$ but ≤ 1), indifference ($\Sigma FIC > 1$ but ≤ 4), and antagonism ($\Sigma FIC > 4$). Sometimes, the additive and indifference categories were combined as indifference. However, results were not consistent between studies. Ozhak-Baysan et al. [29] reported that, among the 28 *Brucella* sp. strains tested, the combination of doxycycline with rifampicin was antagonistic for 25 (89.3%) and indifferent for the remaining three strains. The combination of streptomycin with rifampicin was synergistic, but only one *Brucella* strain was tested. Orhan et al. [36] and Kilic et al. [37] reported two different studies from Turkey, each evaluating antibiotic combinations against 16 human strains of *B. melitensis*. A synergistic effect was reported for the combination of doxycycline with rifampicin for 15/16 (93.7%) strains [36], and for tetracycline with rifampicin for 16/16 (100%) strains [37]. The combination of doxycycline plus streptomycin was synergistic for 11/16 (68.7%) strains [36], while doxycycline plus cotrimoxazole was synergistic for 6/16 (37.5%) strains but antagonistic for the same number of strains [36]. A synergistic effect was found for the combination of cotrimoxazole with rifampicin for 6/16 (37.5%) strains [36] to 14/16 (87.5%) strains [37]. Ciprofloxacin displayed a synergistic effect when combined with cotrimoxazole for 7/16 (43.7%) strains [37], or with azithromycin for 12/16 strains (75%) [36]. Tetracycline plus moxifloxacin combination gave a synergistic effect for only 4/16 (25%) strains [37]. The combination of ciprofloxacin with streptomycin was mainly indifferent [37]. It is to be stressed that Orhan et al. [36] found different results with the same *B. melitensis* strains when using the checkerboard technique. The E-test overevaluated the synergistic effect of most antibiotic combinations compared to the checkerboard technique.

Using kill-time experiments, earlier bactericidal activity was demonstrated with the combination of streptomycin with either a tetracycline (tetracycline or doxycycline), rifampicin, or a fluoroquinolone (including ciprofloxacin) [33,35]. The same was true for the combination of rifampicin with either a fluoroquinolone (especially ciprofloxacin) or a tetracycline [33]. In some studies, the combination of rifampicin with a tetracycline was no more effective than the former antibiotic alone [34]. In contrast, the combination of ciprofloxacin and minocycline was antagonistic [33].

2.2. AST in eukaryotic cell models

Brucella spp. are facultative intracellular bacteria that infect a number of eukaryotic cells, including macrophages, dendritic cells, and trophoblasts of the placenta [38]. These bacteria replicate in acidic endoplasmic reticulum-derived vacuoles. Therefore, *in vivo* efficacy of antibiotics in *Brucella*-infected hosts is likely dependent on their activity against the intracellular and extracellular forms of this pathogen. Whereas MICs determined in cell-free media would allow detection of acquired resistances in specific *Brucella* strains, they cannot predict *in vivo* efficacy of antibiotics on their own. Eukaryotic cell models have been developed to test the activity of antibiotics against intracellular bacteria, including *Brucella* species. Mouse peritoneal macrophages and macrophage cell lines, and human monocyte-derived macrophages and macrophage cell lines (Mono Mac 6), have been most often used. These experimental models are based on *in vitro* infection of eukaryotic cells with a specific strain of *Brucella* sp., then exposure of infected cell monolayers to an antibiotic, and evaluation of residual intracellular viable bacteria to assess the antibiotic activity. The latter is usually determined by colony-forming unit (CFU) counting methodology, but quantitative real-time PCR has been used as a less fastidious alternative, although it does not differentiate viable from nonviable bacteria. Major limitations of these models include difficulties in eliminating nonphagocytized bacteria to ensure proper evaluation of intracellular antibiotic activity, lysis of eukaryotic cells before CFU determination without altering bacterial viability, and defining the most appropriate experimental conditions (especially the time of antibiotic exposure). Also, these models do not evaluate the influence of host–pathogen interactions (especially the host immune response) on intracellular activity of antibiotics.

Richardson et al. [39] first reported that streptomycin (at concentrations up to 50 mg/L) was not bacteriostatic against *B. abortus* grown in bovine cell cultures, while this antibiotic was strongly bactericidal in cell-free media. In contrast, tetracycline displayed the same activity against intracellular and extracellular bacteria. Streptomycin was no more effective when using guinea pig monocytes [40]. Filice et al. [41] demonstrated that rifampicin could induce ultrastructural damages to *B. melitensis* within mouse peritoneal macrophages. In a more recent study, using *B. abortus* strain 2308 and two cell lines (human Mono Mac 6 and J774 murine macrophages), Valderas et al. [42] demonstrated an intracellular bacteriostatic activity for tetracycline and doxycycline (at 1×MIC and 4×MIC in Mono Mac 6 and J774 cells, respectively), for rifampicin (at 0.25×MIC and 1×MIC, respectively), and for ciprofloxacin (at 1×MIC and 4×MIC, respectively). Streptomycin and gentamicin displayed no bacteriostatic activity after 24 h in these cell systems. However, these antibiotics slowly penetrate within eukaryotic cells and reach significant intracellular concentrations only after 3 days of antibiotic–cell contact [43]. A weak intracellular bactericidal activity (≤ 1-log reduction of bacterial titers) was found for rifampicin and ciprofloxacin at 4× and 8× MICs, but not for tetracycline and doxycycline [42]. Akova et al. [11] previously demonstrated the deleterious effect of acidic pH on activity of antibiotics against *Brucella* sp. It may be speculated that most antibiotics lose their bacteriostatic and/or bactericidal activity against intracellular *Brucella* sp. because these bacteria multiply in acidic cell compartments.

2.3. Animal models

Several animal models have been developed to study *in vivo* replication of *Brucella* sp., including mice, rats, guinea pigs, rabbits, and nonhuman primates [44]. The *in vivo* activity of antibiotics against this pathogen has been mainly evaluated in mice, rats, and guinea pigs.

These animals develop persistent bacteremia and a disseminated infection (especially in liver, spleen, and lungs). However, guinea pigs are the most susceptible animals, while rats usually do not develop clinical symptoms. The evaluation of *in vivo* efficacy of antibiotics was primarily based on their ability to eradicate *Brucella* from the spleen of treated animals compared to untreated controls, as determined by numeration of viable bacteria (CFU counts) in spleen tissue collected at the time of sacrifice of infected animals.

Early studies in guinea pigs demonstrated the *in vivo* activity of sulfanilamide in pigs infected with *B. melitensis* [45]. In OF1 mice and Hartley guinea pigs infected with *B. melitensis* or *B. suis*, rifampicin was able to eradicate bacteria from the spleen of most animals, while only partial decrease in spleen bacterial loads were observed with tetracycline [34,46]. In a more recent study, ICR mice were infected with *B. melitensis* 16M and received various antibiotic treatments (21 days orally or 14 days intraperitoneally) 7–14 days postinfection [47]. Rifampin (25 mg/kg/d, ip) and doxycycline (40 mg/kg/d ip) were highly effective to eradicate bacteria from the spleen, while streptomycin (75 mg/kg/d, ip), cotrimoxazole (15 mg/kg/d of TMP, ip), and ciprofloxacin (20 mg/kg/d ip) were not. Doxycycline was less effective when administrated orally at 6–80 mg/kg/d. The same authors later reported a much lower activity of rifampicin at a lower dosage (3 mg/kg/d), but a synergistic effect of the combination of streptomycin with either doxycycline or rifampicin [48]. Spiramycin, a macrolide compound, was tested in Sprague Dawley rats infected with *B. melitensis* [49]. Spiramycin (50 mg/kg/d, 21 days) alone or combined with rifampicin (50 mg/kg/d, 21 days) was found as effective as the combination of doxycycline (40 mg/kg/d, 21 days) with rifampicin. Dirithromycin, another macrolide compound, was less effective (27.3% cure rate) in mice infected with *B. abortus* S544 strain, but highly effective (81.8% cure rate) when combined with rifampicin [50]. In the same model, the fluoroquinolone levofloxacin was poorly effective when used alone (36.4% cure rate), and no more effective than rifampicin alone when combined with this antibiotic (72.7% cure rates in both cases) [50]. In Wistar albino rats infected with *B. abortus* [51], moxifloxacin (21 days) was less effective than rifampicin (cure rates in spleen of 50% and 80%, respectively). In mice infected with *B. melitensis* [52–54], doxycycline was much more effective to prevent bacterial multiplication than the fluoroquinolone compounds ciprofloxacin, moxifloxacin, gatifloxacin, trovafloxacin, and grepafloxacin, when administrated before or within hours after the bacterial challenge. Doxycycline was also effective to control *B. melitensis* infection when administrated 7–14 days following infection, whereas all the tested fluoroquinolones were ineffective. In the same animal model [54], the azalide compound azithromycin was able to control *B. melitensis* infection when administrated 2 h following the bacterial challenge. Altogether, the *Brucella*-infected animal models confirmed *in vivo* activity of rifampicin (the most effective antibiotic in all studies) and doxycycline, administrated alone or in combination. The combination of one of these two antibiotics with streptomycin was also effective. In contrast, the fluoroquinolones, cotrimoxazole, and the macrolides were unable to eradicate *Brucella* in most infected animals. A synergistic effect was found for the combination of a macrolide with rifampicin, but not for that of a fluoroquinolone with rifampicin. It is to be stressed, however, that these animal models greatly varied according to the animal species used, the *Brucella* species tested, the route and inoculum of the bacterial challenge, the dosage and duration of the tested antibiotic treatments, the time of administration of antibiotics compared to the bacterial challenge, and the time of antibiotic treatment evaluation. More standardization is needed to allow comparison of results obtained in different research laboratories.

The *in vivo* efficacy of antibiotics to eradicate *Brucella* has also been evaluated in naturally infected animals. Radwan et al. [55] reported the eradication of *B. melitensis* from 480 naturally infected sheep and goats with the combination of oxytetracycline with streptomycin, as evidenced by cessation of shedding *B. melitensis* from udder secretions and absence of this bacterium in tissues at autopsy after antibiotic treatment.

3. Acquired resistances to antibiotics in *Brucella* species

In vitro selection of rifampicin-resistant mutants has been reported for *B. melitensis, B. abortus,* and *B. suis* [12,34,56]. In *B. suis,* the spontaneous rate of mutations leading to rifampicin resistance was evaluated at 2.5×10^{-9} (for a concentration of 25 mg/L) [34]. Marianelli et al. [56] characterized the genetic mechanisms involved in resistance to rifampicin in the vaccine strain *B. abortus* RB51, and in laboratory mutants derived from two *B. melitensis* isolates. They found missense mutations in two regions of the *rpoB* gene encoding subunit B of RNA polymerase, the bacterial target of rifampicin. These mutations led to a number of amino acid changes: Val154Phe, Asp526Tyr, Asp526Gly, Asp526Asn, His536Leu, His536Tyr, Arg539Ser, Ser541Leu, and Pro574Leu. A number of studies have reported wide ranges of rifampicin MICs (up to 64 mg/L) in human and animal strains of *Brucella* sp., with MIC variations between geographic regions and time periods considered [9,11,15,19,22,23,26,30,33,57,58]. *In vivo* selection of rifampicin-resistant mutants was also reported in a patient who relapsed after treatment with doxycycline and rifampicin [59]. These results have suggested the possibility of acquired resistance to rifampicin in *Brucella* species. However, there is currently no clear characterization of *rpoB* mutations leading to rifampicin resistance in *Brucella* strains isolated from humans or animals. Direct amplification and sequencing of the *rpoB* gene did not reveal any rifampicin resistance mutation in two recent studies from Turkey [60] and Spain [61], in 21 and 62 human strains of *B. melitensis*, respectively.

Very few studies have reported high doxycycline MICs (up to 32 mg/L) in animal and human strains of *Brucella* sp. [11,15,17,57]. In some studies, however, high-level MICs may have been related to the use of a high bacterial inoculum rather than true acquired resistance to tetracyclines [15,17]. Acquired resistance mechanisms to tetracyclines in *Brucella* strains have never been characterized in clinical situation, although the gene encoding the tetracycline resistance protein TetB was found in the genome of *B. abortus* [62]. The same holds true for the aminoglycoside streptomycin, with MICs > 64 mg/L in only two studies [9,15], while high MICs to gentamicin have not been reported so far. High MICs to trimethoprim–sulfamethoxazole combination have also been reported [10,13,17,57,58,63,64], but without characterization of the involved mechanisms. The MICs of macrolides, especially erythromycin [11,16,18,30], are highly variable among *Brucella* strains. For either of these antibiotics, no resistance mechanism has been characterized.

Fluoroquinolone resistance mechanisms have been characterized in *in vitro* selected resistant mutants of *B. melitensis* and *B. abortus* [65–67]. The amino acid substitutions Ala87Val and Asp91Tyr (corresponding to codon positions gyrA83 and gyrA87 in *E. coli* numbering system) were reported. However, efflux pump overexpression was also probably involved in fluoroquinolone resistance in *Brucella* sp. [65,68]. High ciprofloxacin MICs (up to 8 mg/L) have been reported for human and animal strains of *Brucella* sp. [11,15,19,30,57]. No *gyrA* mutation has been reported so far in these strains [61]. However, overexpression of efflux pumps in *Brucella* strains remains difficult to demonstrate, and could partly explain treatment failures observed with fluoroquinolones in brucellosis patients [61]. RND-type efflux pumps have been characterized in *Brucella* sp [69].

4. Correlation between laboratory data and clinical efficacy of antibiotics

In untreated patients, brucellosis may be controlled by the immune system, but relapses and chronic evolution of the disease are frequently observed [1]. The combination of immune defenses and an appropriate antibiotic therapy allows earlier amendment of clinical symptoms and more effective control of infection. The clinical experience regarding the treatment of brucellosis has established some basic principles that remain true today [70]. To reduce the risk of recurrence, at least two antibiotics should be administrated for a minimum of 4–6 weeks. The combination of doxycycline with either rifampicin or an aminoglycoside (streptomycin or gentamicin) is the most effective *in vitro* and is considered the first alternative for the treatment of brucellosis [71]. It is likely that the effectiveness of these antibiotic combinations depends on their activity on both extracellular and intracellular *Brucella,* and their ability to reach the infectious sites and remain active at local conditions (including an acidic pH in eukaryotic cell compartments, but also in organ abscesses). AST in cell-free media is poorly predictive of the *in vivo* activity of antibiotics against *Brucella* sp. However, these models have shown that the aminoglycosides and rifampin display significant bactericidal activity against extracellular *Brucella* [33,35]. Cell models have shown that rifampicin is the only antibiotic with a bactericidal activity against the intracellular form of *Brucella,* whereas the tetracyclines and the fluoroquinolones are mainly bacteriostatic [39,42]. The aminoglycosides had no activity against intracellular *Brucella* [39,42]. However, their activity was evaluated in *Brucella*-infected cell models after 24 h of antibiotic exposure, while these antibiotics significantly penetrate and concentrate in eukaryotic cells only after 3 days [43]. Thus, in patients treated with an aminoglycoside, potential intracellular activity of these antibiotics cannot be ruled out. The animal models confirmed a clear superiority of rifampicin and doxycycline for eradication of *Brucella* sp. from the spleen [34,46,48], while the fluoroquinolones were much less active [50–54]. Altogether, the superiority of the combinations of doxycycline with either an aminoglycoside or rifampicin in brucellosis patients could be related to the synergistic effect of an extracellular bactericidal activity (especially using an aminoglycoside or rifampicin) with an intracellular bactericidal activity (doxycycline or rifampicin, plus an appropriate cell immune response). A prolonged antibiotic therapy is likely needed because of poor bactericidal activity of antibiotics against intracellular *Brucella* and the need for progressive development of an efficient immune response. Hence, brucellosis is usually a more severe disease in immunocompromised patients, often with a chronic evolution [72–74].

Nevertheless, relapse rates of 5%–15% are still reported in immunocompetent patients after administration of appropriate antibiotic therapy, sometimes several decades following the primary infection [73,75]. A first explanation could be the lack of eradication of *Brucella* by antibiotics in these relapsing patients because of interindividual variability in the inflammatory and immune responses to *Brucella* infection. It should be stressed that in animal models, the eradication rates obtained after antibiotic treatment varied from one animal species to the other, and between individuals of a same species [47,48,50–54]. Second, the infectious dose and delay in antibiotic treatment after infection may also greatly influence antibiotic activity. A typical example concerns the fluoroquinolones which were effective to control *Brucella* infection in animal models when administrated before or immediately after the infectious challenge, but not when administrated 1 or 2 weeks later [47,48,50–54]. Third, *in vivo* selection of *Brucella* mutants, resistant to antibiotics in brucellosis patients under antibiotic therapy, could also explain the therapeutic failures and relapses, especially for rifampicin and the fluoroquinolones [59,65–67]. Although *in vitro* studies have suggested that *Brucella* sp. could become resistant to first-line antibiotics used for brucellosis treatment, definite proofs of selection of acquired resistances in the clinical situation are still lacking. Interestingly, similar antibiotic susceptibilities were reported in *B. melitensis* strains isolated before and after antibiotic therapy in brucellosis patients suffering from relapses [28,76], which indicated that treatment failure was not related to development of acquired resistances to antibiotics in this pathogen.

Improving our understanding of treatment failures and relapses in brucellosis patients will necessitate not only a better standardization of assessment of the antibiotic activity using both *in vitro* and *in vivo* approaches, but also the development of new diagnostic tools to explore previous hypotheses directly in infected patients.

5. New therapeutic alternatives

5.1. Novel antibiotics

Tigecycline, a glycylcycline compound derived from minocycline, displays broad ranges of MICs and higher MIC90 *in vitro* than doxycycline against *Brucella* sp. [26,27,29,77]. In contrast, a lower MIC90 was reported for tigecycline (0.125 mg/L) compared to tetracycline (0.25 mg/L) for 60 strains of *B. melitensis* [78]. Using the checkerboard method, Aliskan et al. [79] reported a synergistic effect of the combination of tigecycline with either levofloxacin (50% of the 16 strains tested), rifampicin (31.2%), or gentamicin (18.9%). No synergy was observed with tigecycline in combination with streptomycin or cotrimoxazole. Dizbay et al. [80] reported a higher synergistic effect of antibiotic combinations when tigecycline was used compared to doxycycline. It has been proposed to replace doxycycline by tigecycline in current therapeutic protocols of brucellosis [81–83]. Although tigecycline could be as effective as doxycycline in antibiotic combination therapies, there are currently major limitations for its widespread use in brucellosis patients. At first, tigecycline is tens of times more expensive than doxycycline. Second, it can only be administrated by the parenteral route and thus its use would be restricted to the acute phase of brucellosis and/or in patients hospitalized because of a severe disease. Third, the antibacterial spectrum of tigecycline is much broader than that of doxycycline, including staphylococci (especially methicillin-resistant *S. aureus*), streptococci, enterococci, some anaerobes, and most enterobacterial species (including those secreting extended spectrum beta-lactamases), but not species of the *Proteae* tribe and *Pseudomonas aeruginosa* [83]. Thus, significant alterations of the skin and gut commensal flora would certainly occur in the treated population, with an increased risk of opportunistic infections and development of resistances to the glycylcyclines. Finally, it is not clear if the favorable pharmacokinetic properties of tigecycline in tissues could lead to a significant reduction in duration of treatment or relapse rates. Also, as for tetracyclines, tigecycline is contraindicated in pregnant women and young children.

Among new fluoroquinolones, moxifloxacin did not display higher activity compared to ciprofloxacin *in vitro* [25,29,37] or in animal models [51–54]. The use of a triple combination of doxycycline, rifampicin, and a fluoroquinolone warrants further evaluation, at least for treatment of severe brucellosis cases such as spondylodiscitis, endocarditis, and neurobrucellosis [84–86].

Among the new macrolide compounds, azithromycin displayed *in vitro* bacteriostatic activity against *Brucella* sp. with MIC90 ranging from 0.5 to 8 mg/L [11,26,28,30–32]. A synergistic effect was found when this antibiotic was combined with ciprofloxacin [36]. Azithromycin was also able to control *B. melitensis* infection in the mouse model [54]. However, azithromycin was much less effective than doxycycline to cure brucellosis in Swiss-Webster or BALB/c mice [87]. Although the macrolides are currently not considered suitable for treatment of brucellosis, they could represent a safe alternative in young children and pregnant women. Further evaluation of the *in vitro* and *in vivo* activity of macrolides combined with other antibiotic classes against *Brucella* sp. is warranted.

Medicinal plants have been evaluated for their *in vitro* activity against *B. melitensis.* Using a Mueller Hinton broth dilution method, Motamedi et al. [88] reported that ethanolic and methanolic extracts of six plants displayed anti-*Brucella* activity: *Oliveria decumbens, Salvia sclarea, Ferulago abgulata, Vitex pseudo-negundo, Teucrium pollium,* and *Crocus sativus. O. decumbens* was the most effective with similar MICs and MBCs. Al-Mariri and Safi [89] evaluated the activity of essential oils against 16 *Brucella* strains. They found a bacteriostatic effect for essential oils from two medicinal plants: *Thymus syriacus* and *Origanum syriacum.*

5.2. Intracellular delivery of antibiotics

The aminoglycosides are able to penetrate eukaryotic cells, albeit very slowly, but concentrate in the acidic lysosomal compartment because of their weak base nature [43]. At acidic pH, these antibiotics are partially inactivated because of their protonation. Although intracellular pharmacokinetic studies were mostly conducted using uninfected eukaryotic cells, it is tempting to extrapolate these data to *Brucella*-infected cells. *In vitro* studies have been performed to evaluate the influence of increased uptake of aminoglycosides within eukaryotic cells on their activity against intracellular *Brucella.* These antibiotics (especially streptomycin and gentamicin) were either included in liposomes or attached to nanoparticles. Phagocytosis of liposomal or nanoparticle formulations of aminoglycosides by *Brucella*-infected macrophages resulted in higher intracellular activity compared to free aminoglycosides against *B. melitensis, B. abortus,* or *B. canis* [90–94]. These formulations of the aminoglycosides were also significantly more effective in animal models [90,94,95]. The targeted delivery of aminoglycosides could be a promising therapeutic alternative, both increasing their intracellular activity and reducing their side effects by reducing their concentration in kidneys and the cochleovestibular system. However, there are currently technical limitations in the preparation of liposomal or nanoparticle forms of antibiotics and safety concerns, especially for nanoparticles that limit their use in humans [96].

5.3. Peptide nucleic acids

Peptide nucleic acids (PNAs) are artificially synthesized polymers similar to DNA or RNA that can be used as antisense therapies. They show high specificity in binding to complementary DNAs, resistance to nucleases and proteases, and a high stability over a wide pH range. They readily cross the bacterial cell membranes when coupled with a cell-penetrating peptide. Rajasekaran et al. [97] reported growth inhibition of *B. suis* by PNAs, both in cell-free medium and in murine macrophages. In tryptic soy broth, the inhibitory PNAs were those targeting the genes *kdtA* (coding for a transferase affecting lipid A), *tsf* (elongation factor *Ts*), *polA* (DNA polymerase I), and *rpoB* (subunit B of RNA polymerase). In contrast, in J774A.1 murine macrophages, the inhibitory PNAs targeted the genes *asd* (coding for an aspartate-semialdehyde dehydrogenase involved in diaminopimelic acid synthesis), *gyrA* (subunit A of DNA gyrase), *dnaG* (protein primase that initiates DNA replication), and *polA*. The PNAs were thus able to penetrate the eukaryotic and bacterial membranes, and could represent new therapeutic alternatives for intracellular pathogens such as *Brucella* sp.

5.4. Enhancement of the host response

Multiplication within phagocytic cells is a major virulence factor of *Brucella* species. The host response to *Brucella* infection could be strengthened by restoring the ability of phagocytic cells to control intracellular multiplication of these bacteria and eradicate them via the phagolysosomal pathway, especially using cytokines. Jiang and Baldwin [98] reported the *in vitro* inhibition of *B. abortus* multiplication in BALB/c J774A.1 murine macrophages by gamma interferon (IFN-γ) or to a lesser extent interleukin-2 (IL-2, 100 U/mL). In contrast, IL-1α, IL-4, IL-6, tumor necrosis factor alpha (TNF-α), and granulocyte macrophage–colony-stimulating factor (GM–CSF) had no significant effect on intracellular growth of *B. abortus*. The protective role of IFN-γ was also emphasized by Murphy et al. [99], using IFN-γ gene knockout mice infected with *B. abortus.* When adsorbed to albumin nanoparticles, IFN-γ was even more effective to control *B. abortus* infection in RAW 264.7 macrophages and BALB/c mice [100]. Fahel et al. [101] recently reported in a mouse model of *B. abortus* infection that a higher host resistance to infection was associated with an increased expression of interleukin-12 (IL-12), gamma interferon (IFN-γ), and inducible nitric oxide synthase (iNOS) during the course of infection. This protective Th1 immune response was negatively regulated by 5-Lipooxygenase (5-LO), an enzyme required for the production of the lipid mediators leukotrienes and lipoxins. The use of interferon-gamma has never been reported so far in brucellosis patients.

6. Conclusion

Brucellosis remains a prevalent disease in the world, a major concern in public health and an economic burden in agriculture. Although effective vaccines are available for the livestock, treatment of brucellosis remains challenging in both animals and humans. Recommendations for treatment of common clinical forms of human brucellosis have been addressed, especially by the WHO. However, treatment optimization is still needed for severe forms of the disease and in young children and pregnant women. Moreover, current treatment recommendations could be challenged by the emergence of acquired resistances to first-line drugs in *Brucella* species, although this fear needs to be confirmed with certainty in the clinical situation. Alternative therapeutic options are needed to reduce the human and economic costs associated with this disease. This could be achieved through the development of new molecules but also by an optimized use of currently available antibiotics. However, controlling *Brucella* infection in the livestock remains a priority.

Author details

Max Maurin[1,2*]

Address all correspondence to: MMaurin@chu-grenoble.fr

1 Bacteriology Laboratory, Biology and Pathology Institute, Grenoble University Hospital, France

2 LAPM, UJF/CNRS, Joseph Fourier-Grenoble 1 University, France

References

[1] Pappas G, Akritidis N, Bosilkovski M, Tsianos E. Brucellosis. N Engl J Med. 2005;352:2325-2336.

[2] Franco MP, Mulder M, Gilman RH, Smits HL. Human brucellosis. Lancet Infect Dis. 2007;7:775-786.

[3] CDC. Biosafety in Microbiological and Biomedical Laboratories (BMBL), 5th Edition. 2009. http://www.cdc.gov/biosafety/publications/bmbl5/index.htm

[4] Pappas G, Panagopoulou P, Christou L, Akritidis N. *Brucella* as a biological weapon. Cell Mol Life Sci CMLS. 2006;63:2229-2236.

[5] Yagupsky P, Baron EJ. Laboratory exposures to *Brucellae* and implications for bioterrorism. Emerg Infect Dis. 2005;11:1180-1185.

[6] Singh K. Laboratory-acquired infections. Clin Infect Dis. 2009;49:142-147.

[7] Traxler RM, Lehman MW, Bosserman EA, Guerra MA, Smith TL. A literature review of laboratory-acquired brucellosis. J Clin Microbiol. 2013;51:3055-3062.

[8] Clinical and Laboratory Standards Institute. Performance Standards for Antimicrobial Susceptibility Testing. Twentieth informational Supplement. CLSI document M 100-S20. Wayne, PA, USA. 2010.

[9] Hall WH, Manion RE. *In vitro* susceptibility of *Brucella* to various antibiotics. Appl Microbiol. 1970;20:600-604.

[10] Lonsway DR, Jevitt LA, Uhl JR, Cockerill FR, Anderson ME, Sullivan MM, et al. Effect of carbon dioxide on broth microdilution susceptibility testing of *Brucella* spp. J Clin Microbiol. 2010;48:952-956.

[11] Akova M, Gür D, Livermore DM, Kocagöz T, Akalin HE. In vitro activities of antibiotics alone and in combination against *Brucella melitensis* at neutral and acidic pHs. Antimicrob Agents Chemother. 1999;43:1298-1300.

[12] Shir Y, Michel J. Antibiotic sensitivity of strains of *Brucella*. Pathol Biol (Paris). 1984;32:381-383.

[13] Khan MY, Dizon M, Kiel FW. Comparative in vitro activities of ofloxacin, difloxacin, ciprofloxacin, and other selected antimicrobial agents against *Brucella melitensis*. Antimicrob Agents Chemother. 1989;33:1409-1410.

[14] García-Rodriguez JA, García Sánchez JE, Trujillano I. Lack of effective bactericidal activity of new quinolones against *Brucella* spp. Antimicrob Agents Chemother. 1991;35:756-759.

[15] Al-Mariri A, Safi M. Effect of medium pH on antibiotic activity against Syrian *Brucella* spp. Isolates. Iran J Med Sci. 2013;38:248-254.

[16] Turkmani A, Ioannidis A, Christidou A, Psaroulaki A, Loukaides F, Tselentis Y. *In vitro* susceptibilities of *Brucella melitensis* isolates to eleven antibiotics. Ann Clin Microbiol Antimicrob. 2006;5:24.

[17] Xu X-L, Chen X, Yang P-H, Liu J-Y, Hao X-K. *In vitro* drug resistance of clinical isolated *Brucella* against antimicrobial agents. Asian Pac J Trop Med. 2013;6:921-924.

[18] Mortensen JE, Moore DG, Clarridge JE, Young EJ. Antimicrobial susceptibility of clinical isolates of *Brucella*. Diagn Microbiol Infect Dis. 1986;5:163-169.

[19] Heo E-J, Kang S-I, Kim J-W, Her M, Cho D, Cho Y-S, et al. *In vitro* activities of antimicrobials against *Brucella abortus* isolates from cattle in Korea during 1998-2006. J Microbiol Biotechnol. 2012;22:567-570.

[20] Palenque E, Otero JR, Noriega AR. *In vitro* susceptibility of *Brucella melitensis* to new cephalosporins crossing the blood-brain barrier. Antimicrob Agents Chemother. 1986;29:182-183.

[21] Marianelli C, Graziani C, Santangelo C, Xibilia MT, Imbriani A, Amato R, et al. Molecular epidemiological and antibiotic susceptibility characterization of *Brucella* isolates from humans in Sicily, Italy. J Clin Microbiol. 2007;45:2923-2928.

[22] Abdel-Maksoud M, House B, Wasfy M, Abdel-Rahman B, Pimentel G, Roushdy G, et al. *In vitro* antibiotic susceptibility testing of *Brucella* isolates from Egypt between 1999 and 2007 and evidence of probable rifampin resistance. Ann Clin Microbiol Antimicrob. 2012;11:24.

[23] Bosch J, Liñares J, López de Goicoechea MJ, Ariza J, Cisnal MC, Martin R. *In-vitro* activity of ciprofloxacin, ceftriaxone and five other antimicrobial agents against 95 strains of *Brucella melitensis*. J Antimicrob Chemother. 1986;17:459-461.

[24] Gutiérrez Altés A, Díez Enciso M, Peña García P, Campos Bueno A. *In vitro* activity of N-formimidoyl thienamycin against 98 clinical isolates of *Brucella melitensis* compared with those of cefoxitin, rifampin, tetracycline, and co-trimoxazole. Antimicrob Agents Chemother. 1982;21:501-503.

[25] Trujillano-Martín I, García-Sánchez E, Martínez IM, Fresnadillo MJ, García-Sánchez JE, García-Rodríguez JA. *In vitro* activities of six new fluoroquinolones against *Brucella melitensis*. Antimicrob Agents Chemother. 1999;43:194-195.

[26] Parlak M, Güdücüoğlu H, Bayram Y, Çıkman A, Aypak C, Kılıç S, et al. Identification and determination of antibiotic susceptibilities of *Brucella* strains isolated from patients in van, Turkey by conventional and molecular methods. Int J Med Sci. 2013;10:1406-1411.

[27] Bayram Y, Korkoca H, Aypak C, Parlak M, Cikman A, Kilic S, et al. Antimicrobial susceptibilities of *Brucella* isolates from various clinical specimens. Int J Med Sci. 2011;8:198-202.

[28] Maves RC, Castillo R, Guillen A, Espinosa B, Meza R, Espinoza N, et al. Antimicrobial susceptibility of *Brucella melitensis* isolates in Peru. Antimicrob Agents Chemother. 2011;55:1279-1281.

[29] Ozhak-Baysan B, Ongut G, Ogunc D, Gunseren F, Sepin-Ozen N, Ozturk F, et al. Evaluation of *in vitro* activities of tigecycline and various antibiotics against *Brucella* spp. Pol J Microbiol Pol Tow Mikrobiol Pol Soc Microbiol. 2010;59:55-60.

[30] García-Rodríguez JA, Muñoz Bellido JL, Fresnadillo MJ, Trujillano I. *In vitro* activities of new macrolides and rifapentine against *Brucella* spp. Antimicrob Agents Chemother. 1993;37:911-3.

[31] Qadri SM, Halim MA, Ueno Y, Abumustafa FM, Postle AG. Antibacterial activity of azithromycin against *Brucella melitensis*. Chemotherapy. 1995;41:253-256.

[32] Landínez R, Liñares J, Loza E, Martínez-Beltrán J, Martín R, Baquero F. *In vitro* activity of azithromycin and tetracycline against 358 clinical isolates of *Brucella melitensis*. Eur J Clin Microbiol Infect Dis. 1992;11:265-267.

[33] Rubinstein E, Lang R, Shasha B, Hagar B, Diamanstein L, Joseph G, et al. *In vitro* susceptibility of *Brucella melitensis* to antibiotics. Antimicrob Agents Chemother. 1991;35:1925-1927.

[34] De Rycke J. Effect of rifampicin and tetracycline alone and in combination against *Brucella suis*. Ann Microbiol (Paris). 1980;131B:277-287.

[35] Mateu-de-Antonio EM, Martín M. *In vitro* efficacy of several antimicrobial combinations against *Brucella canis* and *Brucella melitensis* strains isolated from dogs. Vet Microbiol. 1995;45:1-10.

[36] Orhan G, Bayram A, Zer Y, Balci I. Synergy tests by E test and checkerboard methods of antimicrobial combinations against *Brucella melitensis*. J Clin Microbiol. 2005;43:140-143.

[37] Kilic S, Dizbay M, Hizel K, Arman D. *In vitro* synergistic activity of antibiotic combinations against *Brucella melitensis* using E-test methodology. Braz J Microbiol. 2008;39:233-237.

[38] Von Bargen K, Gorvel J-P, Salcedo SP. Internal affairs: investigating the *Brucella intracellular* lifestyle. FEMS Microbiol Rev. 2012;36:533-562.

[39] Richardson M, Holt JN. Synergistic action of streptomycin with other antibiotics of intracellular *Brucella abortus in vitro*. J Bacteriol. 1962;84:638-646.

[40] Goldenbaum EG, Kessel RW, Fukui GM. Effect of chlorpromazine and streptomycin on the survival of *Brucella abortus* in guinea pig monocytes. J Infect Dis. 1966;116:447-454.

[41] Filice G, Carnevale G, Lanzarini P, Castelli F, Gorini G, Benzi-Cipelli R, et al. Intracellular killing of *Brucella melitensis* within mouse peritoneal macrophages: influence of treatment with rifampicin. An ultrastructural study. Microbiologica. 1986;9:189-198.

[42] Valderas MW, Barrow WW. Establishment of a method for evaluating intracellular antibiotic efficacy in *Brucella abortus*-infected Mono Mac 6 monocytes. J Antimicrob Chemother. 2008;61:128-134.

[43] Maurin M, Raoult D. Use of aminoglycosides in treatment of infections due to intracellular bacteria. Antimicrob Agents Chemother. 2001;45:2977-2986.

[44] Silva TMA, Costa EA, Paixão TA, Tsolis RM, Santos RL. Laboratory animal models for brucellosis research. J Biomed Biotechnol. 2011;2011:518323.

[45] Menefee EE, Poston MA. Effects of sulfanilamide on *Brucella melitensis*, var. *melitensis*, *abortus*, and *suis*. J Bacteriol. 1939;37:269-276.

[46] Philippon AM, Plommet MG, Kazmierczak A, Marly JL, Nevot PA. Rifampin in the treatment of experimental brucellosis in mice and guinea pigs. J Infect Dis. 1977;136:481-488.

[47] Shasha B, Lang R, Rubinstein E. Therapy of experimental murine brucellosis with streptomycin, co-trimoxazole, ciprofloxacin, ofloxacin, pefloxacin, doxycycline, and rifampin. Antimicrob Agents Chemother. 1992;36:973-976.

[48] Lang R, Shasha B, Rubinstein E. Therapy of experimental murine brucellosis with streptomycin alone and in combination with ciprofloxacin, doxycycline, and rifampin. Antimicrob Agents Chemother. 1993;37:2333-2336.

[49] Geyik MF, Dikici B, Kokoglu OF, Bosnak M, Celen MK, Hosoglu S, et al. Therapeutic effect of spiramycin in brucellosis. Pediatr Int. 2003;45:31-34.

[50] Arda B, Tunçel M, Yaimazhan T, Gökengin D, Gürel O. Efficacy of oral levofloxacin and dirithromycin alone and in combination with rifampicin in the treatment of experimental murine *Brucella abortus* infection. Int J Antimicrob Agents. 2004;23:204-207.

[51] Sezak N, Kuruuzum Z, Cakir N, Yuce A. Comparison of rifampicin and moxifloxacin efficacy in an experimental model of animal brucellosis. J Chemother. 2008;20:58-62.

[52] Atkins HS, Spencer S, Brew SD, Jenner DC, Russell P, MacMillan AP, et al. Efficacy of ciprofloxacin versus doxycycline as prophylaxis against experimental murine *Brucella melitensis* infection. Int J Antimicrob Agents. 2009;34:474-476.

[53] Atkins HS, Spencer S, Brew SD, Laws TR, Thirlwall RE, MacMillan AP, et al. Efficacy of moxifloxacin or gatifloxacin as prophylaxis against experimental murine *Brucella melitensis* infection. Int J Antimicrob Agents. 2009;34:471-473.

[54] Atkins HS, Spencer S, Brew SD, Jenner DC, Sefton AM, MacMillan AP, et al. Evaluation of azithromycin, trovafloxacin and grepafloxacin as prophylaxis against experimental murine *Brucella melitensis* infection. Int J Antimicrob Agents. 2010;36:66-68.

[55] Radwan AI, Bekairi SI, Mukayel AA. Treatment of *Brucella melitensis* infection in sheep and goats with oxytetracycline combined with streptomycin. Rev Sci Tech Int. 1992;11:845-857.

[56] Marianelli C, Ciuchini F, Tarantino M, Pasquali P, Adone R. Genetic bases of the rifampin resistance phenotype in *Brucella* spp. J Clin Microbiol. 2004;42:5439-5443.

[57] Ilhan Z, Solmaz H, Ekin IH. *In vitro* antimicrobial susceptibility of *Brucella melitensis* isolates from sheep in an area endemic for human brucellosis in Turkey. J Vet Med Sci. 2013;75:1035-1040.

[58] Memish Z, Mah MW, Al Mahmoud S, Al Shaalan M, Khan MY. *Brucella* bacteraemia: clinical and laboratory observations in 160 patients. J Infect. 2000;40:59-63.

[59] De Rautlin de la Roy YM, Grignon B, Grollier G, Coindreau MF, Becq-Giraudon B. Rifampicin resistance in a strain of *Brucella melitensis* after treatment with doxycycline and rifampicin. J Antimicrob Chemother. 1986;18:648-649.

[60] Sayan M, Yumuk Z, Dündar D, Bilenoglu O, Erdenlig S, Yaşar E, et al. Rifampicin resistance phenotyping of *Brucella melitensis* by *rpoB* gene analysis in clinical isolates. J Chemother. 2008;20:431-435.

[61] Valdezate S, Navarro A, Medina-Pascual MJ, Carrasco G, Saéz-Nieto JA. Molecular screening for rifampicin and fluoroquinolone resistance in a clinical population of *Brucella melitensis*. J Antimicrob Chemother. 2010;65:51-53.

[62] Biswas S, Raoult D, Rolain J-M. A bioinformatic approach to understanding antibiotic resistance in intracellular bacteria through whole genome analysis. Int J Antimicrob Agents. 2008;32:207-220.

[63] Baykam N, Esener H, Ergönül O, Eren S, Celikbas AK, Dokuzoguz B. *In vitro* antimicrobial susceptibility of *Brucella* species. Int J Antimicrob Agents. 2004;23:405-407.

[64] Kinsara A, Al-Mowallad A, Osoba AO. Increasing resistance of Brucellae to co-trimoxazole. Antimicrob Agents Chemother. 1999;43:1531.

[65] Ravanel N, Gestin B, Maurin M. *In vitro* selection of fluoroquinolone resistance in *Brucella melitensis*. Int J Antimicrob Agents. 2009;34:76-81.

[66] Turkmani A, Psaroulaki A, Christidou A, Chochlakis D, Tabaa D, Tselentis Y. *In vitro*-selected resistance to fluoroquinolones in two *Brucella* strains associated with mutational changes in *gyrA*. Int J Antimicrob Agents. 2008;32:227-232.

[67] Lázaro FG, Rodríguez-Tarazona RE, García-Rodríguez JA, Muñoz-Bellido JL. Fluoroquinolone-resistant *Brucella melitensis* mutants obtained in vitro. Int J Antimicrob Agents. 2009;34:252-254.

[68] Turkmani A, Psaroulaki A, Christidou A, Samoilis G, Mourad TA, Tabaa D, et al. Uptake of ciprofloxacin and ofloxacin by 2 *Brucella* strains and their fluoroquinolone-resistant variants under different conditions. An in vitro study. Diagn Microbiol Infect Dis. 2007;59:447-451.

[69] Martin FA, Posadas DM, Carrica MC, Cravero SL, O'Callaghan D, Zorreguieta A. Interplay between two RND systems mediating antimicrobial resistance in *Brucella suis*. J Bacteriol. 2009;191:2530-2540.

[70] Pappas G, Papadimitriou P, Christou L, Akritidis N. Future trends in human brucellosis treatment. Expert Opin Investig Drugs. 2006;15:1141-1149.

[71] Skalsky K, Yahav D, Bishara J, Pitlik S, Leibovici L, Paul M. Treatment of human brucellosis: systematic review and meta-analysis of randomised controlled trials. BMJ. 2008;336:701-704.

[72] Akgul O, Ozgocmen S. Infliximab and brucellosis: not the usual suspects, this time. Mod Rheumatol. 2011;21:313-315.

[73] Meneses A, Epaulard O, Maurin M, Gressin R, Pavese P, Brion J-P, et al. Brucella bacteremia reactivation 70 years after the primary infection. Med Mal Infect. 2010;40:238-240.

[74] Al-Anazi KA, Al-Jasser AM. *Brucella* bacteremia in patients with acute leukemia: a case series. J Med Case Reports. 2007;1:144.

[75] Ögredici Ö, Erb S, Langer I, Pilo P, Kerner A, Haack HG, et al. Brucellosis reactivation after 28 years. Emerg Infect Dis. 2010;16:2021-2022.

[76] Ariza J, Bosch J, Gudiol F, Liñares J, Viladrich PF, Martín R. Relevance of in vitro antimicrobial susceptibility of *Brucella melitensis* to relapse rate in human brucellosis. Antimicrob Agents Chemother. 1986;30:958-960.

[77] Tanyel E, Coban AY, Fisgin NT, Tulek N. The effect of tigecycline and ertapenem against clinical isolates of *Brucella melitensis* detected by E-test on different media. Indian J Med Microbiol. 2010;28:370-371.

[78] Kilic S, Dizbay M, Cabadak H. In vitro activity of tigecycline, tetracycline and fluoroquinolones against *Brucella melitensis*. J Chemother. 2008;20:33-37.

[79] Aliskan H, Can F, Demirbilek M, Colakoglu S, Kilic S, Arslan H. Determining *in vitro* synergistic activities of tigecycline with several other antibiotics against *Brucella melitensis* using checkerboard and time-kill assays. J Chemother. 2009;21:24-30.

[80] Dizbay M, Kilic S, Hizel K, Arman D. Tigecycline: its potential for treatment of brucellosis. Scand J Infect Dis. 2007;39:432-434.

[81] Pappas G, Solera J, Akritidis N, Tsianos E. New approaches to the antibiotic treatment of brucellosis. Int J Antimicrob Agents. 2005;26:101-105.

[82] Cocchi S, Bisi L, Codeluppi M, Venturelli C, Di Benedetto F, Ballarin R, et al. Brucellosis in a patient with end-stage liver disease undergoing liver transplantation: successful treatment with tigecycline. Liver Transplant. 2010;16:1215-1216.

[83] Livermore DM. Tigecycline: what is it, and where should it be used? J Antimicrob Chemother. 2005;56:611-614.

[84] Manade VV, Kakrani A, Gadage SN, Misra R. *Brucella* endocarditis in a non-endemic area presenting as pyrexia of unknown origin. BMJ Case Rep. 2014. DOI: 10.1136/bcr-2014-203555

[85] Ioannou S, Karadima D, Pneumaticos S, Athanasiou H, Pontikis J, Zormpala A, et al. Efficacy of prolonged antimicrobial chemotherapy for brucellar spondylodiscitis. Clin Microbiol Infect. 2011;17:756-762.

[86] Ulu-Kilic A, Karakas A, Erdem H, Turker T, Inal AS, Ak O, et al. Update on treatment options for spinal brucellosis. Clin Microbiol Infect. 2014;20:75-82.

[87] Domingo S, Gastearena I, Vitas AI, López-Goñi I, Dios-Viéitez C, Díaz R, et al. Comparative activity of azithromycin and doxycycline against *Brucella* spp. infection in mice. J Antimicrob Chemother. 1995;36:647-656.

[88] Motamedi H, Darabpour E, Gholipour M, Seyyed Nejad SM. *In vitro* assay for the anti-*Brucella* activity of medicinal plants against tetracycline-resistant *Brucella melitensis*. J Zhejiang Univ Sci B. 2010;11:506-511.

[89] Al-Mariri A, Safi M. The antibacterial activity of selected *Labiatae* (*Lamiaceae*) essential oils against *Brucella melitensis*. Iran J Med Sci. 2013;38:44-50.

[90] Fountain MW, Weiss SJ, Fountain AG, Shen A, Lenk RP. Treatment of *Brucella canis* and *Brucella abortus in vitro* and *in vivo* by stable plurilamellar vesicle-encapsulated aminoglycosides. J Infect Dis. 1985;152:529-535.

[91] Vitas AI, Díaz R, Gamazo C. Effect of composition and method of preparation of liposomes on their stability and interaction with murine monocytes infected with *Brucella abortus*. Antimicrob Agents Chemother. 1996;40:146-151.

[92] Prior S, Gander B, Irache JM, Gamazo C. Gentamicin-loaded microspheres for treatment of experimental *Brucella abortus* infection in mice. J Antimicrob Chemother. 2005;55:1032-1036.

[93] Lecároz C, Blanco-Prieto MJ, Burrell MA, Gamazo C. Intracellular killing of *Brucella melitensis* in human macrophages with microsphere-encapsulated gentamicin. J Antimicrob Chemother. 2006;58:549-556.

[94] Imbuluzqueta E, Gamazo C, Lana H, Campanero MÁ, Salas D, Gil AG, et al. Hydrophobic gentamicin-loaded nanoparticles are effective against *Brucella melitensis* infection in mice. Antimicrob Agents Chemother. 2013;57:3326-3333.

[95] Vitas AI, Díaz R, Gamazo C. Protective effect of liposomal gentamicin against systemic acute murine brucellosis. Chemotherapy. 1997;43:204-210.

[96] Abeylath SC, Turos E. Drug delivery approaches to overcome bacterial resistance to beta-lactam antibiotics. Expert Opin Drug Deliv. 2008;5:931-949.

[97] Rajasekaran P, Alexander JC, Seleem MN, Jain N, Sriranganathan N, Wattam AR, et al. Peptide nucleic acids inhibit growth of *Brucella suis* in pure culture and in infected murine macrophages. Int J Antimicrob Agents. 2013;41:358-362.

[98] Jiang X, Baldwin CL. Effects of cytokines on intracellular growth of *Brucella abortus*. Infect Immun. 1993;61:124-134.

[99] Murphy EA, Sathiyaseelan J, Parent MA, Zou B, Baldwin CL. Interferon-gamma is crucial for surviving a *Brucella abortus* infection in both resistant C57BL/6 and susceptible BALB/c mice. Immunology. 2001;103:511-518.

[100] Segura S, Gamazo C, Irache JM, Espuelas S. Gamma interferon loaded onto albumin nanoparticles: *in vitro* and *in vivo* activities against *Brucella abortus*. Antimicrob Agents Chemother. 2007;51:1310-1314.

[101] Fahel JS, de Souza MB, Gomes MTR, Corsetti PP, Carvalho NB, Marinho FAV, et al. 5-Lipoxygenase negatively regulates Th1 response during *Brucella abortus* infection in mice. Infect Immun. 2015;83:1210-1216.

Chapter 10

Recombinant Proteins as Antigens in Serological Diagnosis of Brucellosis

Magda Celina Navarro-Soto, Alberto Morales-Loredo, Genoveva Álvarez-Ojeda, Carlos Ramírez-Pfeiffer, Patricia Tamez-Guerra and Ricardo Gomez-Flores

Additional information is available at the end of the chapter

http://dx.doi.org/10.5772/61762

Abstract

Brucellosis is considered the major zoonosis in developing countries. In susceptible animal species, diagnosis of brucellosis remains a challenge due to the variety of clinical signs that it shares with a wide range of diseases. At present, isolation of *Brucella* is considered the *gold standard* for diagnosis of brucellosis; because of its low sensitivity and becoming potentially hazardous to laboratory technicians, serology is used for the detection of specific antibodies induced by infection. However, since traditional methods commonly show drawbacks and do not differentiate between vaccinated and naturally infected animals, it is necessary to search and test immunoreactive molecules for specific diagnosis of *Brucella*-infected cattle, thus significantly reducing the killing of suspected herds mainly due to vaccination. Advances in biotechnology have allowed exploring the use of recombinant proteins as antigens to avoid the risk involved in the use of viable *Brucella* strains. The benefit of using recombinant proteins, such as outer membrane proteins (OMP) and other non-lipopolysaccharide (non-LPS) molecules as antigens, for serological diagnosis is promising, but there are still many concerns about their application. The aim of the present work is to show advances in the use of recombinant antigens and discuss their advantages and potential use as markers for the serological diagnosis in brucellosis.

Keywords: Serology, *Brucella*, diagnosis, recombinant protein, brucellosis

1. Introduction

1.1. Diagnosis of brucellosis

Brucellosis is a zoonosis caused by bacteria of the genus *Brucella*, which is characterized by gram-negative coccobacilli, intracellular facultative, and slow-growing bacteria that do not have capsule or form spores [1]. Since clinical signs of brucellosis are not pathognomonic, diagnosis is dependent upon demonstration of the presence of *Brucella* spp. by microbiology, polymerase chain reaction (PCR), detection of its antigens, and demonstration of specific antibody or cell-mediated immune responses [2, 3]. At present, isolation of *Brucella* is considered the *gold standard*, but it has low sensitivity and is hazardous to laboratory technicians, therefore, serology is the most common method for the diagnosis of brucellosis.

Brucellosis serology is usually performed using antigens derived from *B. abortus* S19 strain, because the *Brucella* immunodominant antigens associated to the smooth-lipopolysaccharide (S-LPS) are to a large extent shared by all naturally occurring biovars of the so-called "smooth species," *B. abortus, B. melitensis, B. suis, B. neotomae, B. ceti,* and *B. pinnipedialis* [4]. Unfortunately, because of the LPS sharing, conventional methods do not differentiate between the smooth *B.abortus* S19 vaccinated and naturally infected animals; in addition, there could be cross reaction with other gram negative bacteria, such as *Escherichia coli* O157:H7 and *Yersinia enterocolitica,* because of their LPS similarity [7], thus affecting the specificity (Sp) of the test. The rough RB 51 *B. abortus* vaccine lacks the OPS, which avoids false reactions.

Various tests are generally used to improve the final specificity, in which an initial screening assay, such as the buffered *Brucella* antigen, the rose Bengal (RBT),the buffered plate agglutination (BPAT)or the indirect ELISA tests, which possess high sensitivity and relative specificity, are used to select reactive samples, followed by a secondary confirmatory test,with higher specificity than the screening test, such asthe complement fixation test (CFT), rivanol. Other modern tests can also be used including the fluorescence polarization assay (FPA) [3, 5, 8]. ELISA and FPA may be used for diagnosis [20], because of their high performance.On the other hand, since *B. canis* and *B. ovis*, known as "rough species" lack LPS, the CFT, agar gel immunodiffusion (AGID) test, and indirect ELISA (I-ELISA) using soluble surface antigens obtained from *B. ovis,* are preferred [6].

2. Immunodominant antigens

The following immunodominant antigens have been identified within the genus *Brucella*: (a) S-LPS (smooth lipopolysaccharide), (b) R-LPS (rough lipopolysaccharide), (c) outer membrane proteins (OMP), and (d) periplasmic and cytoplasmic proteins [9].

2.1. Brucella spp lipopolysaccharide

Lipopolysaccharide present in smooth species of *Brucella* comprises a glycolipid portion (lipid A) inserted in the outer membrane and a polysaccharide directed outward. The latter is divided into two sections: the core and the O-chain. *Brucella ovis* and *B. canis* naturally lack O-chain (OPS), whereas *B. melitensis, B. abortus,* and *B. suis* might lose it by mutation. S-LPS is markedly immunodominant on the serological response, therefore, most serological tests are focused on detecting antibodies to S-LPS and the use of bacterial suspensions or antigens without OPS leads to misdiagnosis [10].

2.1.1. *Brucella outer membrane proteins*

Although *Brucella* species are genetically closely related, there are differences in pathogenicity and host preference that may be favored, at least in part, by the outer membrane structure [11], mainly composed by LPS and OMPs. Since LPS of rough *Brucella* species (*B. ovis, B. canis,* and *B. abortus RB51*) lacks OPS, OMPs are more exposed on the surface and their role in the virulence of the bacteria has become very important in the search for antigens that can be used in the development of vaccines or diagnostic methods [12]. *Brucella* OMPs were initially identified and classified according to their molecular weight [13]. Thus, membrane proteins that are within group 1 have molecular weights between 88 and 94 kDa, group 2 (omp2a and omp2b) from 36 to 38 kDa, and group 3, comprising omp25 and omp31, from 25 to 27 and 31 to 34 kDa, respectively [14]. In *Brucella,* major OMPs are Omp25 and Omp31 (belonging to group 3), except in *B. abortus* where it has been demonstrated by molecular techniques the missing omp31 gene encoding this protein [15]. One study [16] reported that there is a good reactivity against Omp31 protein extracted from *B. ovis* in sheep sera, experimentally infected with the bacteria and with specific monoclonal anti-Omp31 antibodies, but little reactivity against Omp31 protein recombinant *B. melitensis*. This feature is attributed to the existence of differences in nine nucleotides between *omp31* genes of both *Brucella* strains that strongly modify the antigenic properties of the encoded proteins [5], suggesting that this protein may be useful as antigen for the development of specific tests for the detection of infectious epididymitis caused by *B. ovis* in rams. Moreover, Omp28, also known as CP28 or BP26, has been identified as an immunodominant antigen in infected cattle, sheep, goats, and humans and could be useful for the detection of anti-*Brucella* humoral responses of infected animals [17].

On the other hand, 8 immuno-reactive non-LPS proteins were identified [18] using proteomics and then tested with *Brucella*-positive sera by ELISA and showed no cross-reaction to *Escherichia coli* O157: H7, *Yersinia enterocolitica,* or negative serum to *B. abortus*. Of these proteins, chaperonin GroES (21 kDa) and DnaK (71.2 kDa) showed high immune reactivity and therefore the greatest potential as diagnostic antigens. In addition, 18 immunodominant insoluble proteins of *Brucella abortus* were separated by two-dimensional electrophoresis (2-DE) and their immune-reactivity was tested against the antisera of cattle infected with *B. abortus,* or/and *Yersinia enterocolitica,* or the sera of non-infected cattle using Western blotting. A wide variety of these insoluble proteins were identified by MS/MS analysis as F0F1 ATP synthase subunit b, solute-binding family 5 protein, 28 kDa OMP, Leu/Ile/Val-binding family protein, histidinol dehydrogenase, hypothetical protein, twin-arginine translocation pathway signal sequence domain-containing protein, serine protease family protein, b-hydroxyacyl-(acyl-carrier-protein) dehydratase FabA, short chain dehydrogenase-/reductase carbonic anhydrase, ornithine carbamoyltransferase, leucyl aminopeptidase, cold shock DNA-binding domain-containing protein, Cu/Zn superoxide dismutase, and methionine aminopeptidase [19].

2.2. Recombinant antigens in serology of brucellosis

Advances in biotechnology have allowed exploring the use of recombinant proteins as antigens to avoid the risk involved in the use of viable *Brucella* strains. An extremely useful application of proteomics to the diagnosis of infectious disease relies on the identification of novel diagnostic antigens by screening serum from infected and uninfected individuals against immunoblotted, 2-DE mapped proteomes of infectious agents [20]. Once those antigens are identified, due to easy production of recombinant proteins in prokaryotic systems, a wide variety of non-LPS molecules are cloned and expressed in the *Escherichia coli* system to obtain recombinant immune-reactive proteins. The most studied OMPs belong to group 3 (Omp25 and Omp31); recombinant Omp31 protein (rOmp31) obtained from *Brucella melitensis* expressed in the *Escherichia coli* system showed reactivity in *Brucella* positive sera, but not in *Brucella* negative sera, in a variety of animal species by iELISA. However, the sensitivity and specificity of each affected species showed significant difference [14]. iELISA performed with rOmp31 showed lower sensitivity (85%) and higher specificity (100%), compared with conventional rose Bengal plate test (RBPT), with 92% and 83%, respectively [21]. Other studies found that recombinant *B. melitensis* rOMP28 was immunoreactive to *Brucella* infected cattle, sheep, goat, and dog sera with a sensitivity of 88.7%, specificity of 93.8%, and accuracy of 92.9% by iELISA, demonstrating that it could be used as an antigen for diagnosis of brucellosis in domestic animals [22].

Furthermore, *B. abortus* Omp28 coding gene was cloned and expressed using the pMAL system, and rOmp28 was evaluated for its potential use in the serodiagnosis of bovine brucellosis by iELISA and the latex bead agglutination test (LAT). The sensitivity, specificity, and accuracy were 96.7%, 95.4%, 96.2% in iELISA and 77%, 80.6%, and 78.5% in latex bead agglutination test, respectively [23]. In addition, recombinant BP26 was produced in the *E. coli* system and tested by iELISA, but it resulted less useful than iELISA using the *B. ovis* hot saline (HS) extract as antigen [24, 25]. On the other hand, ribosome recycling factor protein CP24 and *Brucella* lumazine synthase (BLS) showed antigen-antibody interaction by iELISA, using brucellosis positive sera, and therefore it could be considered as a potential alternative diagnostic [26].

Other studies focused in the type IV secretion system (T4SS) encoded by the *virB* locus, located on chromosome II, including *virB1* to *virB12* [27], obtained recombinant VirB5 protein by a prokaryotic expression system, which was used to detect anti-*Brucella* antibodies by ELISA, in both standard brucellosis-positive serum and cattle sera samples; the results showed that recombinant VirB5 protein had good immune-reactivity [27]. In addition, in order to investigate the practical value of VirB5 in clinical applications, serum samples from cattle were screened using the VirB5-ELISA; the sensitivity of the VirB5-ELISA was 88.2% and the specificity was 97.8%. In all test samples, the accuracy reached 94.8%. Thus, these results confirmed the importance of VirB5 as a suitable antigen and VirB5-ELISA as screening test for the serological diagnosis of bovine brucellosis [27]. Another study was developed by Rolan et al. in 2008 [28], evaluating recombinant VirB1, VirB5, VirB11, and VirB12 by antibodies in sera from experimentally infected mice and goats by iELISA. Antibody responses to VirB12 but not to VirB1, VirB5, or VirB11 were detected in mice experimentally inoculated with *B. abortus* and goats experimentally infected with *Brucella melitensis*.

3. Conclusion

At present, FAO-OIE-WHO work together in strategies to prevent a worldwide emergent, re-emergent, and cross-border spread of human and animal infectious diseases [29]. Brucellosis remains a major zoonotic disease in the world and its control and eradication will be possible only with the complete collaboration of all sectors involved in health and animal production. As a significant part of the strategy, *One World-One Health* (OWOH) [30] involves early diagnosis of infected animals. Conventional serological tests have performance differences due to a variety of factors, including sample condition, vaccinated status, wide spread, and others. Therefore, it is necessary to search immune-reactive molecules that prevent faulty results that could compromise campaigns of control and eradication of this disease. The aim of this work is to bring together advances in the use of recombinant antigens, their problems, and perspectives as potential markers for the serological diagnosis in brucellosis. It is known that a test based on recombinant proteins would allow better standardization of the assay, compared with more complex whole-cell antigen preparations currently in use, and hence overcome the limitations associated with the use of LPS-based antigens, but finding results still not optimal (Table 1). Many of the failures in performance found in the analyzed studies might originate due to denaturing conditions in purification or Western blotting that could affect on the tertiary structure of the recombinant protein, and hence to immune-dominant epitopes, or by a low adherence to polystyrene plaque in the ELISA test. In addition, the expression of immune-dominant proteins could be different between *in vitro* and *in vivo* culture conditions and then results obtained would be distinct in sera from animals naturally infected with field strains compared with experimentally infected animals. Therefore, the search of alternative purification techniques to the ones currently used that retains the structural integrity of the protein is essential. Furthermore, standardization of homogeneous diagnostic tests as FPA [31], which minimize the subjective factor involved in the interpretation of results found in agglutination tests, could be helpful in the control and eradication programs worldwide.

Test	Sensitivity (%)	Specificity (%)	Animal specie
RBT[a]	21.0–98.3	68.8–100	Cattle
iELISA[a]	92.5–100	90.6–100	Cattle
CFT[a]	23.0–97.1	30.6–100	Cattle
FPA[a]	99.0–99.3	96.9–100	Cattle
FPA[b]	85.7%	99%	Goat
rOmp31-iELISA[C]	85	100	Goat
*B. melitensis r*OMP28-iELISA[d]	88.7	93.8	Cattle, sheep, goat, and dog
*B. abortus r*Omp28-iELISA[e]	96.7	95.4	Cattle
rVirB5-ELISA[f]	88.2	97.8	Cattle
a. [8]; b; [31]c. [21]; d. [22]; e. [23]; f. [27].			

Table 1. Sensitivity and specificity of serological tests for brucellosis with conventional and recombinant antigens

Author details

Magda Celina Navarro-Soto[1], Alberto Morales-Loredo[2], Genoveva Álvarez-Ojeda[4], Carlos Ramírez-Pfeiffer[3], Patricia Tamez-Guerra[1] and Ricardo Gomez-Flores[1*]

*Address all correspondence to: rgomez60@hotmail.com

1 Universidad Autónoma de Nuevo León, Facultad de Ciencias Biológicas, Laboratorio de Inmunología y Virología, Unidad de Inmunobiología y Acarreadores de Drogas, San Nicolás de los Garza, Nuevo León, México

2 Universidad Autónoma de Nuevo León, Centro de Desarrollo de Agronegocios, Escobedo, Nuevo León, México

3 Universidad México Americana del Norte, Coordinación de Investigación Institucional, Reynosa, Tamaulipas, México

4 Instituto Nacional de Investigaciones Forestales, Agrícolas y Pecuarias. Campo Experimental Río Bravo, Tamaulipas, México

References

[1] Cardoso PG, Macedo GC, Azevedo V, Oliveira SC. Brucella spp noncanonical LPS: structure, biosynthesis, and interaction with host immune system. Microb Cell Fact [Internet]. 2006 Jan [cited 2011 Jul 22];5:13. Available from: http://www.pubmedcentral.nih.gov/articlerender.fcgi?artid=1435926&tool=pmcentrez&rendertype=abstract

[2] Gopaul KK, Koylass MS, Smith CJ, Whatmore AM. Rapid identification of Brucella isolates to the species level by real time PCR based single nucleotide polymorphism (SNP) analysis. BMC Microbiol [Internet]. 2008 Jan [cited 2015 Mar 21];8(1):86. Available from: http://www.biomedcentral.com/1471-2180/8/86

[3] OIE. Bovine brucellosis. Terr Manual Bov Brucell [Internet]. 2012;1:616–50. Available from: http://www.oie.int/fileadmin/Home/eng/Health_standards/tahm/2.04.03_BOVINE_BRUCELL.pdf

[4] Cloeckaert A, Vizcaino N, Paquet JY, Bowden RA, Elzer PH. Major outer membrane proteins of Brucella spp: past, present and future. Vet Microbiol [Internet]. 2002;90:229–47. Available from: http://www.ncbi.nlm.nih.gov/entrez/query.fcgi?cmd=Retrieve&db=PubMed&dopt=Citation&list_uids=12414146

[5] Garin-Bastuji B, Blasco JM, Marín C, Albert D. The diagnosis of brucellosis in sheep and goats, old and new tools. Small Rumin Res [Internet]. 2006 Mar [cited 2015 Mar

21];62(1-2):63–70. Available from: http://www.sciencedirect.com/science/article/pii/S0921448805003378

[6] OIE. Ovine Epididymitis [Internet]. Terrestrial Manual 2009. Ovine Epididymitis (Brucella ovis). 2009 [cited 2015 Jan 1]. p. 1–9. Available from: http://www.oie.int/fileadmin/Home/eng/Health_standards/tahm/2.07.09_OVINE_EPID.pdf

[7] Caroff M, Bundle DR, Perry MB, Cherwonogrodzky JW, Duncan JR. Antigenic S-type lipopolysaccharide of Brucella abortus 1119-3. Infect Immun [Internet]. 1984 Nov 1 [cited 2015 Mar 21];46(2):384–8. Available from: http://iai.asm.org/cgi/content/long/46/2/384

[8] Nielsen K. Diagnosis of brucellosis by serology. Vet Microbiol. 2002. p. 447–59.

[9] Mejía P, Díaz E, Salas E. Identificación de las proteínas de 35 y 38 kDa específicas de Brucella ovis Identification of Brucella ovis-specific proteins of 35 and 38 kDa. Téc Pecu Méx [Internet]. 2004;42(2):277–85. Available from: http://www.tecnicapecuaria.org.mx/trabajos/200405285107.pdf

[10] Guzman-Verri C, Manterola L, Sola-Landa A, Parra A, Cloeckaert A, Garin J, et al. The two-component system BvrR/BvrS essential for Brucella abortus virulence regulates the expression of outer membrane proteins with counterparts in members of the Rhizobiaceae. Proc Natl Acad Sci [Internet]. 2002 Sep 6 [cited 2015 Mar 21];99(19):12375–80. Available from: http://www.pnas.org/cgi/content/long/99/19/12375

[11] Martín-Martín AI, Caro-Hernández P, Sancho P, Tejedor C, Cloeckaert A, Fernández-Lago L, et al. Analysis of the occurrence and distribution of the Omp25/Omp31 family of surface proteins in the six classical Brucella species. Vet Microbiol [Internet]. 2009 May 28 [cited 2012 Jul 19];137(1-2):74–82. Available from: http://www.ncbi.nlm.nih.gov/pubmed/19135812

[12] Caro-Hernández P, Fernández-Lago L, de Miguel M-J, Martín-Martín AI, Cloeckaert A, Grilló M-J, et al. Role of the Omp25/Omp31 family in outer membrane properties and virulence of Brucella ovis. Infect Immun [Internet]. 2007 Aug [cited 2012 Jul 19];75(8):4050–61. Available from: http://www.pubmedcentral.nih.gov/articlerender.fcgi?artid=1952020&tool=pmcentrez&rendertype=abstract

[13] Moreno E, Moriyó I. The Prokaryotes [Internet]. Dworkin M, Falkow S, Rosenberg E, Schleifer K-H, Stackebrandt E, editors. Springer New York; 2006 [cited 2012 Nov 1]. 315-456 p. Available from: http://www.springerlink.com/index/10.1007/0-387-30745-1

[14] Cassataro J, Cassataro J, Velikovsky CA, Velikovsky CA, Barrera S De, Barrera S De, et al. A DNA Vaccine Coding for the. Microbiology. 2005;73(10):6537–46.

[15] Cloeckaert A, Verger J-M, Grayon M, VizcaÃno N. Molecular and immunological characterization of the major outer membrane proteins of Brucella. FEMS Microbiol Lett [Internet]. 1996;145(1):1–8. Available from: http://www.sciencedirect.com/science/article/pii/0378109796003734

[16] Kittelberger R, Cloeckaert A, Ferna L, Mari CM. Minor nucleotide substitutions in the omp31 gene of Brucella ovis result in antigenic differences in the major outer membrane protein that it encodes compared to those of the other Brucella species. 2001;69(11):7020–8.

[17] Gupta VK, Kumari R, Vohra J, Singh SV, Vihan VS. Comparative evaluation of recombinant BP26 protein for serological diagnosis of Brucella melitensis infection in goats. Small Rumin Res. 2010;93:119–25.

[18] Kim J-Y, Sung S-R, Lee K, Lee H-K, Kang S-I, Lee JJ, et al. Immunoproteomics of Brucella abortus RB51 as candidate antigens in serological diagnosis of brucellosis. Vet Immunol Immunopathol [Internet]. 2014 Aug 15 [cited 2015 Mar 22];160(3-4):218–24. Available from: http://www.sciencedirect.com/science/article/pii/S0165242714001226

[19] Ko KY, Kim JW, Her M, Kang S Il, Jung SC, Cho DH, et al. Immunogenic proteins of Brucella abortus to minimize cross reactions in brucellosis diagnosis. Vet Microbiol. 2012;156:374–80.

[20] OIE. Biotechnology in the Diagnosis of Infectious Diseases and Vaccine Development. Terr Man [Internet]. 2009;(138):1–25. Available from: http://web.oie.int/eng/normes/mmanual/2008/pdf/1.1.07_BIOTECHNOLOGY.pdf

[21] Gupta VK, Verma DK, Singh SV, Vihan VS. Serological diagnostic potential of recombinant outer membrane protein (Omp31) from Brucella melitensis in goat and sheep brucellosis. Small Rumin Res [Internet]. 2007 Jul [cited 2015 Mar 21];70(2-3): 260–6. Available from: http://www.sciencedirect.com/science/article/pii/S0921448806000265

[22] Chaudhuri P, Prasad R, Kumar V, Gangaplara A. Recombinant OMP28 antigen-based indirect ELISA for serodiagnosis of bovine brucellosis. Mol Cell Probes [Internet]. 2010 Jun [cited 2015 Mar 21];24(3):142–5. Available from: http://www.sciencedirect.com/science/article/pii/S0890850809000851

[23] Lim JJ, Kim DH, Lee JJ, Kim DG, Min W, Lee HJ, et al. Evaluation of recombinant 28 kDa outer membrane protein of Brucella abortus for the clinical diagnosis of Bovine Brucellosis in Korea. J Vet Med Sci. 2012;74(6):687–91.

[24] Seco-Mediavilla P, Verger J-M, Grayon M, Cloeckaert A, Marín CM, Zygmunt MS, et al. Epitope mapping of the Brucella melitensis BP26 immunogenic protein: usefulness for diagnosis of sheep brucellosis. Clin Diagn Lab Immunol. 2003;10:647–51.

[25] Zygmunt MS, Baucheron S, Vizcaino N, Bowden RA, Cloeckaert A. Single-step purification and evaluation of recombinant BP26 protein for serological diagnosis of Brucella ovis infection in rams. Vet Microbiol. 2002;87:213–20.

[26] Thepsuriyanont P, Intarapuk A, Chanket P, Tunyong W, Kalambaheti T. ELISA for brucellosis detection based on three brucella recombinant proteins. Southeast Asian J Trop Med Public Health. 2014;45:130-141.

[27] Tan W, Wang X, Nie Y, Wang C, Cheng L, Wang X, et al. Recombinant VirB5 protein as a potential serological marker for the diagnosis of bovine brucellosis. Mol Cell Probes [Internet]. 2012 Jun [cited 2015 Mar 21];26(3):127–31. Available from: http://www.sciencedirect.com/science/article/pii/S0890850812000357

[28] Rolán HG, Den Hartigh AB, Kahl-McDonagh M, Ficht T, Adams LG, Tsolis RM. VirB12 is a serological marker of Brucella infection in experimental and natural hosts. Clin Vaccine Immunol. 2008;15:208–14.

[29] FAO/OIE/WHO. The FAO-OIE-WHO Collaboration. A Tipartite Concept [Internet]. 2010;(April):1–8. Available from: http://www.who.int/influenza/resources/documents/tripartite_concept_note_hanoi_042011_en.pdf

[30] Hinchliffe S. More than one world, more than one health: Re-configuring interspecies health. Soc Sci Med [Internet]. 2015 Mar [cited 2015 Mar 22];129:28–35. Available from: http://www.sciencedirect.com/science/article/pii/S0277953614004365.

[31] Ramírez-Pfeiffer C, Díaz-Aparicio E, Gomez-Flores R, Rodríguez-Padilla C, Morales-Loredo A, Álvarez-Ojeda G. Use of the *Brucella melitensis* native hapten to diagnose brucellosis in goats by a rapid, simple, and specific fluorescence polarization assay. Clin Vaccine Immunol. 2008;15:911-915.

Chapter 11

Treatment of Brucellosis

Mitra Ranjbar

Additional information is available at the end of the chapter

http://dx.doi.org/10.5772/61093

Abstract

The goal of brucellosis therapy is to control the illness and prevent complications, relapses and sequelae. Important principles of brucellosis treatment include the use of antibiotics with activity in the acidic intracellular environment (doxycycline, rifampin), use of combination regimens and prolonged duration of treatment.

Keywords: Brucellosis, Treatment

1. Introduction

Human brucellosis is a major zoonosis caused by facultative intracellular Gram-negative bacteria of the genus *Brucella* [1, 2]. Brucellosis is a systemic disease and although less lethal, notoriously hard to eradicate, and relapses are being reported many years after the initial infection. Since global eradication of brucellosis is due to socioeconomic and political factors, it will not be feasible in the near future, and since the evolution of a satisfactory vaccine for human currently seems a utopia, there exists a need for optimal antibiotic treatment schedules [3, 4].

The optimal treatment for brucellosis remains an unsolved medical puzzle, owing to the propensity of the infection for relapses, the universal failure of monotherapy and the absence of multiethnic, randomised trials evaluating possible new regimens for the disease. Current recommended treatment regimens for brucellosis involve the use of two or more antibiotics in order to avoid relapses occurring and to prevent prolonged use of these drugs [4, 5]. The choice of regimen and duration of antimicrobial therapy should be based on whether focal disease is present (e.g. endocarditis, spondylitis, meningitis, paraspinous abscesses) or there are underlying conditions that contraindicate certain antibiotics (e.g. pregnant patients or children under 8 years old) [6]. In this chapter, we will discuss the effects of various antibiotic regimens, monotherapy or in combination with other antibiotics for treating human brucellosis.

1.1. General principles of therapy

Brucella spp. are facultative intracellular pathogens with a unique ability of escaping phagocytosis by human macrophages. Thus, the first major parameter of successful antimicrobial treatment of brucellosis is the use of antibiotics that penetrate into macrophages and are thus active against the pathogen. The second important parameter is the use of antibiotics that are active in the acidic environment of the macrophages infected with *Brucella* spp. [4, 7].

The third major parameter in the successful treatment of brucellosis is the use of combination regimens, as monotherapy has universally been related to unacceptable percentages of relapse. The identity and number of antimicrobial agents used in each combination is the one major subject of debate on the treatment of brucellosis [4, 7].

The fourth major parameter is the evaluation of the duration of treatment, when applied to cases of uncomplicated brucellosis. The fifth major parameter that should be taken into account is the need for a convenient regimen for countries with poor health resources, that is, the need for a cheap, oral regimen, and this is exactly the philosophy that prompted the guidelines modification by WHO in 1986. Finally, the sixth major parameter is the inconcordance between in vitro studies on antimicrobial susceptibility of *Brucella* spp. and in vivo efficacy or resistance [4, 7].

1.2. Therapeutic regimens

Antimicrobial therapy is useful for shortening the natural course of the disease, reducing symptoms, decreasing the incidence of complications and preventing relapse. Appropriate antibiotics should have high in vitro activity and good intracellular penetration. Thus, the use of appropriate antibiotic combinations is required for the successful treatment of brucellosis [1, 8].

2. Specific compounds

Historically, single-agent therapy due to the relapses after treatment has proved inadequate for brucellosis. This is because of the primarily bacteriostatic effect exhibited by most of these agents (predominantly tetracyclines) and to a lesser extent (or not at all) the emergence of resistance [3].

The use of single-agent therapy with rifampin, oxytetracycline or doxycycline showed high relapse rates of 9–25 %. The duration of therapy (either 3, 5 or 8 weeks) showed no statistically significant difference. In addition, the use of monotherapy with trimethoprim–sulfamethoxazole (TMP–SMX) or ciprofloxacin has led to an unacceptable relapse rate of 30 % and up to 83 %, respectively. Thus, monotherapy is not accepted as a treatment strategy for brucellosis [9].

2.1. Tetracyclines

Tetracyclines are the cornerstone of successful antibiotic regimens for the treatment of brucellosis. The two regimens suggested by WHO both include a tetracycline, and most of the subsequently proposed regimens also include a member of this antibiotic class. Tetracyclines are inexpensive antimicrobial agents, easy to obtain and easy to adhere to; side effects are unusual and of mild severity; and dosage, in the form of doxycycline administered twice daily – the tetracycline currently employed in almost all regimens – is convenient. There is strong evidence that the tetracyclines (especially doxycycline and minocycline) are the most effective drugs for brucellosis treatment. The rate of treatment failure in tetracyclines is 1–5 %, the relapse rate is 5–10 % and the cure rate exceeds 80 % when an appropriate duration is used [4, 6].

Doxycycline exhibits excellent activity in the acidic phagolysosomal environment where the compound interfaces with *Brucellae*, and its bactericidal activity has been repeatedly proven. Doxycycline has also been used as adjunctive monotherapy in cases of residual focal brucellosis for a protracted period, although there are no official data supporting its effectiveness when used as a single agent after an initial combination with another compound. The suggested adult dose of doxycycline employed in the various therapeutic combinations is 100 mg b.i.d. [4, 6].

Of the other tetracyclines, minocycline has also been favoured as the tetracycline of choice in several trials. Moreover, tigecycline is a glycylcycline antibiotic, related to tetracyclines, that exhibits a similar but fivefold enhanced mode of action compared with tetracyclines while also avoiding the emergence of antimicrobial resistance. The enhanced effectiveness of tigecycline may allow for its use as a single agent in brucellosis, even with decrease in treatment duration. Studies have shown that tigecycline can be a therapeutic alternative option for the treatment of brucellosis [3].

2.2. Streptomycin and other aminoglycosides

Streptomycin has been the second cornerstone in the treatment of brucellosis for the last 50 years and remains a popular antibiotic choice, especially by senior specialists. The need for parenteral administration, the significant percentage of toxicity (mainly ototoxicity) and difficulty in obtaining the drug in certain countries are parameters responsible for a lack of interest in the use of streptomycin in the last 25 years, especially as an acceptable all-oral regimen had been applied in clinical practice [4, 9].

Streptomycin is an example of the discrepancy between in vitro studies and in vivo effectiveness, as it has been proven that the drug does not survive in the acidic phagolysosomic environment, but it has also been proven that it is the only compound exhibiting bactericidal activity in the first 24 h after administration. Streptomycin is usually administered at a dose of 15 mg/kg body weight/day for 2 or 3 weeks. Further administration would significantly increase the rate of unwanted effects [4, 6].

The need of combining an equally effective, but less toxic, compound with doxycycline switched interest to other members of the antibiotic class of aminoglycosides. Of these, gentamicin is the most extensively studied compound, and various studies have proven that its combination with doxycycline is an excellent regimen. The suggested dose is gentamicin 5 mg/kg/day, administered intravenously or intramuscularly, and the usual period of administration does not exceed 1 week. Netilmicin has also been employed in various combination regimens, but it is less well studied than gentamicin [2, 4, 6].

2.3. Rifampicin

In the early 1970s, it was determined that rifampicin in combined treatment regimens is effective for brucellosis, and by the early 1980s, this compound gradually replaced streptomycin as the complementary agent of choice to doxycycline in the treatment of the disease, culminating in the 1986 WHO guidelines, which advocated its use in the optimal treatment of the disease. Moreover, various therapeutic combinations have recently preferred the use of rifampicin over doxycycline, making rifampicin the cornerstone of modern antibiotic treatment [4, 6].

Rifampicin survives in the acidic environment of the infected macrophages and exhibits bactericidal activity 48 h after administration. One potential problem that could arise with the use of rifampicin-containing regimens for the treatment of brucellosis involves the concurrent high incidence of tuberculosis in areas endemic for brucellosis, due to the pertaining socioeconomic status. Fear that extended use of rifampicin would increase population resistance to the compound in the treatment of tuberculosis exists but has not been validated in clinical practice. The suggested dose for rifampicin in the treatment of brucellosis is 600–1200 mg/day [4, 6].

2.4. Macrolides

Ideally, macrolides should exhibit excellent efficacy against a facultative intracellular pathogen, as in various other zoonotic infections and various atypical respiratory pathogens. Thus, the newer macrolides and azithromycin, a relative compound of the class of azalides, were considered ideal candidates for the treatment of brucellosis, in certain combination regimens. Erythromycin was used instead of tetracycline in combination with streptomycin as early as 1961; however, the high doses necessary for achieving a clinical response similar to that of the combination of tetracycline and streptomycin were accompanied by unacceptable high rates of adverse reactions [4, 10].

The use of azithromycin in combination with gentamicin was also evaluated in a small clinical trial but resulted in a disappointingly high percentage of treatment failure (either relapse, frank failure or withdrawal due to side effects). Although the planned treatment duration was only 21 days, the cases of frank failure preclude the favourable approach to the use of azithromycin in brucellosis. Azithromycin does not survive in the acidic environment of the infected macrophages [4, 10].

2.5. Quinolones

The evolution of fluoroquinolones and the successful use of these compounds in various infections, including certain zoonotic diseases and numerous intracellular pathogens, led to the development of what amounted to a scientific obsession in proving their efficacy in the treatment of brucellosis [4, 11].

Laboratory and clinical studies regarding using quinolone in the treatment of human brucellosis suggest that there is a lack of evidence supporting the use of quinolones in the initial therapeutic regimen. In vitro studies show that activity of quinolones decreased at pH 5 compared to pH 7 and there is lack of synergistic activity with the older antibiotics against brucellosis. Trials with ciprofloxacin as a single agent for the treatment of brucellosis have yielded disappointingly high percentages of treatment failure. However, recent studies with the combination of ofloxacin and rifampicin have yielded promising results [4, 11, 12].

Newer quinolones have also been interesting candidates. A trial of moxifloxacin monotherapy is underway in our institution. Their use in various combination regimens is promising and should be evaluated but will eventually be hampered, as with ofloxacin and ciprofloxacin, by cost restrictions, in the presence of a significantly more cost-effective combination regimen such as the one advocated by WHO [1, 11].

2.6. Trimethoprim–sulfamethoxazole

Trimethoprim–sulfamethoxazole has long been a popular agent in the treatment of brucellosis and remains the most popular choice for monotherapy trials. It has been extensively studied in the paediatric population, and its clinical efficacy, when compared to in vitro studies of *Brucellae* susceptibility, underlines the inconcordance between in vitro studies and clinical reality. However, trimethoprim–sulfamethoxazole cannot be viewed at present as more than a convenient third drug in a complex therapeutic regimen for focal brucellosis [4, 6].

2.7. β-Lactams

β-Lactams are active in vitro, and ampicillin was a popular therapeutic choice in the early 1950s. The in vitro susceptibility, however, does not translate to in vivo efficacy, due to the specific in vivo environmental conditions [4, 6].

The efficacy of ceftriaxone in the treatment of a variety of infectious diseases led certain investigators to study its possible use as a monotherapy in the treatment of brucellosis. The results of some studies indicate failure of ceftriaxone in the treatment of acute brucellosis. There are reports of excellent in vitro activity of cefotaxime and meropenem for treatment of brucellosis, but these agents have not been tested clinically [4, 13].

3. Combined regimens

Treatment of brucellosis is still far from ideal, the major problem being identification of the most practical and affordable double or triple antimicrobial combination to prevent relapse which is very common after treatment with single agents [13].

In 1971, the World Health Organization (WHO) suggested a 21-day regimen of tetracycline plus streptomycin as the treatment of choice for treatment of human brucellosis. Although this regimen was successful in reducing the early symptoms, it failed to treat the disease completely, and immediate relapse was seen in some patients. Accordingly, in 1986, the joint Food and Agriculture Organization of the United Nations (FAO)/WHO Expert Committee on Brucellosis suggested two new regimens: rifampicin (600 to 900 mg/day orally) plus doxycycline (200 mg/day orally) for 6 weeks and doxycycline (200 mg/day orally) for 45 days plus streptomycin (1 g/day intramuscularly) for 2 to 3 weeks. However, later studies showed a treatable but high rate of relapse for the mentioned regimens [3, 5].

The rifampicin plus doxycycline regimen is the most popular treatment for brucellosis and favourable to the more effective regimen of streptomycin plus doxycycline, possibly due to its lower price and ease of administration. Streptomycin requires parenteral administration in a hospital setting or in an appropriately set up primary care network. The plasma levels of doxycycline in patients treated with rifampin were significantly lower than those in the plasma of patients treated with doxycycline and streptomycin. Furthermore, bacterial clearance in patients treated with rifampin was significantly higher than that in patients treated with doxycycline and streptomycin [4, 5].

According to the suggestions of WHO, only the combination of doxycycline with gentamicin can be considered an acceptable (albeit not ideal) novel regimen for brucellosis [3]. Giving doxycycline plus gentamicin to people with brucellosis may reduce the incidence of total treatment failure compared to administration of doxycycline plus streptomycin. Thus, the combination of oral doxycycline plus gentamicin appears to be as effective as the traditional therapy of streptomycin plus doxycycline [2, 5, 14].

A longer duration of gentamicin plus doxycycline or netilmicin plus doxycycline for at least 14 days followed by doxycycline alone for a further 30–60 days is associated with less therapeutic failure and a lower relapse rate than a regimen containing aminoglycoside for only 7 days [15].

Significant geographical variations in clinical practice, even among different areas of the same country, exist, and in general, the treatment regimen of choice reflects the traditional approach by each institution and the clinical experience of each specialist. The combination of doxycycline for 45 days with gentamicin for the first 5–7 days is gaining acceptance as a first-line treatment regimen, whereas multiple regimens are also applied in various countries. This is particularly important in endemic areas, where many patients exhibit a mild form of the disease and diagnosis and prescription can be readily made at the emergency department. Thus, the all-oral regimen of doxycycline and rifampicin for a period of 45 days still seems a reasonable, inexpensive and convenient first-line treatment for most endemic areas [4, 9].

http://dx.doi.org/10.5772/61093

Alternative treatments for brucellosis include other antibiotics, such as fluoroquinolones and co-trimoxazole and their combinations with rifampicin. Combinations of streptomycin with trimethoprim–sulfamethoxazole, or rifampicin with trimethoprim–sulfamethoxazole, are variably reported in some series [4, 16]. Some studies have suggested that fluoroquinolones in combination with rifampin or doxycycline can be used for the treatment of acute uncomplicated brucellosis as an alternative to the doxycycline plus rifampin combination [12, 13].

The use of ofloxacin plus rifampicin for the treatment of human brucellosis is as effective as the standard doxycycline plus rifampicin regimen. Although ofloxacin in combination with rifampicin decreased the duration of the therapy and provided shorter course of fever, these superiorities are not sufficient for declaring this treatment as treatment of choice. The cost of ofloxacin plus rifampicin treatment is higher than doxycycline plus rifampicin treatment [12, 17].

The use of triple antimicrobial therapy is not widely implemented except in selected situations and in patients with focal disease. However, triple combinations, utilising trimethoprim–sulfamethoxazole or both streptomycin and rifampicin in addition to a tetracycline, remain popular in certain endemic regions [3, 14].

Amikacin plus doxycycline and rifampicin regimen for the treatment of human brucellosis had a higher efficacy and more rapid action in terms of relief of symptoms compared to the doxycycline in combination with rifampicin regimen, and no significant difference in drug side effects and disease relapse existed in the patients of either group; adding amikacin to the doxycycline plus rifampicin standard treatment regimen seems beneficial [18].

Nevertheless, there are still a number of obstacles to overcome, such as the need for parenteral administration of aminoglycosides, the danger of inducing emergence of resistance to rifampicin in countries where tuberculosis poses a problem, the treatment compliance in a disease in which symptoms disappear a few days after initiating treatment, the difficulty of patient follow-up in underdeveloped rural areas and the relapses, which are observed approximately in 10 % of the patients [19].

4. Duration of treatment

Various efforts have been made to evaluate the ideal treatment duration for brucellosis; studies with doxycycline plus an adjunct for a total duration of 30 days have yielded a higher percentage of relapses, and the addition of gentamicin or newer quinolones, or application of triple regimens, has not consistently exhibited an advantage or equality in the efficacy of shorter periods of treatment. In the treatment of brucellosis, the rule is that a longer treatment duration causes fewer relapses, and many cases with residual complaints after regimen completion can be effectively treated with a protracted course of doxycycline alone. Many specialists treat patients for a shorter period, but the lack of data on the geographical distribution of biotypes of *Brucella melitensis* and the virulence of both *B. melitensis* and *B. abortus* and inadequate data on diagnosis and follow-up preclude any permanent conclusions. A total of 45 days of treatment seems to be the golden equilibrium of acceptable success, compliance and lack of significant side effects [4, 14].

5. Special issues

Treatment protocols for brucellosis may differ in children aged less than 8 years and pregnant women, because of adverse reactions of some medications, including inhibition of bone growth due to tetracycline treatment in children and teratogenic potential of some drugs, such as streptomycin [5].

Patients with localisations such as spondylitis, endocarditis, neurobrucellosis and abscess formations in body organs may require hospitalisation for possible surgery, and triple antibiotics (doxycycline, aminoglycoside and rifampicin) should be used for a longer period of up to 6 months. Urgent valve replacement or drainage of abscesses may also be required with antibiotics (Table 1) [15, 20, 21].

5.1. Paediatric population

Children often have fewer or milder symptoms than adult patients. Doxycycline and tetracycline are not recommended for children younger than 8 years of age because of irreversible staining of permanent teeth. Thus, the use of tetracyclines in children is prohibited, and the suggested combinations for children include rifampicin plus trimethoprim–sulfamethoxazole or rifampicin plus streptomycin or another aminoglycoside. The preferred treatment regimen for brucellosis in children is rifampicin plus TMP–SMZ for 6–8 weeks. An alternative regimen is rifampicin or TMP–SMZ for 8 weeks plus gentamicin 5 mg/kg/day for the first 5 days. Treatment over prolonged periods (>6 months) with TMP–SMZ has produced favourable results in some cases [4, 6, 22].

5.2. Pregnancy

Among pregnant women with clinical evidence of brucellosis, high rates of spontaneous abortion, premature delivery and intrauterine infection with foetal death have been described. Women who received early diagnosis and adequate treatment had successful maternal and foetal outcomes. The use of tetracyclines and streptomycin should be avoided for treatment of human brucellosis during pregnancy. Rifampicin is the mainstay of treatment in pregnancy. Recent reports suggest that, among antibiotic use permitted during pregnancy, there is no superior combination with rifampicin in treatment outcome [4, 6]. TMP–SMZ should not be used in pregnancy, either before 13 weeks because of the risk of teratogenic effects or after 36 weeks because of the risk of kernicterus [6, 23]. Furthermore, some studies indicated that ceftriaxone/rifampicin treatment can be the most effective treatment for pregnant women with brucellosis [24].

5.3. Treatment of focal diseases

Focal disease in brucellosis includes endocarditis, myocarditis, pericarditis, aortic root abscess and vertebral infection. A prolonged course of 6–52 weeks was traditionally recommended for focal disease such as endocarditis, spondylitis or neurobrucellosis. The occurrence of focal disease in brucellosis was reported to be epididymo-orchitis (7.5 %), meningitis (3.6 %), endocarditis (1.5 %), bone and joint symptoms (55 %) and septic arthritis (5–10 %) [9, 25, 26].

5.3.1. Osteoarticular brucellosis and spondylitis

Osteoarticular complications of brucellosis are the most common and in cases of spondylitis, often the most troublesome. Whereas sacroiliitis and peripheral arthritis rapidly resolve with the administration of antibiotic regimens employed in the treatment of uncomplicated brucellosis, spondylitis often requires protracted antibiotic administration or combined medical and surgical treatment. Patients with focal spinal disease may have higher rates of treatment failure if they are treated with doxycycline plus rifampicin for 6 weeks. Thus, such patients may require a longer course of therapy for more than 5 months [4, 14, 27].

Many patients with spondylitis experience residual complaints and some have been treated with various regimens for protracted periods, sometimes exceeding 12 months. Limited data support the inclusion of an aminoglycoside in the treatment regimen of spondylitis patients. Spondylitis may be the one aspect of brucellosis where quinolones may prove cost-effective; their ability to penetrate and achieve significant concentrations in bone and soft tissues allows their use in brucellar spondylitis for maximising response. An initial report of a combination of doxycycline and ciprofloxacin for a period of 3 months has been encouraging [4, 14, 28].

5.3.2. Brucella endocarditis

Brucella endocarditis is another ominous, but fortunately extremely rare, complication (2–5 %). As a rule, brucellar endocarditis is treated surgically, and the duration of postsurgical antibiotic treatment ranges 3–15 months, usually utilising at least three of the active compounds against brucellosis [4, 14].

Cases of isolated conservative treatment of brucellar endocarditis exist, and conservative treatment can be considered an option in the absence of prosthetic valves, the absence of congestive heart failure and the presence of only mild extravalvular heart involvement and assuming that antibiotic administration starts immediately after diagnosis [4, 14]. Most patients with brucellar endocarditis are usually treated with the use of a combination of tetracycline and doxycycline, rifampin and an aminoglycoside or TMP–SMX for a mean duration of 3 months. Surgical interventions are more likely to be required for treatment of patients with heart failure, valvular destruction and abscesses [9, 14].

5.4. Chronic brucellosis

There is no consensus on the definition of chronic brucellosis, and thus, there is no background for establishing guidelines for treatment. Protracted courses of the usual regimens should be advocated, but treatment options are largely subject to specialist preferences and individualised patient parameters. One important aspect of the so-called chronic brucellosis is the possibility of an underlying immune-mediated mechanism in its pathogenesis: numerous anecdotal reports of the use of corticosteroids in patients with 'chronic' brucellosis exist but cannot be substantiated. Others suggest that the clinical entity that is characterised as chronic brucellosis is in fact a result of impaired cellular immunity; thus, the use of interferon has been advocated, but this approach cannot be substantiated either [4, 6].

Patient group	Recommended therapy	Alternative therapy
Acute brucellosis (adults and children "/>8 years old)	Doxycycline 100 mg PO twice daily for 45 days plus either streptomycin 15 mg/kg IM daily for 14–21 days, gentamicin 3–5 mg/kg IV or IM daily for 7–14 days or doxycycline 100 mg PO twice daily for 45 days plus rifampicin 600–900 mg PO daily for 45 days	Rifampicin 600 mg PO daily for 42 days plus quinolone (ofloxacin 400 mg PO twice daily or ciprofloxacin 750 mg PO twice daily) for 42 days or doxycycline 100 mg PO twice daily plus TMP–SMZ one double-strength tablet twice daily for 2 months or monotherapy with doxycycline or minocycline PO daily for 6–8 weeks
Children <8 years old	TMP–SMZ 5 mg/kg (of trimethoprim component) PO twice daily for 45 days plus gentamicin 5–6 mg/kg IV daily for 7 days or rifampicin 15 mg/kg PO daily for 45 days plus gentamicin 5–6 mg/kg IV or IM daily for 7 days	
Brucellosis during pregnancy	Rifampicin 600–900 mg PO daily for 45 days	Rifampicin 600 mg PO daily for 45 days plus TMP–SMZ one double- strength tablet twice daily for 45 days
Focal infections (endocarditis, spondylitis, meningitis, paraspinous abscesses)[b]	Doxycycline 100 mg PO twice daily and rifampicin 600 mg PO daily for 6–52 weeks plus either streptomycin 1 g IM daily or gentamicin 3–5 mg/kg IV or IM daily for 14–21 days	Consider TMP–SMZ, ciprofloxacin 750 mg PO twice daily or ofloxacin 400 mg PO twice daily as a substitute for doxycycline or rifampicin

IM, intramuscularly; IV intravenously; PO, orally; TMP–SMZ, trimethoprim–sulfamethoxazole

[a]The choice of regimen/duration should be based on the presence of focal disease and whether there are underlying conditions that may contraindicate certain antibiotic therapy. Aminoglycoside and quinolone dosage should be adjusted in patients with poor renal function.

[b]Patients with focal disease, such as spondylitis or endocarditis, may require long courses of therapy depending on the clinical evolution. Surgery should be considered for patients with endocarditis, cerebral or epidural abscess, spleen or hepatic abscess or other abscesses that are antibiotic resistant.

Table 1. Recommended treatment for brucellosis according to patient group[a]

6. Future targets

6.1. Re-evaluating current alternatives

Because the current officially endorsed regimens are not ideal, other approaches using currently existing antibiotics should be further validated. Gentamicin has been recently validated in a large sample with excellent results, yet its parenteral administration does not service the requested convenience, and the agent should be further evaluated only for seriously complicated, hospitalisation-requiring cases. On the other hand, co-trimoxazole-containing regimens can be considered as convenient (all-oral) regimens that may be of significantly lower cost than traditional combinations in certain developing countries. The emergence of community-acquired resistance should be studied for rifampicin; its potential overuse/abuse may reflect on increasing rifampicin resistance in *Mycobacterium tuberculosis* because both brucellosis and tuberculosis can simultaneously be endemic/exist in the same countries in many parts of the world [4, 7].

6.2. Optimising antibiotic delivery

An interesting new approach, still in preclinical evaluation, is the optimisation of antibiotic delivery in the macrophages by using antibiotic-containing microparticles. The development of gentamicin-loaded poly-(D,L-lactide-co-glycolide) (PLGA) microspheres and studies of their release patterns are promising in this field because optimisation of encapsulation efficiency and gentamicin loading may lead to prolonged antibiotic release. Gentamicin-containing PLGA microspheres can be successfully phagocytosed by infected THP-1 human monocytes, and the antibiotic reaches *Brucella*-specific compartments and reduces the intracellular *Brucella* infection [7, 14].

6.3. Novel compounds

Following development, many agents have generated hope as a possible monotherapeutic treatment of human brucellosis with most of these hopes proving to be futile in clinical practice. Most of these new agents are costly, intravenously administered antibiotics that would be neither practical nor cost-effective for the disease. There is one new agent that is unique enough to generate theoretical interest of its possible future role in brucellosis treatment. Tigecycline is a novel glycylcycline antibiotic, a 9-t-butylglycylamido minocycline, which inhibits bacterial protein synthesis with 3- and 20-fold greater potency than that of minocycline and tetracycline, respectively, partly attributed to its binding to additional ribosomal subunit targets. Tetracyclines are the mainstay of most antibiotic regimens for brucellosis, and replacing doxycycline with a more potent analogue might not only increase efficacy but might offer further advantages by possibly reducing treatment duration [7, 14].

7. Conclusion

Brucellosis, the most common bacterial zoonosis in the world, is still endemic in many developing countries. The optimal duration of antibiotic treatment in patients with brucellosis is unclear, even for the most common clinical presentation of acute, uncomplicated brucellosis without focal disease [4, 6].

Most cases with uncomplicated brucellosis in adults can be readily treated with the combination of doxycycline and rifampicin (in a dose adjusted to body weight) for 45 days. The use of doxycycline for 45 days in combination with streptomycin for 14 days (or gentamicin for 5–7 days) is a reasonable alternative approach. For patients with treatment failure or repeated relapses, an array of second-line agents, such as quinolones, or trimethoprim-sulfamethoxazole can be utilised [4, 14].

For patients with complicated disease, therapeutic intervention demands a careful evaluation of the patient and a thorough therapeutic plan. Patients with spondylitis should possibly receive a quinolone in the initial regimen, for a protracted period [4, 14].

Attempts at monotherapy should be reserved for therapeutic trials or cases where traditional therapeutic regimens have failed. Chronic brucellosis should be ideally classified as a clinical entity and treated for a protracted period with one of the accepted regimens [4, 6].

Author details

Mitra Ranjbar*

Address all correspondence to: mitraranjbar@yahoo.com

Department of Infectious Diseases, Iran University of Medical Sciences, Tehran, Iran

References

[1] Madkour MM. Brucellosis: Overview. In: Madkour MM, editor. Madkour's Brucellosis, 2nd ed. Berlin: Springer; 2001. p. 1-14.

[2] Hasanjani Roushan MR, Mohraz M, Hajiahmadi M, et al. Efficacy of gentamicin plus doxycycline versus streptomycin plus doxycycline in the treatment of brucellosis in humans. Clin Infect Dis 2006; 42:1075.

[3] Pappas G, Solera J, Akritidis N, Tsianos E. New approaches to the antibiotic treatment of brucellosis. International journal of antimicrobial agents. 2005; 26(2):101-5.

[4] Pappas G, Akritidis N, Tsianos E. Effective treatments in the management of brucellosis. Expert opinion on pharmacotherapy. 2005; 6(2):201-9.

[5] Yousefi-Nooraie R, Mortaz-Hejri S, Mehrani M, Sadeghipour P. Antibiotics for treating human brucellosis. The Cochrane Library. 2012.

[6] Solera J. Update on brucellosis: therapeutic challenges. International journal of antimicrobial agents. 2010; 36:18-20.

[7] Pappas G, Papadimitriou P, Christou L, Akritidis N. Future trends in human brucellosis treatment. 2006; 15(10):1141-9.

[8] Hashemi SH, Gachkar L, Keramat F, Mamani M, Hajilooi M, Janbakhsh A, et al. Comparison of doxycycline-streptomycin, doxycycline-rifampin, and ofloxacin-rifampin in the treatment of brucellosis: a randomized clinical trial. International journal of infectious diseases. 2012; 16(4):247-51.

[9] Al-Tawfiq J, Memish Z. Antibiotic susceptibility and treatment of brucellosis. Recent patents on anti-infective drug discovery. 2013; 8(1):51-4.

[10] Solera J, Beato JL, Martínez-Alfaro E, Segura JC, de Tomas E. Azithromycin and gentamicin therapy for the treatment of humans with brucellosis. Clinical infectious diseases. 2001; 32(3):506-9.

[11] Falagas ME, Bliziotis IA. Quinolones for treatment of human brucellosis: critical review of the evidence from microbiological and clinical studies. Antimicrobial agents and chemotherapy. 2006; 50(1):22-33.

[12] Keramat F, Ranjbar M, Mamani M, Hashemi SH, Zeraati F. A comparative trial of three therapeutic regimens: ciprofloxacin-rifampin, ciprofloxacin-doxycycline and doxycycline-rifampin in the treatment of brucellosis. Tropical doctor. 2009; 39(4): 207-10.

[13] Ariza J, Bosilkovski M, Cascio A, Colmenero JD, Corbel MJ, Falagas ME, et al. Perspectives for the treatment of brucellosis in the 21st century: the Ioannina recommendations. PLOS medicine. 2007; 4(12):317.

[14] Al-Tawfiq JA. Therapeutic options for human brucellosis. Anti-infective therapy. 2008; 6(1):109-20.

[15] Cook GC, Zumla A. Manson's tropical diseases. Elsevier Health Sciences; 2008.

[16] Skalsky K, Yahav D, Bishara J, Pitlik S, Leibovici L, Paul M. Treatment of human brucellosis: systematic review and meta-analysis of randomised controlled trials. BMJ. 2008; 336(7646):701-4.

[17] Karabay O, Sencan I, Kayas D, Şahin I. Ofloxacin plus rifampicin versus doxycycline plus rifampicin in the treatment of brucellosis: a randomized clinical trial [ISRCTN11871179]. BMC infectious diseases. 2004; 4(1):18.

[18] Ranjbar M, Keramat F, Mamani M, Kia AR, Hashemi SH, Nojomi M. Comparison between doxycycline–rifampin–amikacin and doxycycline–rifampin regimens in the treatment of brucellosis. International journal of infectious diseases. 2007; 11(2):152-6.

[19] del Pozo JSG, Solera J. Systematic review and meta-analysis of randomized clinical trials in the treatment of human brucellosis. PloS one. 2012; 7(2):32090.

[20] Ulu-Kilic A, Karakas A, Erdem H, Turker T, Inal A, Ak O, et al. Update on treatment options for spinal brucellosis. Clinical microbiology and infection. 2014; 20(2):75-82.

[21] Mile B, Valerija K, Krsto G, Ivan V, Ilir D, Nikola L. Doxycycline-rifampin versus doxycycline-rifampin-gentamicin in treatment of human brucellosis. Tropical doctor. 2012; 42(1):13-7.

[22] Roushan MRH, Amiri MJS. Update on childhood brucellosis. Recent patents on anti-infective drug discovery. 2013; 8(1):42-6.

[23] Al-Tawfiq J, Memish ZA. Pregnancy associated brucellosis. Recent patents on anti-infective drug discovery. 2013; 8(1):47-50.

[24] Gulsun S, Aslan S, Satici O, Gul T. Brucellosis in pregnancy. Tropical doctor. 2011; 41(2):82-4.

[25] Herrick JA, Lederman RJ, Sullivan B, Powers JH, Palmore TN. Brucella arteritis: clinical manifestations, treatment, and prognosis. The Lancet infectious diseases. 2014; 14(6):520-6.

[26] Yilmaz M, Arslan F, Baskan O, Mert A. Splenic abscess due to brucellosis: a case report and a review of the literature. International journal of infectious diseases. 2014; 20:68-70.

[27] Hashemi SH, Keramat F, Ranjbar M, Mamani M, Farzam A, Jamal-Omidi S. Osteoarticular complications of brucellosis in Hamedan, an endemic area in the west of Iran. International journal of infectious diseases. 2007; 11(6):496-500.

[28] Alp E, Doganay M. Current therapeutic strategy in spinal brucellosis. International journal of infectious diseases. 2008; 12(6):573-7.

Chapter 12

Treatment of Human Brucellosis — Review of Evidence from Clinical Trials

Julián Solís García del Pozo and Javier Solera

Additional information is available at the end of the chapter

http://dx.doi.org/10.5772/61223

Abstract

Unresolved issues remain surrounding the treatment of human brucellosis. The present work aims to provide useful information to help clinicians make decisions when treating brucellosis patients. Information based on scientific evidence from clinical trials published over the past 30 years has been compiled and presented in an updated form, covering both focal and non-focal, or uncomplicated, human brucellosis. This chapter shows that, despite the studies published in recent years, areas such as the role of monotherapy or treatment in cases of focal disease, have not been adequately addressed in clinical trials, and demonstrates the need for further research.

Keywords: Human brucellosis, antimicrobial therapy, clinical trials, review

1. Introduction

Infection caused by *Brucella spp.* affects humans and different animal species. The infection of animals is particularly significant in rural areas of developing countries because in addition to the implications for human health, there are also serious economic implications [1]. Human brucellosis remains a major human health problem in countries of the Middle East, North Africa, and the Balkan Peninsula [2, 3]. Many of these countries lack adequate health care coverage that can ensure a correct management of all detected cases.

Furthermore, the treatment of human brucellosis continues to present complications such as the need for parenteral administration of aminoglycosides, the risk of inducing rifampicin resistance in countries where tuberculosis poses a problem, and treatment compliance in a disease in which symptoms disappear a few days after initiating therapy. Additionally, patient follow-up in underdeveloped rural areas is difficult and approximately 10% of patients relapse

[4]. Moreover, there is insufficient scientific evidence on the management of special patient groups such as pregnant women or patients with focal infection.

In order to properly understand the current state of knowledge on antimicrobial treatment for human brucellosis, it is important to be familiar with the clinical trials conducted on the treatment of this infection, including those dealing with special populations (children, pregnant women) or with focal complications (spondylitis, endocarditis, or neurobrucellosis).

In the last four years, several systematic reviews [4-6] and some new clinical trials [7-9] have been published. Most of these studies have focused on patients with uncomplicated human brucellosis. The present work aims to provide useful information extracted from published clinical trials on human brucellosis in the past 30 years, such as establishing the most effective evidence-based treatment regimens and identifying those treatment issues that remain unclear or insufficiently addressed. This is an important step toward achieving the goal of aiding clinicians in decision-making processes when treating brucellosis patients.

2. Which treatment regimens were most widely tested in clinical trials?

A search for clinical trials in patients with acute brucellosis published in the last 30 years was conducted in MEDLINE, using the terms "Brucella (or human brucellosis) and therapy (or treatment) and clinical trial." A total of 33 comparative clinical trials were found. The search was completed by the literature cited in these clinical studies.

Interest in this topic is also reflected by the fact that in the last 20 years, there have been at least five systematic reviews on the treatment of uncomplicated human brucellosis [4-6, 10, 11]. These reviews help us to summarize the evidence available to date. Table 1 shows the comparative clinical trials conducted on patients with uncomplicated brucellosis. [COMP: insert Table 1]

Author [Ref]	Year	Country	Therapeutic regimen and duration (days)	Follow-up duration (months)	Type of study
Ariza [12]	1985	Spain	TETR ó DX (30) + STP (21) vs DX (30) + RF (30)	6-24	R
Ariza [34]	1985	Spain	TETR (21) + STP (14) vs TMP/SMX (45)	6-36	R
Colmenero [13]	1989	Spain	DX (30) + STP (21) vs DX (45) + RF (45)	6	R
Acocella [14]	1989	Multinational	TETR (21) + STP (14) vs DX (45) + STP (14) vs DX (45) + RF (45)	12	R
Lang [15]	1990	Israel	CPX (42) vs DX (42) + RF (42)	12	R
Solera [16]	1991	Spain	DX (45) + STP (14) vs DX (45) + RF (45)	12	R
Lang [31]	1992	Israel	Ceftriaxone (≥14) vs DX (28) + STP (14)	6	R
Ariza [17]	1992	Spain	DX (45) + STP (15) vs DX (45) + RF (45)	15.7	R, DB

http://dx.doi.org/10.5772/61223

Author [Ref]	Year	Country	Therapeutic regimen and duration (days)	Follow-up duration (months)	Type of study
Montejo [18]	1993	Spain	DX (42) + STP (14) vs DX (42) + STP (21) vs DX (28) + RF (28) vs DX (42) + RF (42) vs DX (42) vs TMP/SMX (180)	12	R
Akova [19]	1993	Turkey	DX (42) + RF (42) vs OFX (42) + RF (42)	14.6	R
Colmenero [20]	1994	Spain	DX (42) + STP (21) vs DX (42) + RF (42)	6	R
Solera [21]	1995	Spain	DX (45) + STP (14) vs DX (45) + RF (45)	12	R
Kalo [22]	1996	Albania	DX (42) + RF (42) vs DX (42) + CPX (42)	6	R
Solera [42]	1997	Spain	DX (30) + G (7) vs DX (45) + G (7)	12	NR
Agalar [23]	1999	Turkey	DX (45) + RF (45) vs CPX (30) + RF (30)	12	R
Saltoglu [24]	2002	Turkey	DX (45) + RF(45) vs OFX (45) + RF (45)	6	R
Karabay [25]	2004	Turkey	DX (45) + RF (45) vs OFX (30) + RF (30)	~5	R
Hasanjani Roushan [43]	2004	Iran	TMP/SMX (60) + RF (60) vs DX (60) + TMP/SMX (60)	12	R
Solera [44]	2004	Spain	DX (30) + G (7) vs DX (45) + G (7)	8.7	R, DB
Ersoy [26]	2005	Turkey	DX (42) + STP (21) vs DX (42) + RF (42) vs OFX (42) + RF (42)	6-18	R
Hasanjani Roushan [32]	2006	Iran	DX (45) + STP (14) vs DX (45) + G (7)	12	R
Ranjbar [27]	2007	Iran	DX (56-84) + RF (56-84) + AMK (7) vs DX (56) + RF (56)	6	R
Alavi [28]	2007	Iran	DX (56) + RF (56) vs DX (56) + TMP/SMX (56)	6	R
Keramat [29]	2009	Iran	DX (56-84) + RF (56-84) vs DX (56-84) + CPX (56-84) vs CPX (56-84) + RF (56-84)	6	R
Hasanjani Roushan [33]	2010	Iran	DX (45) + STP (14) vs DX (56) + G (5)	12	R
Mile [7]	2012	Macedonia	DX (45) + RF (45) vs DX (45) + RF (45) + G (7-10)	≥6	NR
Hashemi [30]	2012	Iran	OFX (42) + RF (42) vs DX (42) + STP (21) vs DX (42) + RF (42)	6	R
Sofian [9]	2014	Iran	DX (42) + RF (42) + STP (7) vs DX (56) +RF (56) + STP (7)	24	R

Abbreviations: DX = doxycycline; RF = rifampicin; TETR = tetracycline; STP = streptomycin; TMP/SMX = cotrimoxazole; CPX = ciprofloxacin; OFX = ofloxacin; G = gentamicin; AMK = amikacin; R = randomized; NR = non-randomized; DB = double-blind.

Table 1. Comparative clinical trials in uncomplicated human brucellosis

The therapeutic regimens most tested were those including two drugs. In uncomplicated human brucellosis, the combination most often used in two-drug trials was that of doxycycline and rifampicin, included in 20 clinical trials [7, 12-30], followed by the regimen including doxycycline and streptomycin, in 13 clinical trials [12-14, 16-18, 20, 21, 26, 30-33]. In 12 of these 13 trials, the combination of doxycycline and streptomycin was compared to the combination of doxycycline and rifampicin. In another nine clinical trials, an antimicrobial regimen including quinolones was tested [15, 19, 22-26, 29, 30]. In one of them, quinolone was evaluated as monotherapy [15] and in the other eight, quinolone in combination with another antimicrobial agent, usually rifampicin. In all cases in which quinolones were used, they were compared with doxycycline and rifampicin.

There were only three trials including triple-drug therapy [7, 9, 27], which in all cases consisted of a combination of doxycycline, rifampicin, and an aminoglycoside. In two of these studies, triple-drug therapy was compared with doxycycline and rifampicin. In the remaining study, two different durations of the same triple-drug therapy were compared.

Four studies included trials with only a single antimicrobial agent. One trial was performed using ceftriaxone [31] and another one using ciprofloxacin [15]. In another two, the antimicrobial agent evaluated was cotrimoxazole [18, 34]. Only one clinical trial utilizing monotherapy with doxycycline has been conducted over the last 30 years [18]. The last study involving monotherapy was published by Montejo et al. in 1993 [18]. Since then, there have been no clinical trials conducted on human brucellosis assessing treatment with single antimicrobial agents.

3. Which therapeutic regimens based on a combination of two antimicrobial agents produced the highest cure rates?

The percentage of relapses and treatment failures obtained in clinical trials assessing the most commonly used regimens, are shown in Table 2. The data in Table 2 support the conclusion that the combination of doxycycline and streptomycin produces the highest cure rates and therefore the lowest rates of treatment failures and relapses. [COMP: insert Table 2]

Reference	*N*	**Relapses**	**Therapeutic failures**	**Comments**
			DOXYCYCLINE + STREPTOMYCIN	
12	28	2	0	Some patients were treated with tetracycline. Treatment duration was 30 days for doxycycline and 21 days for streptomycin.
14	53	0	2	
13	59	3	2	Treatment duration was 30 days for doxycycline and 21 days for streptomycin.

http://dx.doi.org/10.5772/61223

Reference	*N*	Relapses	Therapeutic failures	Comments
16	38	2	1	
31	10	0	0	Treatment duration was 28 days for doxycycline and 14 days for streptomycin..
17	51	3	2	
18	84	4	0	40 patients with 14 days of streptomycin and another 44 patients with 21 days of streptomycin were included.
20	10	0	0	
21	94	5	2	
26	32	3	1	Treatment with streptomycin was maintained for 21 days.
32	94	3	4	
33	82	5	4	
30	65	3	3	Treatment with streptomycin was maintained for 21 days.
Total	839	37 (4.4%)	26 (3.1%)	
			DOXYCYCLINE + RIFAMPICIN	
12	18	7	0	The treatment duration was 30 days.
13	52	7	0	
14	63	3	0	
15	4	0	0	
16	38	9	3	
17	44	6	2	
18	111	19	2	65 of these patients received treatment for 4 weeks and the remaining patients for 6 weeks.
19	30	1	0	
20	10	1	1	
21	100	16	8	
22	12	1	0	
23	20	2	0	
24	30	2	NR	
25	14	2	0	
26	45	6	1	
27	110	9	13	Treatment was maintained for 8 weeks.
28	51	6	5	Treatment was maintained for 8 weeks.
29	61	2	2	
7	94	13	5	
30	62	9	10	
Total	969	121 (21.8%)	52 (5.4%)	

Reference	*N*	Relapses	Therapeutic failures	Comments
		QUINOLONE + RIFAMPICIN ÓR DOXYCYCLINE		
19	31	1	1	Quinolone + rifampicin
22	12	1	0	Quinolone + doxycycline
23	20	3	0	Quinolone + rifampicin. Treatment duration was 30 days.
24	27	2	NR	Quinolone + rifampicin
25	15	2	0	Quinolone + rifampicin. Treatment duration was 30 days.
26	41	5	1	Quinolone + rifampicin
29	117	10	10	In 55 patients, ciprofloxacin plus doxycycline regimen was used. In another 62 patients, ciprofloxacin plus rifampicin regimen was used. The treatment duration ranged from 56 to 84 days.
30	64	5	4	Quinolone + rifampicin
Total	327	29 (8.9%)	16 (4.9%)	

Table 2. Relapses and treatment failures in different therapeutic regimens used in clinical trials

4. Is triple-drug antimicrobial therapy better than the combination of two antimicrobial agents for the treatment of uncomplicated brucellosis?

Only three clinical trials using a triple-drug antimicrobial therapy for the treatment of uncomplicated human brucellosis have been published (Table 3). All these trials used a combination of doxycycline, rifampicin, and an aminoglycoside during the initial days of treatment. [COMP: insert Table 3]

The first of these trials was published by Ranjbar et al. in 2007 [27]. In this trial, a treatment regimen with doxycycline and rifampicin was used for a period ranging from 8 to 12 weeks, with amikacin for the first seven days. This regimen was compared to a combination of doxycycline and rifampicin, also lasting for 8-12 weeks. The authors suggested that triple-drug therapy was beneficial with respect to the dual-drug therapy, based on greater efficiency in terms of relief of symptoms, with borderline significance ($p = 0.04$; 95% Confidence Interval = 0.008 to 0.15). In terms of relapse, no significant differences between the two treatment groups ($p = 0.4$) were obtained.

The second trial was conducted by Mile et al. [7]. It was a non-randomized study comparing the efficacy and tolerance of a doxycycline-rifampicin regimen administered for 45 days (94 patients), versus doxycycline-rifampicin regimen given for 45 days plus gentamicin for the first 7-10 days (87 patients). The doxycycline-rifampicin-gentamicin regimen demonstrated a significantly lower relapse rate in comparison to the doxycycline-rifampicin combination ($p = 0.034$). Interestingly, in this second study, treatment failure rates were similar in both groups and no significant differences were found in overall cure rate ($p = 0.097$).

Reference	*N*	Relapses	Treatment failures	Comments
		DOXYCYCLINE + RIFAMPICIN + AMINOGLYCOSIDE		
27	110	6	4	The duration of treatment ranged from 8 to 12 weeks. The aminoglycoside amikacin was used for 7 days.
7	87	4	5	The treatment duration was 45 days. The aminoglycoside gentamicin was used for the first 7-10 days.
9	72	10	0	The treatment duration was 6 weeks. The aminoglycoside streptomycin was used for the first 7 days.
9	72	7	0	The treatment duration was 8 weeks. The aminoglycoside streptomycin was used for the first 7 days.
Total	341	27 (7.9%)	9 (2.6%)	

Table 3. Relapses and treatment failures with triple-drug therapy in clinical trials on human brucellosis

The third study was published in 2014 by Sofian et al. [9]. It was a randomized, controlled trial to compare the triple-drug regimen of doxycycline and rifampicin for six weeks plus streptomycin for the first seven days, versus doxycycline and rifampicin for eight weeks plus streptomycin for seven days. This trial found no significant difference between six weeks and eight weeks of treatment ($p = 0.42$).

On the basis of these trials, it cannot be concluded that treatment with three drugs is currently a better therapeutic regimen than treatment with two drugs. There are several arguments to support this conclusion. Firstly, only two of these trials compared triple-drug therapy with dual-drug therapy, and the results between these two trials were contradictory. Whereas in the first trial, triple-drug therapy was better in terms of relief of symptoms but not in terms of relapse rates, in the second trial, the contrary occurs, with triple-drug therapy more effective in preventing relapses but not in short-term treatment success. Moreover, failure and relapse rates obtained in these trials with triple-drug therapy were no lower than those obtained in other dual-drug therapy trials using doxycycline and streptomycin (Tables 2 and 3). Furthermore, triple-drug therapy renders treatment more complicated, with increased costs. In addition, the effects resulting from the difficulty of administering this treatment in developing countries should also be considered [4]. Therefore, until more data are available, we cannot conclude that triple-drug therapy is better than two-drug treatment.

5. Is monotherapy a valid alternative?

Human brucellosis is a disease with low mortality rates and good response to different therapeutic regimens. Most cases occur in developing countries with limited resources. This fact has led some authors to consider the use of more simple and inexpensive therapeutic regimens based on monotherapy.

Only four of the studies included in Table 1 tested therapeutic regimens based on monotherapy in uncomplicated adult human brucellosis. Monotherapy with cotrimoxazole for 45 days was evaluated by Ariza et al., and they obtained a high relapse rate (46.6%) [34]. Montejo et al. were able to reduce the recurrence rate with cotrimoxazole to 3.1%, but at the cost of prolonging the treatment for 6 months [18], which also increases the probability of side effects or of the patient's abandonment of treatment.

Lang et al. performed two monotherapy trials with a small number of patients. In the first of these trials, six patients treated with a six-week regimen of oral ciprofloxacin were included [15]. Of these patients, five relapsed. In the second clinical trial, eight patients were treated with intramuscular ceftriaxone for at least two weeks [31]. Only two patients in this group responded to treatment.

However, unlike in the previously described trials, in the study conducted by Montejo et al. [18], the results obtained with doxycycline monotherapy were better, showing a relapse rate of 14.1%, which was only slightly higher than that obtained in the same study with the combination of doxycycline and rifampicin for 45 days (11%). These results were also better than those obtained with rifampicin and doxycycline for 30 days (21.5% relapse rate). Doxycycline monotherapy appears to yield similar outcomes to those obtained by some of the trials using both doxycycline and rifampicin that are reflected in Table 2.

Therefore, it has been postulated that monotherapy with doxycycline can be a cost-effective treatment in patients without focal disease and with low risk of relapse. Solera et al. [35] identified as predictors of relapse a baseline temperature more than 38.3°C, duration of symptoms to be less than 10 days before starting the treatment, and baseline positive blood cultures. In patients with none or one of these factors, the risk of recurrence is low, and doxycycline monotherapy might be an appropriate treatment. Further clinical trials are needed to confirm this hypothesis.

6. Which treatment regimens were used in clinical trials on brucellosis in children?

There were three trials conducted in children with brucellosis. Firstly, the trial by Lubani et al. [36] was performed using a variety of therapeutic regimens. Excluding cotrimoxazole monotherapy, which showed a high rate of relapse (30%), the rest of the treatment regimens in the study (including monotherapy regimens) demonstrated good results with low relapse and treatment failure rates. The authors of this trial recommend cotrimoxazole and gentamicin-containing regimens for patients aged 8 years or younger, for whom tetracyclines are contraindicated.

Khuri-Bulos et al. [37] conducted a study in which 113 children were treated with a six-week combination of trimethoprim-sulfamethoxazole (10 to 12 mg/kg trimethoprim, 50 to 60 mg/kg sulfamethoxazole) and rifampicin (15 to 20 mg/kg in two divided doses). The treatment was well-tolerated, and only four children relapsed during the six-month follow-up.

Hasanjani Roushan et al. [38] published a study on two different durations for a regimen including cotrimoxazole and rifampicin (42 versus 56 days of treatment). After a year of follow-up, the authors observed a similar cure rate in the two treatment groups (89.1% and 95.5% cure rate for 42 and 56 days, respectively; $p = 0.204$). The authors reached the conclusion that a six-week treatment duration was sufficient to treat brucellosis.

Considering these data, it can be stated that childhood brucellosis responds to treatment regimens that include cotrimoxazole, gentamicin, and rifampicin, with a low failure rate and relapse. Although recommended regimens are those including cotrimoxazole or rifampicin for 45 days plus gentamicin in the first seven days [1], clinical trials also showed a good treatment response rate to cotrimoxazole plus rifampicin for six weeks.

7. Which treatment regimens were used in clinical trials for the treatment of brucella spondylitis?

There were two clinical trials on patients with brucellar spondylitis. The first was performed by Bayindir et al. [39]. In this study, 102 patients suffering from a lumbar brucellar spondylitis were randomized to receive five different regimens of antibiotic therapy: streptomycin (15 days) plus tetracycline (45 days), doxycycline (45 days) plus streptomycin (15 days), doxycycline plus rifampicin (45 days), ofloxacin plus rifampicin (45 days), and finally doxycycline plus rifampicin (45 days) plus streptomycin (15 days). The only group in which there were no relapses or treatment failures was the one that received triple-drug therapy with doxycycline, rifampicin, and streptomycin. Thus, this treatment was recommended by the study authors according to their results.

The other trial, conducted by Alp et al. [40], included 31 patients with spinal brucellosis who were consecutively assigned to one of two treatment regimens tested. These treatments were either a combination of doxycycline and streptomycin, or a combination of ciprofloxacin with rifampicin. Treatment was continued for an average of 12 weeks. The authors concluded that the success rate with each combination was the same, but based on the lower cost of treatment, the authors recommended the combination of streptomycin and doxycycline.

According to these two trials, it may be concluded that triple-drug therapy successfully treats brucellar spondylitis with a short course of just 45 days of antibiotics versus dual-drug therapy. However, despite the greater methodological difficulties of the second trial described here, therapy with doxycycline and streptomycin could be an alternative if treatment time is prolonged.

8. Which treatment regimens were used in clinical trials on brucellosis in pregnancy?

No clinical trials on the treatment of brucellosis during pregnancy were found. Therefore, the therapy in this group of patients is mainly based on expert recommendations and observational studies. Tetracycline and streptomycin should be avoided during pregnancy. The regimen of choice includes rifampicin 900 mg daily for six weeks. Trimethoprim-sulfamethoxazole could be combined with rifampicin, but should not be used before 13 weeks of pregnancy because of teratogenic risk nor after 36 weeks due to risk of kernicterus [1, 3].

9. Which treatment regimens were used in clinical trials for the treatment of Brucella endocarditis?

Likewise, no clinical studies were found on patients suffering from Brucella endocarditis and, as with brucellosis during pregnancy, the therapy in this group of patients is mainly based on expert recommendations and observational studies. Antibiotics used in these cases include doxycycline, rifampicin, and aminoglycosides in triple-drug therapy and sometimes cotrimoxazole [1, 3]. Brucella endocarditis requires prolonged treatment for 2 to 10 months and must be maintained on the basis of clinical, laboratory, and echocardiographic data. In cases of persistent infection, prosthetic valve infection, heart failure, abscesses or periannular extension of infection, surgery is indicated [3].

10. Which treatment regimens were used in clinical trials for the treatment of neurobrucellosis?

Involvement of the nervous system in Brucella infection may have different manifestations such as meningoencephalitis, myelitis, radiculitis, peripheral neuropathies, subarachnoid hemorrhage, or psychiatric manifestations [41]. There is no consensus on antibiotic therapy for neurobrucellosis. No clinical trials on patients suffering from neurobrucellosis have been found. Dual- or triple-combination therapy with doxycycline, rifampicin, trimethoprim-sulfamethoxazole, and aminoglycosides has been recommended [3, 41]. Neurobrucellosis may require prolonged courses of treatment over several months.

11. What systematic reviews have been conducted on the treatment of human brucellosis?

Until now, five systematic reviews on the treatment of human brucellosis have been conducted [4-6, 10, 11] (Table 4). The first was published in 1997 and was performed with the aim of comparing a doxycycline plus streptomycin regimen with a doxycycline plus rifampicin regimen [10]. The authors concluded that the doxycycline-rifampicin treatment presented a greater number of relapses and a lower number of cures than streptomycin-doxycycline treatment.

The next published systematic review was performed by Skalski et al. [11], which recommended triple-drug therapy as one of the most appropriate regimens. However, as indicated by Yousefi-Nooraie et al. [5], the review had some methodological limitations, such as combining trials based on different drug classes (e.g., comparing quinolone with non-quinolone-based regimens) or comparing studies on brucellar spondylitis with studies on non-complicated brucellosis, despite differences in the treatment duration of these studies.

Since then, three other systematic reviews have been published [4-6]. Despite some differences in the methodology used among the three, the conclusion they all reached was that the combination of doxycycline-aminoglycoside [especially doxycycline (six weeks) plus streptomycin (two or three weeks)] in uncomplicated adult brucellosis was more effective than a doxycycline plus rifampicin (six-week) regimen.

Author [Ref]	Year	Conclusions
Solera [10]	1994	"In human brucellosis, treatment with rifampicin and doxycycline presents a greater number of recurrences and a lower number of cures than the classical treatment with streptomycin and tetracycline drugs."
Skalsky [11]	2008	"There are significant differences in effectiveness between currently recommended treatment regimens for brucellosis. The preferred treatment should be with dual or triple regimens including an aminoglycoside."
Solís García del Pozo [4]	2012	"Although the preferred treatment in uncomplicated human brucellosis is a doxycycline-aminoglycoside combination, other treatments based on oral regimens or monotherapy should not be rejected until they are better studied. Triple therapy should not be considered the current treatment of choice."
Yousefi-Nooraie [5]	2012	"A doxycycline (six weeks) plus streptomycin (two or three weeks) regimen is more effective than a doxycycline plus rifampicin (six weeks) regimen. Quinolone plus rifampicin (six weeks) is slightly better tolerated than doxycycline plus rifampicin, and low quality evidence did not show any difference in overall effectiveness."
Alavi [6]	2013	"In uncomplicated brucellosis in adult patients, a doxycycline-aminoglycoside combination is the first choice, with doxycycline-rifampin and doxycycline-cotrimoxazole as alternative regimens. The other oral regimens including quinolones may be considered as alternatives. Cotrimoxazole plus rifampin for six weeks may be the regimen of choice for the treatment of patients younger than 8 years old. Gentamicin for 5 days plus cotrimoxazole for six weeks may be a suitable alternative regimen."

Table 4. Main conclusions of the systematic reviews published on treatment of human brucellosis

12. Conclusions

Over the past few years, several trials and systematic reviews on the treatment of human brucellosis have been published. However, unresolved issues remain surrounding the treatment of this disease that may be important for patient management, such as the role of monotherapy in low risk patients, or treatment for special groups such as those with focal disease. These unresolved issues have not been adequately addressed in clinical trials. Further research on the treatment of this zoonosis is necessary to provide the clinician with the best scientific evidence upon which to base clinical decisions.

Author details

Julián Solís García del Pozo[1*] and Javier Solera[2]

*Address all correspondence to: julianeloysolis@gmail.com

1 Internal Medicine Department, Hospital de Villarrobledo, Villarrobledo (Albacete), Spain

2 Internal Medicine Department, Complejo Hospitalario Universitario de Albacete, Albacete, Spain

References

[1] Solera J. Update on brucellosis: Therapeutic challenges. *Int J Antimicrob Agents*. 2010; 36 (Suppl 1); S18-S20. DOI: 10.1016/j.ijantimicag.2010.06.015

[2] Ariza J, Bosilkovski M, Cascio A, et al. Perspectives for the treatment of brucellosis in the 21st century: The Ioannina recommendations. *PLoS Med*. 2007; 4: e317. DOI: 10.1371/journal.pmed.0040317

[3] Rodríguez Zapata M, Solera Santos J. Brucelosis. *Medicine-Programa de formación medica continuada*. 2014; 11: 3045-53. DOI: 10.1016/S0304-5412(14)70738-3

[4] Solís García del Pozo J, Solera J. Systematic review and meta-analysis of randomized clinical trials in the treatment of human brucellosis. *PLoS One*. 2012; 7(2): e32090. DOI: 10.1371/journal.pone.0032090

[5] Yousefi-Nooraie R, Mortaz-Hejri S, Mehrani M, Sadeghipour P. Antibiotics for treating human brucellosis. *Cochrane Database Syst Rev*. 2012; 17: 10:CD007179. DOI: 10.1002/14651858.CD007179.pub2

[6] Alavi SM, Alavi L. Treatment of brucellosis: A systematic review of studies in recent twenty years. *Caspian J Intern Med*. 2013; 4: 636-41.

[7] Mile B, Valerija K, Krsto G, et al. Doxycycline-rifampin versus doxycycline-rifampin-gentamicin in treatment of human brucellosis. *Trop Doct*. 2012; 42: 13-7. DOI: 10.1258/td.2011.110284

[8] Hashemi SH, Gachkar L, Keramat F, et al. Comparison of doxycycline-streptomycin, doxycycline-rifampin, and ofloxacin-rifampin in the treatment of brucellosis: A

randomized clinical trial. *Int J Infect Dis*. 2012; 16: e247-51. DOI: 10.1016/j.ijid.2011.12.003

[9] Sofian M, Velayati AA, Aghakhani A, et al. Comparison of two durations of triple-drug therapy in patients with uncomplicated brucellosis: A randomized controlled trial. *Scand J Infect Dis*. 2014; 46: 573-7. DOI: 10.3109/00365548.2014.918275

[10] Solera J, Martínez-Alfaro E, Sáez L. [Meta-analysis of the efficacy of the combination of rifampicin and doxycycline in the treatment of human brucellosis]. *Med Clin (Barc)*. 1994; 21 (102): 731-8.

[11] Skalsky K, Yahav D, Bishara J, et al. Treatment of human brucellosis: Systematic review and meta-analysis of randomised controlled trials. *BMJ*. 2008; 336: 701-4. DOI: 10.1136/bmj.39497.500903.25

[12] Ariza J, Gudiol F, Pallarés R, Rufí G, Fernández-Viladrich P. Comparative trial of rifampin-doxycycline versus tetracycline-streptomycin in the therapy of human brucellosis. *Antimicrob Agents Chemother*. 1985; 28: 548-51. DOI: 10.1128/AAC.28.4.548

[13] Colmenero Castillo JD, Hernandez Marquez S, Reguera Iglesias JM, et al. Comparative trial of doxycycline plus streptomycin versus doxycycline plus rifampin for the therapy of human brucellosis. *Chemotherapy*. 1989; 35: 146-52.

[14] Acocella G, Bertrand A, Beytout J, et al. Comparison of three different regimens in the treatment of acute brucellosis: A multicenter multinational study. *J Antimicrob Chemother*. 1989; 23: 433-9. DOI: 10.1093/jac/23.3.433

[15] Lang R, Raz R, Sacks T, Shapiro M. Failure of prolonged treatment with ciprofloxacin in acute infections due to Brucella melitensis. *J Antimicrob Chemother*. 1990; 26: 841-6. DOI: 10.1093/jac/26.6.841

[16] Solera J, Medrano F, Rodríguez M, Geijo P, Paulino J. [A comparative therapeutic and multicenter trial of rifampicin and doxycycline versus streptomycin and doxycycline in human brucellosis]. *Med Clin (Barc)*. 1991; 96: 649-53.

[17] Ariza J, Gudiol F, Pallares R, et al. Treatment of human brucellosis with doxycycline plus rifampin or doxycycline plus streptomycin. A randomized, double-blind study. *Ann Intern Med*. 1992; 117: 25-30. DOI: 10.7326/0003-4819-117-1-25

[18] Montejo JM, Alberola I, Glez-Zarate P, et al. Open, randomized therapeutic trial of six antimicrobial regimens in the treatment of human brucellosis. *Clin Infect Dis*. 1993; 16: 671-6. DOI: 10.1093/clind/16.5.671

[19] Akova M, Uzun O, Akalin HE, et al. Quinolones in treatment of human brucellosis: Comparative trial of ofloxacin-rifampin versus doxycycline-rifampin. *Antimicrob Agents Chemother*. 1993; 37: 1831-4. DOI: 10.1128/AAC.37.9.1831

[20] Colmenero JD, Fernández-Gallardo LC, Agúndez JA, et al. Possible implications of doxycycline-rifampin interaction for treatment of brucellosis. *Antimicrob Agents Chemother*. 1994; 38: 2798-802. DOI: 10.1128/AAC.38.12.2798

[21] Solera J, Rodríguez-Zapata M, Geijo P, et al. Doxycycline-rifampin versus doxycycline-streptomycin in treatment of human brucellosis due to Brucella melitensis. The GECMEI Group. Grupo de Estudio de Castilla-la Mancha de Enfermedades Infecciosas. *Antimicrob Agents Chemother*. 1995; 39: 2061-7. DOI: 10.1128/AAC.39.9.2061

[22] Kalo T, Novi S, Nushi A, Dedja S. Ciprofloxacin plus doxycycline versus rifampin plus doxycycline in the treatment of acute brucellosis. *Méd Mal Infect*. 1996; 26: 587-9.

[23] Agalar C, Usubutun S, Turkyilmaz R. Ciprofloxacin and rifampicin versus doxycycline and rifampicin in the treatment of brucellosis. *Eur J Clin Microbiol Infect Dis*. 1999; 18: 535-8.

[24] Saltoglu N, Tasova Y, Inal AS, Seki T, Aksu HS. Efficacy of rifampicin plus doxycycline versus rifampicin plus quinolone in the treatment of brucellosis. *Saudi Med J*. 2002; 23: 921-4.

[25] Karabay O, Sencan I, Kayas D, Sahin I. Ofloxacin plus rifampicin versus doxycycline plus rifampicin in the treatment of brucellosis: A randomized clinical trial. *BMC Infect Dis*. 2004; 4: 18. DOI: 10.1186/1471-2334-4-18

[26] Ersoy Y, Sonmez E, Tevfik MR, But AD. Comparison of three different combination therapies in the treatment of human brucellosis. *Trop Doct*. 2005; 35: 210-2. DOI: 10.1258/004947505774938765

[27] Ranjbar M, Keramat F, Mamani M, et al. Comparison between doxycycline-rifampin-amikacin and doxycycline-rifampin regimens in the treatment of brucellosis. *Int J Infect Dis*. 2007; 11: 152-6. DOI: 10.1016/j.ijid.2005.11.007

[28] Alavi SM, Rajabzadeh AR. Comparison of two chemotherapy regimen: Doxycycline-rifampicin and doxycycline cotromoxazol in the brucellosis patients. Ahvaz, Iran, 2004-2006. *Pak J Med Sci*. 2007; 23: 889-92.

[29] Keramat F, Ranjbar M, Mamani M, Hashemi SH, Zeraati F. A comparative trial of three therapeutic regimens: Ciprofloxacin-rifampin, ciprofloxacin-doxycycline and doxycycline-rifampin in the treatment of brucellosis. *Trop Doct*. 2009; 39: 207-10. DOI: 10.1258/td.2009.090030

[30] Hashemi SH, Gachkar L, Keramat F, et al. Comparison of doxycycline-streptomycin, doxycycline-rifampin, and ofloxacin-rifampin in the treatment of brucellosis: A randomized clinical trial. *Int J Infect Dis*. 2012; 16: e247-51. DOI: 10.1016/j.ijid.2011.12.003

[31] Lang R, Dagan R, Potasman I, Einhorn M, Raz R. Failure of ceftriaxone in the treatment of acute brucellosis. *Clin Infect Dis*. 1992; 14: 506-9. DOI: 10.1093/clinids/14.2.506

[32] Hasanjani Roushan MR, Mohraz M, Hajiahmadi M, Ramzani A, Valayati AA. Efficacy of gentamicin plus doxycycline versus streptomycin plus doxycycline in the treatment of brucellosis in humans. *Clin Infect Dis*. 2006; 42: 1075-80. DOI: 10.1086/501359

[33] Hasanjani Roushan MR, Amiri MJ, Janmohammadi N, et al. Comparison of the efficacy of gentamicin for 5 days plus doxycycline for 8 weeks versus streptomycin for 2

weeks plus doxycycline for 45 days in the treatment of human brucellosis: A randomized clinical trial. *J Antimicrob Chemother*. 2010; 65: 1028-35. DOI: 10.1093/jac/dkq064

[34] Ariza J, Gudiol F, Pallarés R, Rufí G, Fernández-Viladrich P. Comparative trial of co-trimoxazole versus tetracycline-streptomycin in treating human brucellosis. *J Infect Dis*. 1985; 152: 1358-9. DOI: 10.1093/infdis/152.6.1358

[35] Solera J, Martínez-Alfaro E, Espinosa A, et al. Multivariate model for predicting relapse in human brucellosis. *J Infect*. 1998; 36: 85-92. DOI: 10.1016/S0163-4453(98)93342-4

[36] Lubani MM, Dudin KI, Sharda DC, et al. A multicenter therapeutic study of 1100 children with brucellosis. *Pediatr Infect Dis J*. 1989; 8: 75-8.

[37] Khuri-Bulos NA, Daoud AH, Azab SM. Treatment of childhood brucellosis: Results of a prospective trial on 113 children. *Pediatr Infect Dis J*. 1993; 12: 377-81.

[38] Hasanjani Roushan MR, Mohraz M, Janmohammadi N, Hajiahmadi M. Efficacy of cotrimoxazole and rifampin for 6-8 weeks of therapy in childhood brucellosis. *Pediatr Infect Dis J*. 2006; 25: 544-5. DOI: 10.1097/01.inf.0000219403.91975.ce

[39] Bayindir Y, Sonmez E, Aladag A, Buyukberber N. Comparison of five antimicrobial regimens for the treatment of brucellar spondylitis: A prospective, randomized study. *J Chemother*. 2003; 15: 466-71.

[40] Alp E, Koc RK, Durak AC, et al. Doxycycline plus streptomycin versus ciprofloxacin plus rifampicin in spinal brucellosis. *BMC Infect Dis*. 2006; 6: 72. DOI: 10.1186/1471-2334-6-72

[41] Guven T, Ugurlu K, Ergonul O, et al. Neurobrucellosis: Clinical and diagnostic features. *Clin Infect Dis*. 2013; 56(10): 1407-12. DOI: 10.1093/cid/cit072

[42] Solera J, Espinosa A, Martínez-Alfaro E, et al. Treatment of human brucellosis with doxycycline and gentamicin. *Antimicrob Agents Chemother*. 1997; 41(1): 80-4.

[43] Hasanjani Roushan MR, Gangi SM, Ahmadi SA. Comparison of the efficacy of two months of treatment with co-trimoxazole plus doxycycline vs. co-trimoxazole plus rifampin in brucellosis. *Swiss Med Wkly*. 2004; 134: 564-8.

[44] Solera J, Geijo P, Largo J, et al; Grupo de Estudio de Castilla-la Mancha de Enfermedades Infecciosas. A randomized, double-blind study to assess the optimal duration of doxycycline treatment for human brucellosis. Clin Infect Dis. 2004; 39: 1776-82. DOI: 10.1086/426024

Chapter 13

Control of Animal Brucellosis — The Most Effective Tool to Prevent Human Brucellosis

Marta Pérez-Sancho, Teresa García-Seco, Lucas Domínguez and Julio Álvarez

Additional information is available at the end of the chapter

http://dx.doi.org/10.5772/61222

Abstract

The World Health Organization classifies brucellosis as one of the seven neglected endemic zoonosis which contribute to the perpetuation of poverty in developing countries. Although most of the developed countries are free from this important zoonosis, brucellosis has still a widespread distribution in the Mediterranean region, the Middle East, Central Asia, and parts of Latin America, making it a global problem. Nearly half a million of new cases of human brucellosis are reported each year around the world, in which animals (or products of animal origin) are the most likely source of infection. *Brucella melitensis,* the main etiologic agent of small ruminant brucellosis, is the most prevalent specie involved in cases of human disease in most parts of the world. Additionally, *Brucella abortus* (main responsible of bovine brucellosis) and *Brucella suis* (the most common etiological agent of porcine brucellosis) are often associated with human brucellosis. In animal production, brucellosis has a strong economic impact due not only to its direct consequences (e.g., reproductive failures) but also to indirect loses (e.g., trade restrictions). The problem of brucellosis could be considered a clear example of the need for a "One World, One Health" strategy, given that the only approach to achieve its control and subsequent eradication is the cooperation between public and animal health authorities. The prevention of human brucellosis cannot be achieved without the control of the disease in the animals, as exemplified by the impact that the early measures adopted in the beginning of the 20th century forbidding the consumption of goat milk had on the prevalence of the disease in the British soldiers in Malta. When the prevalence of the disease in the animal population is high or when eradication cannot be achieved due to other factors (e.g., lack of economic resources), its control in livestock must be the first objective. When deciding the optimal approach to tackle the disease, the prevalence of animal brucellosis is not the only parameter to consider by the decision makers since other epidemiological and economic aspects should be considered in order to implement the most adequate control strategy in each region. Cooperation between all stakeholders involved is a cornerstone in the success of any control strategy. Strict biosafety and management measures, vaccination, and test-and-slaughter strategy are recognized as the most effective strategies to control this pathology in livestock. The adequate combination of these measures depends on several factors that will determine the success of the eradication efforts. The present chapter will review the abovementioned measures for the control and eradication of brucellosis in livestock, focusing on the advantages and drawbacks of the diagnosis tools and immunization strategies currently available and evaluating new approaches based on the advance on the knowledge of different aspects of this disease and its etiological agents.

---

1. Introduction

Animal brucellosis is one of the most important challenges faced by animal health authorities and producers worldwide due to the large number of host species that can be affected, limitations of the currently available diagnostic and prophylactic tools, and complex epidemiology. Yet, control and eventual eradication of animal brucellosis is the only way to ultimately win the battle against human brucellosis. Although the present chapter is focused on the current approaches for the control of *B. melitensis* in small ruminants (small ruminant brucellosis, SRB), *B. abortus* in cattle (bovine brucellosis, BB), and *B. suis* (biovars 1, 2, and 3) in swine (porcine brucellosis, PB), the complex and dynamic nature of the epidemiology of animal brucellosis must be borne in mind when analyzing a given epidemiological setting since sometimes certain *Brucella* species can be found in host species other than their preferred ones (for example, *B. abortus* may be the etiological agent of brucellosis in sheep [1, 2]). A perfect example of this complex situation is shown by the increasing importance of *B. melitensis* in cattle in some Mediterranean countries, e.g., Saudi Arabia, Egypt, and Kuwait [3-5].

The need for a control of animal brucellosis has been a major concern since the first report describing the implication of animals in the epidemiology of the disease in 1905 [6]. Although brucellosis had been known for centuries as a chronic recurrent febrile disease mostly present in the Mediterranean region, it was not until the end of the 19th century when it was recognized as a dramatic disease wreaking havoc among the British army stationed in Malta. In 1887, Sir David Bruce (a British surgeon whose surname would later give name to the genus) isolated the etiological agent (firstly named as *Micrococcus melitensis*) of the infectious disease that was affecting an increasing number of soldiers in the island [7]. In 1904, the great concern raised by the impact of brucellosis in Malta contributed to the constitution of the "Mediterranean Fever Commission (MFC)," with Sir Bruce as the president of the organization. One of the main aims of the commission was to identify the sources of infection of the disease, an objective that was finally achieved by serendipity [8]: Sir Themistocles Zammit, a Maltese doctor member of MFC, included goats for experiments due to the temporary shortage of monkeys, traditionally used for in vivo studies. Surprisingly, agglutinins and bacteria were detected in the blood and milk of infected goats, thus suggesting these small ruminants were susceptible to the disease and a potential source of infection [6]. The ban on the consumption of Maltese goat milk among British soldiers was the first step for the control of this dramatic zoonosis in the island [9], one of the first preventive measures to control the transmission of *Brucella* from animals to humans.

Brucellosis can be considered a paradigm of the need for a "One World, One Health" strategy given that the only approach to achieve the control and subsequent eradication of this zoonotic disease is the cooperation between the industry, producers, and public and animal health authorities [10]. Human-to-human transmission, although possible and occasionally reported due to transplantation, sexual contact, and lactation [11-14], has an insignificant impact on the epidemiology of the disease since humans are traditionally considered dead-end hosts [15]. The major sources of infection for human are therefore infected animals, not only due to direct contact but also - and most importantly - through the consumption of raw dairy products [3]. Traditionally, the main etiological agent of human brucellosis is *B. melitensis*, although a relevant role of *B. abortus* and *B. suis* (mainly biovars 1 and 3) has also been described. Although approximately 500,000 new human cases of brucellosis are reported every year around the world [16, 17], underdiagnosis/underreporting of human brucellosis is a major issue in many regions [18, 19]. The control of the disease in humans is impaired by the lack of available vaccines [20], thus leaving the control of animal brucellosis as the most effective strategy to prevent human infection [19, 21, 22]. In fact, surveillance systems for human brucellosis can act as sentinel tools of the situation of the disease in animals since the occurrence of human cases can be one of the first indicators of the presence of disease in the animal population [23], and likewise, a decreasing trend in the number of human cases may suggest that brucellosis control campaigns are effective [24, 25].

However, and despite its crucial importance from the public health perspective, the justification for the control of animal brucellosis rests not only on its zoonotic nature but also in the severe losses that its presence entails. Economic costs derived from the presence of *Brucella* infection in animals are derived from the direct consequences of the disease (abortion, infertility, reduction of milk production, orchitis, epididymitis, etc.) and the indirect losses (replacement of reactors, costs associated to control/eradications programs, movement restrictions, trade limitations, etc. [23, 26]). In addition, brucellosis has been recognized as a neglected zoonotic disease that contributes to the perpetuation of the poverty in endemic regions of low-income countries, compromising their economic development [27, 28]. Moreover, costs due to human brucellosis, as the investments on treatments, prevention of the disease, and loss of productivity are other overheads attributable to animal brucellosis.

2. Control and eradication strategies for animal brucellosis

Despite the huge efforts invested on the control of animal brucellosis, results have not always matched the expectations, particularly in the case of ovine and caprine brucellosis, in which control has proven to be more challenging than that of bovine brucellosis due to *B. abortus*. This situation may be the consequence of the combined effect of several factors, including those inherent to the disease regardless of the etiological agent/infected host [existence of a prolonged latent period often associated with lack of serological responses [29] and limited sensitivity of some diagnostic tests in certain epidemiological situations [30, 31] and also other factors associated with the etiological agent (environmental resistance of *B. melitensis* and *B.*

abortus [32]) and the host (traditional farming practices as communal pastures and transhumance practices, typical of small ruminants [33, 34]).

Still, three major strategies have been demonstrated as effective tools to control brucellosis in domestic animals when used in combination:

1. Strict biosecurity at the farm level
2. Test and slaughter programs
3. Immunization of the susceptible population

The sole implementation of one of these measures is however much less effective since optimal results are obtained when at least two of them are applied jointly. Still, the best strategy will depend on the epidemiological situation in a given setting, the availability of resources, etc. [26]. Moreover, in addition to these "classical" strategies, other complementary tools should be considered to ensure the success of the program (animal identification, animal movement control, economic compensations, etc.) [33].

The present chapter will review the tools currently available to achieve the control and eradication of brucellosis in livestock (bovine, porcine, and small ruminant brucellosis), focusing on the advantages and drawbacks of the diagnostic tools and the immunization strategies the two main pillars in which control programs are based. New approaches based on the advance in the knowledge of different aspects of the disease and of their etiological agents will also be reviewed. Finally, the factors that should be considered when selecting the most suitable strategy for control of small ruminant, bovine, and porcine brucellosis and that often determine the success of the control/eradication efforts will be discussed.

2.1. Management and biosecurity

Management and hygienic measures against *Brucella* infection must be focused in diminishing the possibility of contact with viable *Brucella*, including both infected animals and contaminated environments.

The most frequent routes of entry of *Brucella* in a free farm are the following:

- Purchase of infected animals that can shed the bacteria to the environment, therefore exposing susceptible individuals. In ruminants, up to 10^{10}-10^{13} CFU/g of tissue and membranes of aborted fetus can be excreted during the clinical phase of the disease [35]. In swine, infected boar may excrete 10^{4}-10^{5} CFU/ml of semen, thus turning venereal transmission one of the most important routes of infection for *B. suis*, particularly in brucellosis-free settings in which artificial insemination can constitute an important risk factor [32].

- Contact with infected material, pastures, etc., due to the high environmental resistance of *Brucella* spp., which leads to its persistence outside the host for long periods, allowing a variety of transmission routes of *Brucella* (conjunctival, oral, and respiratory).

Thus, the use of appropriate biosecurity measures is of critical importance to prevent the entrance of the disease in a naïve epidemiological unit. These strategies include the implementation of quarantine before the introduction of new animals, the separation of animals with an unknown/uncertain status, the control of animal movements, the adequate management of replacement, the isolation of pregnant females before parturition (particularly primiparous animals), and the strict quality/sanitary control of semen. In case of artificial insemination, avoid or limit the contact between livestock and wildlife in environments where wild animals have been seen to be a source of infection [23, 29, 36, 37].

In infected settings, in addition to the biosecurity recommendations cited above, hygienic measures are essential to limit and control the bacterial load in the environment, decreasing the possibility of contact with viable *Brucella* spp., and should be systematically implemented. Removal of abortion products, full cleaning and disinfection of premises, elimination of infected manure, and incineration of infected material are some examples of measures to attain this objective.

Certain management/farming practices (traditionally used in small flocks from endemic region of low-income countries), such as nomadism, mixing animals from different origins at grazing, and use of shared pastures, may favor transmission of the bacteria, thus hindering the effectiveness of control strategies [38, 39].

2.2. Test and slaughter programs

The main aim of this approach is the early detection and removal of possible sources of infection (infectious animals), thus avoiding circulation of *Brucella*. Despite the effectiveness of the diagnostic strategy used, there is always a certain risk of having infected animals that may remain as silent carriers [40] maintaining the pathogen in the flock and, if there is a drop in the immunity of the herd, may lead to an abortion storm. This strategy is most useful in low-prevalence settings where economic resources and veterinary expertise are available for its support [41]. Test and slaughter strategies may also be useful for the management of outbreaks, particularly when numbers of animals make the implementation of stamping-out measures unfeasible [42]. Although the tests used for the detection of infection can be classified according to different criteria, this section is organized based on its ability to detect the pathogen (direct tests) or the immune response induced in the infected host (indirect tests that can be further subdivided on account of the immune response they target, humoral or cellular). In some cases, the only measure that achieves complete elimination of the bacteria on the flock is the stamping out followed by a thorough cleaning and disinfection and replacement with *Brucella*-free animals [43].

2.2.1. Indirect diagnostic tests

Most of these techniques (especially those using inactivated whole-cell suspensions of *Brucella* as antigens) were developed for the diagnosis of bovine brucellosis in the first place and were further adapted later for its application in small ruminants and swine considering that the principle of all techniques is the same regardless of the *Brucella* species/host: all the major tests are based on the detection of antibodies against the smooth lipopolysaccharide (S-LPS; the immunodominant antigen of smooth *Brucella* species: *B. abortus*, *B. melitensis*, and *B. suis*) [44].

The outer-polysaccharide chain (O-PS), the main antigen moiety of smooth *Brucella* LPS, shows a different proportion of α-1,2 and α-1,3 linkages dividing strains in two groups: A-strains or M-strains, depending on the quantitative distribution of A and M antigens in the smooth species. Thus, the suitability of *Brucella* antigens recovered from M-dominant strains (such as *B. abortus* biovar 1, typically used for rose bengal test (RBT), complement fixation test (CFT), and some ELISA techniques) for the diagnosis of brucellosis due A-dominant strains (e.g., *B. melitensis* biovar 1) has been questioned [45]. In fact, some authors have shown that RB and CFT may present an impaired diagnostic performance when used on small ruminants (particularly in goats) compared with that observed in cattle [46]. However, other studies have demonstrated that the use of *B. abortus* antigens for performing RB and other serological techniques allows an appropriate sensitivity for its use in *B. melitensis* diagnosis in small ruminants [47, 48]. A possible explanation for this finding would be the existence of common epitopes (C-antigen) present in the LPS of A- and M-dominant *Brucella* strains [49].

The accuracy of the diagnostic tests in the control/eradication programs of brucellosis is an essential component in the success of test and control strategies [50]. Although the diagnostic performance of most of the currently available diagnostic techniques has been demonstrated to be adequate, there are some epidemiological situations in which serological diagnosis may have some limitations. For example, silent carriers of the disease (e.g., infants infected congenitally *in utero* or by ingestion of contaminated colostrum/milk) may remain seronegative until a reproductive failure occurs [51]. In addition, positive results may not always be indicative of an active infection [52] since the occurrence of diagnostic interferences associated with exposure to other Gram-negative bacteria has been extensively demonstrated [53]. These microorganisms have LPS molecules similar to the *Brucella*-LPS in the outer membrane and may induce the production of cross-reacting antibodies, thus leading to false-positive results in the traditional serological techniques for brucellosis diagnosis. Different bacteria (including *Escherichia coli* O:116, *E. coli* O:157, and *Vibrio cholerae* O:1) have been recognized as a potential cause of this diagnostic interference, but *Yersinia enterocolitica* serotype O:9 is considered the main agent compromising the diagnostic specificity of serological tests [54]. This is a major challenge in the case of swine brucellosis [32, 55], especially when biovar 2 occurs, because its LPS antigenic structure is more similar to *Y. enterocolitica* than to other biovars of *B. suis* [56]. Most of these cross-reacting antibodies belong to the M isotype, and therefore the implementation of serological techniques based on the predominant detection of IgG1 is potentially more useful [53].

The diagnostic specificity of serological tests may also be compromised by the occurrence of false-positive reactions caused by antibodies induced by vaccine strains (mainly the smooth *B. melitensis* Rev. 1 and *B. abortus* S19, the most widely used strains for immunization against small ruminants and bovine brucellosis, respectively).

There is not a single serological test that can detect 100% of the infected population, and even used in combination may miss up to 30% of the infected animals using some serological tests [45], although its sensitivity at the herd level is much higher. In fact, in the frame of control and eradication programs, serological results are often interpreted at the herd level [46]; hence, the presence of one reactor involves the possible exposure to *Brucella* spp. of all animals of the flock that are therefore considered suspected and put under restriction measures until the infection is considered cleared in the herd/flock.

However, limitations in terms of the specificity of serological tests (such as those stated before) lead to the need of confirming the infection using other tools (epidemiological evidences of exposures and, preferably, isolation of the bacteria) at the herd level. Culture is considered the gold standard technique for the confirmation of the infection due to its high specificity [57], although this method is not free of drawbacks (see below).

The existence of international standards for diagnostic tests, vaccines requirements, reporting data systems, etc., is a cornerstone in the implementation of adequate control/eradication programs for animal brucellosis, making possible the harmonization of animal health systems worldwide [58]. For animal brucellosis, the OIE is the main standard-setting body publishing.

Factors including cost, time between sampling and achievement of test results, resource requirements, and ease of performance are other aspects that need to be considered in the choice of the best serological methods for the diagnosis of animal brucellosis in a given setting [50].

2.2.1.1. Indirect diagnostic tests based of humoral immune response against Brucella spp.

Rose bengal test (RBT)

RBT is a slide agglutination technique based on the use of cells of *B. abortus* S99 or S1119-3 stained with 1% rose bengal as the antigen [59]. It mainly detects IgM and IgG1 [30] mostly produced against LPS from smooth *Brucella* [60]. The antigen is buffered at an acidic pH (3.65 ± 0.5) in order to limit the agglutination due to IgM increasing the specificity of the technique [53]. The main advantage of this test is its high sensitivity, which makes it very suitable as a first screening test for determining the presence/absence of infection at the herd level [59, 61, 62]. The sensitivity (Se) and specificity (Sp) of this test have been extensively evaluated in different epidemiological scenarios in cattle (with Se estimates ranging from 53% to 100% and Sp from 79% to 100% [63-70]), small ruminants [Se ranges between 75.8% and 100% and Sp between 68.4% and 100% [66, 67, 71-73]), and pigs (Se estimates from 66% to 100% and Sp from 45.5% to 100% [32, 55, 74-76]). Its few technical requirements, speed for obtaining results, and low cost coupled with its performance have made this diagnostic tool one of the most widely used tests for the diagnosis of animal brucellosis. Its main disadvantages are related to its limited specificity in certain conditions, often due to cross-reacting antibodies derived from previous vaccination or exposure to other Gram-negative bacteria [77]. In many countries, the RBT is used as a first screening tool so that positive reactions are subsequently confirmed with an additional technique applied in series if no evidences of infection exist in the epidemiological unit. Due to its reliability, the RBT is one of the techniques described for international trade in cattle, small ruminants, and swine [59, 62].

Complement Fixation Test (CFT)

This test is based on the ability of the complement (obtained from guinea pig serum) to lyse erythrocytes (traditionally sheep erythrocytes sensitized with hemolysin) in the absence of an antibody-antigen complex. When *Brucella*-specific antibodies are present in the serum being analyzed, they bind to the *Brucella* antigens (whole cells) provided externally, forming antigen-antibody complexes that then bind to the complement [78]. In this case, the amount of complement in the reaction decreases, preventing its attachment to the hemolysin and the subsequent lysis of the erythrocytes that are added in the final stage. Procedures for performing this technique are described in the OIE Manual of Diagnostic Tests and Vaccines for Terrestrial Animals [59, 61, 62]. Many studies have evaluated the sensitivity and specificity of this technique, showing a slightly to moderately better overall performance in general compared with the RBT (Se estimates vary from 80.6% to 98.79% in small ruminants [66, 67, 79] and from 53% to 100% in cattle [63, 68, 69], and Sp values range between 65.5% and 100% in small ruminants [66, 67, 79] and between 80% and 100% in cattle [63, 68, 69]). Due to its high performance, the CFT has been broadly used as a confirmatory technique in the programs of eradication and control of brucellosis in cattle and small ruminants (for confirmation of RBT-positive results) and is prescribed for international trade. However, under field conditions, the CFT may show a lower sensitivity than RBT, which makes it a very reliable test at the herd level but more limited at the individual level [35, 80]. The sensitivity of this test is also directly related to the stage of infection of the animal being tested, with higher values for animals in an acute phase than in chronically infected ruminants [81]. The disadvantages of this technique are derived from the subjectivity of its interpretation (especially for low titers), the complexity of its performance, and the unavoidable variability of reagents, procedures, etc., that makes comparison of results difficult [82]. Moreover, false positives may also occur in animals sensitized with *Y. enterocolitica* O:9 [83] and in those immunized with smooth vaccines (Rev. 1 in small ruminants or S19 in cattle [59, 80]) as in the case of RBT. The natural anticomplementary activity of sheep serum must also be considered because it can lead to the occurrence of false-positive reactions [23]. Furthermore, the swine complement interacts with the guinea pig complement used in the test, resulting in a procomplementary activity that may reduce its sensitivity in pigs [32, 84-86]. Nevertheless, the CFT is still contemplated by the OIE as a diagnostic technique of election for swine [61], with a wide range of specificity estimates (from 40% to 100% depending on the study [32, 87, 88]).

Enzyme-Linked Immunosorbent Assay (ELISA)

Since the first ELISA-based technique in the diagnosis of brucellosis [89], many studies have assessed its usefulness. ELISAs based on the use of LPS as the main antigen are considered the most useful and are widely employed. This has led to the commercialization of many ELISA kits (including indirect and competition ELISAs) for its use in domestic species. Based on currently available information, the sensitivity of ELISA-based techniques is similar or greater than that of RB and FC tests, although the actual values may vary depending on the study (from 67% to 100% in small ruminants [71, 72, 90, 91], from 67.9% to 100% in cattle [63, 65, 68, 69], and from 68.5% to 100% in pigs [32, 55, 74, 75]). The specificity of these tests is also considered very high (from 94.5% to 100% in small ruminants [71, 73, 91, 92], from 90.5% to 100% in cattle [63, 65, 68, 69], and from 76% to 100% in pigs [32, 55, 74, 75]). For these reasons,

ELISAs are considered by the OIE adequate tests for the diagnosis of bovine, small ruminants, and porcine brucellosis [59, 61, 62], with the advantages of the possible automation of the technique, its reproducibility, and its objective interpretation (since a quantitative value is obtained as the final result). However, ELISAs based on LPS may suffer from the same diagnostic interference problems due to vaccine antibodies [53] and false-positive serological reactors (FPRS) associated with the presence of antibodies against *Y. enterocolitica* O:9 or other Gram-negative bacteria (mainly in swine [55] and cattle [70]) as those described for RBT and FCT. Due to these diagnostic limitations, the use of other antigens (e.g., proteins of outer or cytoplasmic membrane) has been evaluated for the development of new ELISA techniques for brucellosis diagnosis. However, in general, the serological response induced by these non-LPS antigens is considered to be heterogeneous and delayed compared with that observed using LPS antigen, which may affect the performance of diagnostic tests in the context of a control and eradication program. Still, extensive research has been carried out in this regard, with numerous studies focusing on the development of ELISAs based on proteins that could help to differentiate vaccinated from infected cattle, sheep, and goats (see section Development of Diagnostic Techniques for the Differentiation of Infected and Vaccinated Animals (DIVA)). Other studies have focused on protein targets that may allow the differentiation of *Brucella*-infected animals from those exposed to other bacteria, usually *Y. enterocolitica* O:9, mainly in pigs and cattle (BP26 protein, cytoplasmic protein extracts). However, these tests have generally shown a lower sensitivity than the ELISAs based on the LPS [70, 76].

Other indirect diagnostic tests based on the humoral immune response against *Brucella* spp.

Besides the abovementioned serological techniques, other tests have been developed for the diagnosis of *Brucella* spp. in animals. Among those, one of the most frequently used techniques is the fluorescence polarization assay (FPA), considered by the OIE as a valid technique for international trade in cattle, small ruminants, and pigs [59, 61, 62]. This test has similar or superior diagnostic performance compared with conventional techniques (CFT/RBT), being technically easier to perform [50, 75, 79, 93, 94]. Thus, in bovine, its use is recommended instead the CFT [59]. Another technique that has been widely used in certain countries is the standard agglutination test (SAT). This assay shows, however, a lower sensitivity and specificity than others, such as RBT and FCT in small ruminants [46, 95-97]. Still, its usefulness in these animal species has been demonstrated [98]. In cattle, SAT has been widely employed in brucellosis eradication programs as a confirmatory test [63, 99]. However, the OIE does not recommend nowadays the use of SAT for international trade in cattle [59] due to its lower specificity compared to CFT [59]. Nevertheless, SAT (and also the FPA) has demonstrated a higher sensitivity compared with the CFT for the detection of recently infected animals [100]. In swine, SAT has also been widely used [101, 102], and it is currently referred as a confirmatory technique in the EU international trade in pigs, although the OIE highlights that it may show a limited specificity due to the presence of nonspecific IgM antibodies in swine serum [61]. Finally, the milk ring test (MRT) has demonstrated its usefulness to detect specific antibodies against *Brucella* spp. in bovine milk samples used at herd level [59, 103], although its sensitivity may be impaired when it is used in large herds, and its use in small flocks is not recommended due to the expected low specificity [59, 62].

2.2.1.2. Indirect diagnostic tests based on the cellular immune response against Brucella spp.

Brucellin Skin Test (BST)

This diagnostic test involves the intradermal injection of a mixture of cytosolic proteins generally extracted from a *B. melitensis* rough strain (e.g., *B. melitensis* B115-Brucellin INRA) [104] that will induce a delayed hypersensitivity reaction (Type IV) [35] if the animal has previously contacted the bacteria. Recent studies have studied the usefulness of *B. abortus ΔmanBcore* as an alternative source of antigens for the BST for swine brucellosis diagnosis [87, 105]. The inoculation is usually performed in the lower eyelid in small ruminants [62], in the caudal fold, in the skin of the flank or the side of the neck in cattle [59], and in the base of the ear or the side of the tail in pigs [61]. Free-LPS antigens are required to prevent the subsequent induction of cross-reacting antibodies that may interfere with the traditional serological tests [81]. The main characteristic of BST is its high specificity, which makes it a useful tool to elucidate problems due to FPSR caused by *Y. enterocolitica* O:9 [106, 107], especially in brucellosis-free areas [25, 44], and as a complementary technique to serological tests [108]. However, occasional false-positive reactions due to *Ochrobactrum anthropi* infection have also been described [109]. In addition, its use is exclusively indicated in unvaccinated animals. This technique may be of particular interest to detect animals in the early and chronic stages of infection [23, 108], but its limited sensitivity makes its interpretation at the individual level difficult. Still, it is considered a suitable tool for *Brucella* diagnosis at herd level. Herd history, clinical signs, and serological or bacteriological results should be considered in the interpretation of the BST results. In ruminants, BST is recognized as an alternative technique for international trade [62]. In the case of swine brucellosis, it is not currently regarded as an official test, although its usefulness is supported by the EFSA and the OIE as a complementary diagnostic test [32, 61].

Interferon Gamma (IFN-γ) Detection

The interferon gamma is one of the most important cytokines involved in the cellular immune response against *Brucella* [110-112]. The usefulness of the in vitro quantification of IFN-γ produced by cells from naturally infected animals for monitoring the cellular immune response against this pathogen has been studied in cattle [113], porcine [107], and sheep [114, 115]. The levels of IFN-γ measured in samples stimulated with a *Brucella*-specific antigen (and that should be especially high in cases of previous contact with *Brucella* spp.) are typically quantified using an ELISA. This technique has been suggested as a complementary test to the serological techniques routinely used for the diagnosis of brucellosis in ruminants in the case of false-positive reactors due to its specificity [113], although there is still some controversy about its usefulness as a routine diagnostic technique for brucellosis.

2.2.2. Direct diagnostic tests

These techniques are based on the direct detection of the etiologic agent or its genetic material in clinical samples from infected animals. *Brucella* isolation is the gold standard for confirmation of infection [59, 61, 62, 116], and its use is recommended to improve the efficiency of eradication plans [25]. The use of specific staining methods (e.g., Stamp's method) in clinical specimens may reveal the existence of *Brucella* in clinical samples, although the limited sensitivity and specificity (especially due to the potential presence of other abortifacient pathogens such as *Chlamydia abortus* and *Coxiella burnetii* [62] that may lead to false-positive results) of this diagnostic approach can compromise its usefulness for the routine laboratory diagnosis of brucellosis.

2.2.2.1. *Bacteriology*

The World Health Organization classifies the *Brucella* genus bacteria as a risk agent III [62], and therefore high laboratory and training requirements are needed to handle the pathogen and potentially contaminated samples. The preferred samples for the direct detection of *Brucella* spp. are as follows: (i) in live animals: vaginal swab, milk, placenta, and fetus aborted samples (especially lung, spleen, and stomach contents) and (ii) postmortem: the reticuloendothelial system, udder, uterus, testis, and epididymis [25, 59, 61, 62, 117]. The possible contamination of clinical samples requires the use of selective media, frequently Thayer-Martin and Farrel media, for the isolation of *Brucella* spp. [59, 61, 62]. However, the presence of some components in the Farrel medium may have an inhibitory effect on some *B. abortus* and *B. melitensis* strains as well as in the *B. suis* biovar 2 [118]. Thus, the combination of more than one selective culture media and inoculation of at least two plates of each sample, including also a nonselective media for the isolation of *B. suis* biovar 2, may help to increase the chance of isolation of the pathogen [119]. The addition of serum or blood (usually from horse) to the media promotes the growth of *Brucella* spp. [82] and is necessary in the case of *B. abortus* biovar 2 [59]. Moreover, some strains of *B. abortus* (biovars 1-4 and 9) need a 5-10% CO_2 atmosphere [59]. Microbiological culture has a limited sensitivity in certain epidemiological situations, such as chronically infected animals that have typically low bacterial load in their samples. For this reason, negative culture result should not be considered as definitive evidence to rule out *Brucella* infection in an animal/herd [29, 120]. In fact, the sensitivity of culture is highly variable, depending on the stage of infection, the specimens analyzed, and the number of samples cultured [100, 102, 118, 121-123].

2.2.2.2. *Molecular detection*

DNA-based techniques allow the detection of nonviable *Brucella* or highly contaminated samples that may be challenging if handled using a traditionally culture-based diagnostic approach. In addition, molecular techniques may be applied at large scale through the use of automated equipment. PCR techniques are also routinely used for identification of *Brucella*-compatible isolates cultured from clinical samples. A considerable number of molecular techniques based on the PCR amplification of *Brucella* spp. DNA has been described, although often these techniques have not been fully validated on field samples as direct detection tests, hampering their implementation as routine techniques for *Brucella* detection [124]. Despite the high homology of DNA among *Brucella* species, different PCR protocols to identify different species/biovar and even vaccine/field strains have been described [125-133]. The efficiency in the DNA extraction procedure (which depends on the nature of the sample [134]) determines substantially the results of the PCR assays [135-137].

2.3. Immunization

Since Eduard Jenner described the first vaccine against smallpox in 1796, the immunization against infectious agents has become a cornerstone in the control of many of the most important infectious diseases. As general rule, vaccination efforts are often focused in the most susceptible individuals in order to stimulate a protective immune response against the pathogen of interest. However, in the case of animal brucellosis, vaccination campaigns target a less susceptible population (nulliparous nonpregnant young sheep, goats, and cows), while vaccination of the most susceptible subset is avoided due to the side effects of vaccination of pregnant animals (abortion, bacteria excretion, environmental contamination, etc.) [26].

The characteristics of the "ideal vaccine against brucellosis" include the following: (i) to induce a solid and long-lasting protection against the infection by different *Brucella* species without the need of re-vaccinations, (ii) to be innocuous regardless of the reproductive stage of the animal (so that there is no induction of abortion in pregnant animals, and mass vaccination can be applied if needed), (iii) to have no or very residual virulence for human and be susceptible to the antibiotics typically used to treat human brucellosis, (iv) to avoid the induction of cross-reacting antibodies in the serological techniques traditionally used in control/eradication programs, (v) to be affordable, and (vi) to possess stability at different environmental temperatures [138, 139]. Unfortunately, this ideal vaccine is far from those currently available for the control of animal brucellosis. For example, in the case of small ruminant brucellosis, Rev. 1 has been recognized as the most effective vaccine currently available considering its efficacy to prevent the abortion and transmission of *B. melitensis*, but it cannot be applied in pregnant females and is pathogenic for humans, among other nondesirable side effects [139]. The smooth S19 strain is the most widely employed vaccine in the case of bovine brucellosis, and even though it is currently considered the reference strain, it presents similar limitations as the Rev. 1 despite its demonstrated efficacy. For these reasons, the rough strain RB51 is increasingly used in some regions of the world as an alternative for vaccination against bovine brucellosis since its use does not induce the production of cross-reacting antibodies, even though its efficacy is still under discussion in certain epidemiological situations [140]. In general, the inability to vaccinate pregnant animals is a major disadvantage in animal brucellosis vaccination since it complicates achieving a quick increase in the proportion of the resistant subset of the population, which could lead to an average benefit-cost ratio of 3.2 (2.27-4.37) by reducing (52%) the transmission between animals by means of mass vaccination [21].

The success of the use of live vaccines for immunization against animal brucellosis is based on a balance between an adequate colonization of the host, triggering a solid protection against infection with other *Brucella* field strains, and a limited replication that minimizes the residual virulence of these vaccine strains [141]. Although immunological mechanisms induced by living vaccine have not been completely elucidated, live vaccines should stimulate the innate immunity, activate CD8+ and CD4+ cells, and generate an adequate population of memory cells, among other mechanisms, to induce a solid protection [139].

Most of the drawbacks associated with the use of live vaccines could be overcome with the use of killed bacteria or subunit vaccines; however, the ability of these inactivated vaccines to

http://dx.doi.org/10.5772/61222

provide a solid and long-lasting immune response against *Brucella* has been traditionally considered lower than that triggered by live attenuated vaccines. New approaches are being investigated to elude the main drawbacks of inactivated vaccines to induce protective immunity in domestic livestock.

In the following section, the main drawbacks of currently available vaccines (Rev. 1 for SRB and S19/RB51 for BB) are described, as well as some of the new approaches followed to solve some of these shortcomings.

2.3.1. Residual virulence of attenuated live vaccines

The pathogenicity of Rev. 1 and S19, evident in its ability to induce abortion, has been a limitation since they were first used. However, in the case of Rev. 1, some authors have reported significant differences in its residual virulence. In a study performed to assess the immunogenicity and residual virulence of Rev. 1 strains recovered from different geographic origins, important differences between strains were identified [142], which may explain, at least in part, the diversity of results sometimes reported using this strain. For this reason, according to the OIE recommendations, strict quality controls must be maintained during the Rev. 1 production process in order to confirm that all batches have the typical characteristic of the original *B. melitensis* biovar 1 Rev. 1 strain. Residual virulence of Rev. 1 and S19 is reflected in the following sections.

2.3.1.1. Abortifacient effect

The ability of Rev. 1 to induce abortions was reported in the first studies, around the middle of the last century [143]. This adverse effect is especially significant when females are immunized around midpregnancy [144]. The abortifacient effect of the S19 strain has been demonstrated, although it is considered reduced and lower than that observed after Rev. 1 vaccination in general [140]. The appearance of a small percentage of vaccinated animals that may remain persistently infected with the S19 strain has also been described and may lead to abortions in adulthood [145]. In addition, vaccination may involve the excretion of the vaccine strain in milk and vaginal secretions [146, 147]. Even so, although the possible excretion of Rev. 1 during the lactation has been demonstrated, there is some disagreement about the relevance of this phenomenon [148].

Different strategies have been explored in order to avoid the abortifacient effect of Rev. 1 and S19, as described in the following sections.

Restriction of vaccination to replacement females (nulliparous, nonpregnant)

The protection induced by vaccination at full doses in 3-6-month-old animals using Rev. 1 [149, 150] and in 3-8-month-old animals using S19 [59, 151] is sufficient to induce a long-lasting protection. However, this control strategy may be problematic in certain epidemiological situations (e.g., high prevalence of brucellosis when mass vaccination is the only strategy to control the disease [24]).

Application of reduced doses of vaccine

Different studies have demonstrated the suitability of the immunization with reduced doses as an alternative to full dosages of vaccines, assuming that the afforded immunity was adequate and/or the abortion rate associated with the vaccination was significantly lower [59, 152-154]. However, field results obtained after the application of Rev. 1/S19 at reduced doses has led to a divergence of opinions among different experts about its usefulness and implications: many authors have reported a significant number of reproductive failures/vaccine excretion [155-157], advising against the use of this strategy in brucellosis control programs. In addition, some authors have showed that this immunization strategy using Rev. 1/S19 induces an inadequate protection against *B. melitensis*/*B. abortus* infection [156-159]. Additionally, reduced doses may not avoid the induction of persistent antibody titters when Rev. 1 and S19 are applied in adult animals, leading to a diagnostic interference problem with traditional serological techniques [59, 153, 156]. However, other experts have argued in favor of the efficacy of this approach as part of some brucellosis control programs [160-163]. In the case of S19, some experiments have shown that the best protection was obtained by subcutaneous vaccination of calves at full doses followed by conjunctival administration of a booster reduced dose [164].

Modification of route of vaccination

Although the application of Rev. 1 by the conjunctival route has been demonstrated to reduce the number of reproductive failures induced after subcutaneously immunization of pregnant females, the safety of this immunization strategy is not enough to be used regardless of the physiological stage of females [144, 146]. In bovine, S19 conjunctival vaccination does not avoid completely abortions in pregnant females [155], although it is considered that the conjunctival administration in reduced doses (5×10^9 microorganisms) is an alternative route in adult vaccination due to the reduction of abortion rates [59].

2.3.1.2. Other side effects

In addition to the induction of reproductive failures, other adverse effects, as transient periods of fever and anorexia or swelling at the vaccination site, have been reported after Rev. 1 vaccination [31]. Some studies have showed a risk of environmental contamination with the vaccine strain after Rev. 1 vaccination of young females, suggesting these animals are shedding the Rev. 1 strain and could therefore be a source of infection for other susceptible individuals [165, 166]. However, other authors have reported that conjunctival vaccination of nonpregnant animals immunized is safe for the environment [167, 168]. Some occasional contradictory effects (as orchitis) in billy goat and ram have also been reported [169, 170]. Regarding to the S19 vaccine, other side effects reported include the appearance of arthropathies associated with type III hypersensitivity reactions [171], persistent orchitis in males [153], and significant reduction in milk production and udder infections [140, 172].

2.3.2. Zoonotic potential and antibiotic resistance of attenuated living vaccines

A limited number of human brucellosis due to Rev. 1 [173, 174] and S19 [175-177] infection has been reported. The risk of infection for human and environmental contamination is nevertheless reduced if the adequate biosafety practices during handling these live vaccines are followed. Rev. 1 and RB51 carry antibiotic resistance genes to streptomycin and rifampicin, respectively, which are used in the treatment of human brucellosis. In the case of S19, resistance to penicillin G (associated with an increased virulence in mice) has been evidenced [178].

2.3.3. *Instability of vaccine strains*

The possible instability of Rev. 1 is due to its tendency to dissociate into a rough phenotype, reducing its effectiveness in the field [138]. Several strategies such as the addition of 5% of serum (from horse, cattle, or rabbit) on the solid medium used for Rev. 1 production have been demonstrated to be useful to prevent this dissociation [179]. Biological quality and efficacy of S19 may be affected by inadequate subculture or maintenance conditions [180]. In the field, the main strategy to prevent this instability is the strict control of refrigeration temperatures for storage during all the process until the moment of inoculation (what could be problematic in certain circumstances, leading to the application of low-quality vaccines) [181]. In addition, preliminary observations also suggest that a reversion to a more pathogenic phenotype of the Rev. 1 strain is also possible [166], although the genetic stability and homogeneity of Rev. 1 strains is considered demonstrated [182].

2.3.4. *Diagnostic interference in serological techniques*

The smooth LPS antibodies induced after Rev. 1 and S19 vaccination are indistinguishable from those triggered after infection with a smooth field *Brucella* strain. The Rev. 1-derived antibodies may be detected even 4 years after vaccination depending on the age of the animal at vaccination, the immunization doses, and the serological technique being used [183]. For this reason, vaccination using smooth Rev. 1 and S19 creates a diagnostic interference problem when test-and-slaughter (T&S) programs based on the use of traditional serological techniques are in place, complicating the combination of these two strategies. The following sections present three possible approaches to overcome this diagnostic interference problem.

2.3.4.1. *Reduction of the serological response induced by Rev. 1 vaccination*

- Application of reduced doses of vaccine (see section Application of Reduced Doses of Vaccine)

- Restriction of vaccination to replacement females [nulliparous, nonpregnant; see section ′Restriction of Vaccination to Replacement Females (Nulliparous, Nonpregnant)].

- Modification of the route of vaccination

The subcutaneous route, traditionally used for the immunization with Rev. 1 and S19 in small ruminants and cattle, respectively, triggers a solid and long-lasting serological response (at least up to 20 months after vaccination in goats [184] and 22 months in cattle [185]). However, in the last 30 years, the usefulness of the alternative use of the conjunctival route has been demonstrated in cattle [164, 186] and small ruminants [187]. Vaccination of young animals using Rev. 1 inoculated by the conjunctival route induces a limited serological response but is able to trigger an adequate protection for at least the two first pregnancies following vaccination) [188]. The serological response induced by conjunctival Rev. 1 vaccination is more long-lasting in adults, therefore leading to the potential occurrence of diagnostic interference problems [187], although these would be still more limited than those observed after its application by the subcutaneous route [189].

In the case of the S19 vaccination, the OIE suggests an alternative immunization protocol based on the application of 5×10^9 CFUs conjunctively in bovines regardless of the age of the animal [59]. Thus, as mentioned above, the vaccination protocol based on subcutaneous application of S19 during calfhood and conjunctival revaccination using reduced doses in adult animals has been proved as a suitable strategy for the control of BB in endemic populations, which avoids the need for slaughter of false-positive reactors [164]

2.3.4.2. Development of diagnostic techniques for the Differentiation of Infected and Vaccinated Animals (DIVA)

Different studies have been carried out to identify immunogenic non-LPS components that could allow the development of diagnostic techniques able to detect the serological response induced by *Brucella* field strains only. Some studies have showed promising results, but most of the authors also report limitations (such as less intense and more heterogeneous antibody response, lack of information about diagnostic performance under field conditions, etc.) that make their routine implementation on animal brucellosis control/eradication campaigns difficult. In the case of S19, the use of competition ELISAs coated with S-LPS allows the removal of most false-positive responses due to vaccination-derived cross-reacting antibodies [59, 93, 190, 191].

The use of several non-LPS *Brucella* components as the main antigen for DIVA serological techniques has been described, including the following:

- *Proteins.* The detection of immunogenic proteins involved in the humoral immune response of the host in the outer membrane of *Brucella* was the first step in the development of alternative serological methods for brucellosis diagnosis. In the case of *B. melitensis,* CP28 (also called BP26) was recognized as a good candidate to distinguish between Rev. 1 vaccinated and infected animals [192]. Several indirect [193, 194] and competitive [195] ELISAs have been developed to assess the suitability of CP28 as a diagnostic target for small ruminant brucellosis diagnosis, showing a lower diagnostic performance than that detected using ELISAs based on the LPS antibodies response [196]. In the case of *B. abortus,* different protein antigens (*N*-formylperosamine *O*-polysaccharide-protein conjugate [197], an extract of cytoplasmic proteins of *Brucella* and an 18-kDa cytoplasmic protein [198]) have been described as suitable candidates for the development of new immunological tests for screening and infection confirmatory diagnosis. Additionally, Pajuaba *et al.* showed that the AHRPO protein (protein A-horseradish peroxidase) is an adequate conjugate for the development of an indirect ELISA (that uses *B. abortus* S-LPS as an antigen) to differentiate S19 vaccinated and *B. abortus*-infected animals due to a preferential detection of the IgG2 isotype, a valuable marker of *Brucella* infection [199].

- *Polysaccharides.* The native hapten, one of the polysaccharides present in the surface of smooth *Brucella* strains, has also been used as a potential antigen in an agar gel immunodiffusion (AGID) test to solve the potential diagnostic interference problem. When antibodies against this polysaccharide are present (samples from *B. abortus*/*B. melitensis*-infected ruminants), a ring of precipitations appears in the agar [200, 201]. If samples from vaccinated (and uninfected) animals are analyzed several months after vaccination, no antibodies against the polysaccharide would be detected. In adult cattle, subcutaneous vaccination with reduced doses does not produce positive reactions (except for those animals that are infected and excrete the bacteria in milk [202]). The AGID test has demonstrated its usefulness to solve diagnostic interference problems in bovine and small ruminants [77, 203, 204], although some authors have also reported a sensitivity too limited for its wide-scale application [53]. This technique has also been demonstrated to be suitable to elucidate cases of FPSR due to *Y. enterocolitica* infection in cattle [70].

2.3.4.3. Use of rough vaccine strains (lack of O-PS or O-PS defective strains)

Rough *Brucella* strains are naturally devoid of the O-PS, which confers them a more granular and dull surface compared with those carrying complete S-LPS (smooth strains). Due to the lack of antigenic O-PS, these rough mutants may not induce anti-O-PS antibodies and, therefore, do not cause diagnostic interferences in most serodiagnostic tests. The rough phenotype can be observed by crystal violet staining (rough strains uptake the staining turning to red/violet) or autoagglutination in acriflavine solution [140]. In 1997, a WHO Consultation on the Development of New/Improved Brucellosis Vaccines encouraged the need of studies on live attenuated rough vaccines as an alternative to smooth strains for immunization against brucellosis [205]. Mutant rough *Brucella* strains are obtained by (i) natural dissociation of smooth (S) to rough (R) phenotype and subsequent repeated in vivo or in vitro passages of R mutants or (ii) genetic modification of the sequence of genes involved in the synthesis/transportation of component(s) of the smooth LPS [140]. Despite the potential advantages associated with the use of rough strains as vaccine candidates, some potential undesirable traits may make their application in the field difficult:

- The attenuation of R mutants has been associated to modifications in the outer membrane of *Brucella* and, therefore, possible changes in their interaction with components of the immune system of the host [206]. If the attenuation is too high, the rapid clearance of the R mutants in the host may lead to an insufficient protection [140]. However, natural rough *Brucella* species (*B. canis* and *B. ovis*) are virulent for their preferred hosts, and in fact, the role of LPS in the pathogenesis of *Brucella* is controversial: although the protection against *Brucella* is mainly mediated by the cellular immune response (triggered primarily by bacterial antigenic proteins), the humoral response (antibodies) may also have a role in the resistance against *Brucella*, as demonstrated by passive immunity experiment with sera against the LPS [207-209] and even with antibodies against the rough *B. melitensis* B115 strain [210] (see section Control of Small Ruminant Brucellosis).

- The diagnostic interference associated to the smooth phenotype of *Brucella* may not be totally avoided with the use of rough strains since animals vaccinated with R strains have showed occasional reactions to the S-LPS ELISA [211].

- The possible zoonotic potential of rough *Brucella* strains may limit their large-scale use. In the case of human brucellosis due to rough *Brucella* strains, traditional serological techniques, based on the detection of antibodies against S-LPS, may not detect the infection leading to misdiagnosis [140]. A possible alternative in this case would be the use of specific techniques for the detection of antibody response against rough *Brucella*, such as the CFT developed for the detection of rough B115 *B. melitensis* infection in sheep [212].

In the case of bovine brucellosis, the suitability of several rough vaccines (45/20, *pgm* mutant, RB51, *Brucella abortus* strain 82) for the control of the infection due to *B. abortus* has been evaluated [213-216]. However, RB51 vaccine could be considered the main representative example of the potential usefulness of rough *Brucella* vaccines in the battle against animal brucellosis. RB51 (R: rough; B: *Brucella*; 51: identification number of the laboratory of origin) is a stable rough rifampicin resistant *B. abortus* strain produced after repeated passages of *B. abortus* strain 2308 on trypticase soy supplemented with 1.5% agar and varying concentrations of rifampin or penicillin [215]. No O-PS antibodies were detected in rabbits, goats, and cattle after immunization with this strain [215, 217, 218], although some authors have reported low level of M-like O-chain in vaccinated species [219] and certain apparent anamnestic responses have been reported [220]. The induction of none to very limited vaccine-mediated abortions has been reported in cattle [221, 222], although contradictory evidences have also been reported [223]. In cattle, RB51 triggered an adequate protection against infection with virulent *B. abortus* strains [151, 224, 225], but certain concerns have been raised regarding its suitability in certain epidemiological situations in the field (see section Control of Bovine Brucellosis). RB51 has also been evaluated as a tool for the control of small ruminant and swine brucellosis. In the case of *B. suis*, some authors have demonstrated its usefulness preventing abortion in swine [226], although recent studies have demonstrated the inefficacy of parental RB51 vaccination to induce humoral or cell-mediated immune responses or to protect against abortion in a virulent challenge with *B suis* in domestic pigs [85]. Protection induced by RB51 vaccination against *B. melitensis* was also insufficient to consider it as a potential candidate in the prevention of ovine brucellosis [227], although the results regarding the suitability of this vaccine strain for the immunization of goats are controversial [140, 228, 229].

Many attempts have been conducted to achieve a stable immunogenic rough vaccine against *B. melitensis* using genetic engineering [VTRM1- *rfbU* mutant, *rpoB* mutant, *wa***, and *wzm* mutant, B115) [206, 211, 230-232]. In the case of swine brucellosis, a recent study of Stoffreger *et al.* has demonstrated that a rough *B. suis* strain (353-1), isolated from urine of a feral boar and prepared by propagation from the original isolation on Tryptose agar containing 5% bovine serum (TSA) at 37°C and 5% CO_2, can induce a significant immune response and confer a partial level of protection from a challenge with a virulent *B. suis* [233]. However, no rough vaccine candidate is currently recognized as a suitable alternative for immunization of sheep/goats and swine in the framework of an animal brucellosis control program.

3. Control of bovine brucellosis

The OIE has established the following requirements for a country/zone to be considered as free from this disease: (i) BB is declared notifiable; (ii) an official veterinary control is established in the entire bovine population, in which flock prevalence of disease is lower than 0.2%; (iii) no vaccination has been performed in the last 3 years (at least); (iv) all herds are subjected to periodical serological testing; (v) all reactors are culled; and (vi) new animals introduced in the region belong to officially brucellosis-free (OBF) herds (or free of brucellosis with vaccination). Some countries (France, Germany, Norway, Sweden, The Netherlands, Japan, Canada, Australia, and New Zealand, among others [59]) are considered to be OBF, but the disease is still present in many others despite the implementation of control/eradication programs. In general, measures against BB are based on vaccination (when the prevalence is high, in the initial steps of the control strategies) and test-and-slaughter programs (or herd depopulation when the disease prevalence is already very low and economic and technical resources are available) in the final stages of the eradication process prior to the achievement of the OBF status. These measures (vaccination, test and slaughter programs, and herd depopulation) alone cannot however be fully effective in eradicating the disease without the additional implementation of other complementary prevention measures, such as control of animal movements, use of surveillance systems, adequate laboratory support, etc.

Even though the role of wildlife reservoirs in the epidemiology of bovine brucellosis is considered minimal in most countries in the world, several wild species in certain scenarios can act as reservoirs of the disease for cattle, such as wild bison elk in the Greater Yellowstone Area (USA) [234]. In these situations, wild populations should be considered in the design of BB control programs.

In the case of BB, two vaccines are available for the control of *B. abortus* in cattle: the S19 (smooth) and the RB51 (rough) strains, which have demonstrated their effectiveness in the reduction of the number of abortion, transmission, excretion, etc., in certain epidemiological situations [235].

The S19 strain has been the main vaccine used against bovine brucellosis in many countries for more than 50 years. Numerous studies have demonstrated the usefulness of S19 calfhood vaccination with full doses (10^{10} CFUs) to protect them against *B. abortus* infection during their whole productive lifespan [236]. However, as mentioned before, its smooth nature may lead to the induction of O-PS antibodies that may persist until the adulthood, causing a diagnostic interference problem. Nevertheless, adult vaccination may be occasionally recommended in certain scenarios (high prevalence settings in which a rapid impact on disease spread is needed, large herds in which test-and-slaughter strategies are not feasible). Still, adult vaccination remains an emergency measure since the induction of vaccine antibodies and the possible abortifacient effect of S19 in pregnant cows are two very important side effects that would be associated with it. The use of reduced doses of S19 vaccine (10^{9} CFUs) in adults can partially limit those side effects, but its full usefulness is debatable [214, 237]. Immunization with RB51 vaccine (rough strain with a minimal expression of O-PS) for the control of *B. abortus* infection has emerged as an alternative to S19/stamping out in certain scenarios [238]. However, its true usefulness and its ability to induce a degree of protection equivalent to that induced with the S19 vaccine are still under discussion. The safety and protection afforded by RB51 against infection with *B. abortus* have been demonstrated in experimental conditions [224, 239, 240], but some of these results are still considered controversial [140]. Field evidences suggest RB51 could be considered a useful complementary tool for BB control [151, 238, 241], but the impossibility of comparing the progress achieved by strategies with and without RB51 vaccination under the exact same conditions in most cases impairs the evaluation of the relative contribution of RB51 vaccination to the overall success of an eradication program [242]. Recent studies have showed a potential beneficial effect of an RB51 booster vaccination in adult cattle after S19 calfhood vaccination to control *B. abortus* infection [243].

Even though *B. abortus* is undoubtedly the main concern when dealing with infection in cattle, *B. melitensis* is also a potential etiologic agent of brucellosis in bovine. The control of *B. melitensis* infection in cattle is hampered by the lack of information on important aspects of its epidemiology [244]. Outbreaks due to *B. melitensis* in cattle are often attributed to the presence of infected small ruminants in the surrounding area [245], suggesting that the key for the control of this pathogen in bovine will be the control of the disease in ovine and caprine flocks, as for human brucellosis.

4. Control of small ruminant brucellosis

Even though the most important factors that have to be considered for the control of SRB have been well characterized, socioeconomic factors have influenced the choice of the most suitable control measures in most of the endemic areas. For example, the existence of pastoral ecosystems, a traditional management practice in low-income areas where *B. melitensis* is endemic, has contributed to the perpetuation of the disease due to the difficulty of detecting the disease in the early stages of infection and of implementing control measures [246]. In addition, management practices favoring the mixing of animals with different origins (for example, the existence of communal grazing pastures) modify the traditional concept of minimal epidemiological unit of intervention (an essential key to consider by decision makers of animal brucellosis control programs). The minimal epidemiological unit is defined as "any number of animals that are held, kept or handled in such a manner that they share the same risk of exposure to brucellosis" [247] and can therefore include the flock or supraflock levels.

Although extremely important, the prevalence of brucellosis is not the only issue to consider for decision makers: the organization of the veterinary services, the availability of a suitable animal identification system and of the economic and technical resources that these measures require, the involvement of producers, veterinarians, and administrative authorities, etc., are all key aspects that must be evaluated [24]. When the prevalence of brucellosis is high and/or the socioeconomic resources are limited, the vaccination is the most suitable tool for the control of the disease. Despite its drawbacks, Rev. 1 is the best currently available vaccine to immunize sheep and goats against *B. melitensis*. In order to minimize the diagnostic interference problem due to Rev. 1 cross-reacting antibodies, a restricted vaccination strategy has been implemented in most of the regions where test and slaughter policy is applied as part of the SRB control program. The vaccine is administered by the conjunctival route in young (<6 months) female animals at doses of 0.5-2 × 10^9 CFU/animal (also controlling the impact of the abortifacient effect of Rev. 1). Some authors [24, 31] have suggested that restricted vaccination may be insufficient in certain epidemiological situations (such as high prevalence regions or where nomadism is practiced) and mass vaccination should be implemented instead. The immunization at full doses by the conjunctival route during the prebreeding period and late lambing season would be the most suitable approach for whole flock vaccination because it may prevent reproductive failures due to Rev. 1 vaccination [156]. Blasco *et al.* [24] have described two methods to carry the whole flock vaccination in the case of sheep and goats: (i) mass vaccination of males and females every two years avoiding lambing period (and considering 15-25% annual replacement) and (ii) restricted vaccination of replacement animals (at least 8-10 years) except the first year when all animals would be immunized regardless of their age. When the prevalence has decreased, a restricted Rev. 1 strategy could be then implemented. In general, a vaccination program against SRB should last at least 8-10 years in order to assure an adequate vaccine coverage [24]. The correct identification of vaccinated animals is an important factor to achieve this vaccination coverage that will grant an adequate immunity at the flock level [33].

Despite the success achieved thanks to Rev. 1 vaccination in many regions of the world, the drawbacks associated with its use have prompted the study of alternative vaccines against *B. melitensis*: DNA vaccines, subunits vaccines, outer membrane vesicles, smooth *B. melitensis* mutants (BP26, P39, Omp25, and *ΔpurE201*), nondividing but metabolically active gamma-irradiated *Brucella melitensis*, and attenuated live rough vaccines [230, 231, 248-254]. Among rough vaccines against SRB, the B115 strain has demonstrated to induce a solid protection not only against *B. melitensis* but also against *B. ovis* and *B. abortus* in the murine model. An abortifacient effect was demonstrated in sheep after subcutaneous vaccination with B115, although the interference diagnostic problem was drastically reduced [255]. Still, the possible occurrence of reversions of its phenotype (rough to smooth) in vivo could affect its attenuation, thus highlighting the need of further studies to better determine the stability of B115 in sheep before giving it further consideration as a possible candidate for SRB vaccination.

When certain epidemiological indicators (disease prevalence, number of cases of human brucellosis, etc.) suggest the control of brucellosis has been achieved, the next step is to success in the eradication of the disease [24]. A restricted Rev. 1 immunization strategy should be implemented exclusively when the prevalence is already low after 6-12 years of whole-flock vaccination, a strict control of animal movements and an accurate animal identification system exist, and veterinary services and economic resources are available. The change from mass vaccination to restricted vaccination is a critical step in the control/eradication programs since it may suppose the culling of a high number of false seropositive adult vaccinated animals, even if conjunctival vaccination is performed. Two different approaches have been proposed to minimize this shortcoming [24]: (i) lack of testing for two years after the change from mass to restricted vaccination (after which a strict test and slaughter policy would be implemented, where all CFT-positive animals are culled and their flocks of origin retested until 100% of animals are seronegative at least two consecutive tests) and (ii) the implementation of a serological test capable of differentiate vaccinated from infected small ruminants as part of the test-and-slaughter strategy as soon as the whole flock vaccination is stopped (such as the radial immunodiffusion tests whose usefulness has been discussed before). The restricted vaccination should be maintained after the achievement of a close to zero brucellosis prevalence. After that, if the epidemiological situation is maintained and the risk of reintroduction of *B. melitensis* has been minimized, the prohibition of vaccination and the implementation of an eradication program based exclusively on test and slaughter policy could be proposed. Vaccination coverage, the implementation of other complementary measures, and the availability of an effective monitoring strategy should be considered by decision makers to establish the moment of vaccination ban [34]. The availability of economic and technical resources (economic compensation for farmers, strict animal movement control, etc.) is a cornerstone to ensure the success of a test-and-slaughter strategy in regions with close to zero disease prevalence.

5. Control of swine brucellosis

Porcine brucellosis is a notifiable OIE-listed disease [256]. However, in many countries, no specific control and eradication programs are implemented, and there is no obligation to conduct monitoring/surveillance strategies on the swine population for *Brucella* infection. Therefore, the actual prevalence of porcine brucellosis in many areas is not exactly known and probably is often underestimated. For example, in the case of EU Members States, the estimates of the prevalence of swine brucellosis vary depending on the region, but the current situation of *B. suis* in swine population is not totally recognized due to the lack of systematic epidemiologic data [32]. One of the main differences in the control and eradication of this pathology in swine compared to ruminant brucellosis is the lack of availability of safe and effective vaccines against *B. suis* as Rev. 1 for *B. melitensis* and S19/RB51 for *B. abortus* [32, 61]. Nowadays, the only country where vaccination against swine brucellosis is applied is China, where a national control program against this disease (mainly caused by *B. suis* biovar 1) was initiated due to the high rate of human brucellosis cases and the economic losses in animal production. In addition to animal vaccination, other strategies such as culling of all aborted females, separation and removal of infected animals, and quarantine policies were also implemented [257]. Since 1981, pigs have been immunized in China with a live attenuated *B. suis*S2 vaccine. In some brucellosis-infected areas with low prevalence, vaccination was only applied to young livestock so that test-and-slaughter programs could also be implemented. In other areas in which this was not feasible, an intermittent vaccination policy was applied, and the vaccinated animals were not tested to avoid the diagnostic interference problems caused by the use of this vaccine. The S2 vaccine can be administered by parenteral route or *per os*, although it should be applied at high doses (20×10^{10} FCU/animals) in two doses [257]. One of the side effects of this vaccine is that it can cause abortions in pregnant sows, and despite its wide use in China for decades, OIE does not recommend its use for the control of swine brucellosis, partly due to the absence of trials demonstrating its efficacy and safety in controlled conditions [61].

In general terms, although in most countries there are no specific plans for the control and eradication of porcine brucellosis, the most frequent approach for swine brucellosis control is the test and slaughter strategy, similar to that used in ruminants. Thus, eradication requires the identification of infected animals, the progressive elimination of reactors from the herd, and their replacement with noninfected animals (testing all animals and applying a quarantine period) [32]. The application of whole-herd slaughter when reactors are detected should be considered as one strategy that would reduce the risk of circulation within the drove and its spread to other holdings due to undetected infected animals. However, this measure is often not feasible because of the economic implications for farmers. On the other hand, whole-herd depopulation and repopulation with noninfected animals must be implemented in countries considered free of the disease [258]. An example of a country where this measure is used as part of its control an eradication program is the USA, where *B. suis* has been eradicated from commercial pigs [259], thanks to the great efforts invested in the last decades. In 1972, the U.S. Department of Agriculture National Brucellosis Eradication Program implemented in ruminants was expanded to cover swine herds, based on the serological testing and removal of reactors. Depending on the epidemiological situation, three strategies were implemented [260]: (i) whole-herd depopulation of infected herds and repopulation, recommended for commercial herds and seed stock producers who wish to eliminate swine brucellosis from their population rapidly, and often the solution in the final efforts at eradication; (ii) exceptionally, in herds with only one or a few reactors (and no clinical signs of swine brucellosis), frequent test and removal of reactors, although this option was not generally recommended; and (iii) offspring segregation: this plan was recommended where valuable bloodlines had to be saved and weaned pigs (usually negative when tested at weaning) were allowed to be moved to separate, clean premises (animals had to be retested at least once prior to breeding to tested, clean boars).

As part of a control program, certain conditions and testing are required to classify a herd as swine brucellosis free. Thus, herds may be validated as swine brucellosis free by conducting a complete herd test with negative results. Validation may be maintained by periodical testing of the whole herd with negative results. Besides USA, some other countries in America (such as Cuba and Panama) [261], where porcine brucellosis is present, have also implemented control and eradication programs based on these same approaches. Some countries and regions offer the farmers the option of implementing voluntary programs covered by the authorities in order to certify the flocks as swine brucellosis-free herds. These voluntary programs are based on the same principles as those used in the eradication and control programs, consisting of periodic serological testing of all animals in the herd and removal of reactors. This measure has been implemented in Argentina, being mandatory for local genetic suppliers and breeding animals destined for sale, fairs, auctions, and exhibitions [262]. Another example of voluntary program is in Australia, accepted by all states and nowadays implemented in Queensland, where *B. suis* is an enzootic disease of feral pigs [263]. Farms included in the Australian voluntary program should buy breeding stock only from herds registered in this scheme. If infection is detected in the herd, then the accreditation is withdrawn until all reactors are removed and the herd tested back to accreditation standards [264]. Another fundamental key for the control of swine brucellosis is the control of artificial insemination centers because they may be an important source of infection to many animals [265]. Therefore, control measures implemented in these centers are especially restrictive and have specific regulations for each country or region. These measures are based on serological testing and quarantine of all introduced animals (that must come from accredited *B. suis*-free farms), continuous serological monitoring of the whole population of the center, and preparation of semen doses following certain requirements [32].

Control of wildlife reservoirs is an important part of the swine brucellosis control and eradication in regions where the disease is widespread in wildlife and may get in contact with the commercial swine population. For example, in USA, where swine brucellosis remains endemic in feral swine [266], the control of PB in this wild species is included in the current program of control and eradication, with specific measures regarding the restriction of feral swine movement between states, including test and slaughter and control contact with domestic pigs. According to the OIE, treatment with antibiotics is not being implemented anywhere as a control measure [256]. Despite its potential application to control an outbreak at the farm level [267], antibiotic therapy is currently strongly discouraged because it does not allow the total clearance of the infection and involves the use of high doses with a considerable cost and poses some additional problems due to the limits of maximum residue in animals destined to human consumption.

Author details

Marta Pérez-Sancho[1*], Teresa García-Seco[1], Lucas Domínguez[1] and Julio Álvarez[2]

*Address all correspondence to: maperezs@visavet.ucm.es

1 Neglected and Emerging Diseases Unit, VISAVET Health Surveillance Centre, Universidad Complutense de Madrid, Madrid, Spain

2 Department of Veterinary Population Medicine, College of Veterinary Medicine, University of Minnesota, St. Paul, USA

References

[1] Allsup TN. Abortion in sheep associated with *Brucella abortus* infection. Veterinary Record. 1969;84(5):104-108.

[2] Stoenner HG. Isolation of *Brucella abortus* from sheep. Journal of the American Veterinary Medical Association 1951;118(887):101-102.

[3] Corbel MJ. Brucellosis: an overview. Emerging Infectious Diseases. 1997;3(2):213-221; PM:9204307.

[4] Refai M. Incidence and control of brucellosis in the Near East region. Veterinary Microbiology. 2002;90(1-4):81-110.

[5] Samaha H, Al-Rowaily M, Khoudair RM, and Ashour HM. Multicenter study of brucellosis in Egypt. Emerging Infectious Diseases. 2008;14(12):1916-1918.

[6] Zammit TA. A preliminary note on the examination of the blood of goats suffering from Mediterranean fever, Part III Proceedings of the Royal Society of London 1905; 76B:377-378.

[7] Bruce D. Note on the discovery of a microorganism in Malta Fever. Practitioner. 1887;39:161-170.

[8] Vassallo DJ. The corps disease: brucellosis and its historical association with the Royal Army Medical Corps. Journal of the Royal Army Medical Corps. 1992;138(3): 140-150.

[9] Nicoletti P. A short history of brucellosis. Veterinary Microbiology. 2002;90(1-4):5-9.

[10] Plumb GE, Olsen SC, and Buttke D. Brucellosis: 'One Health' challenges and opportunities. Revue Scientifique et Technique (International Office of Epizootics). 2013;32(1):271-278.

[11] Arroyo CI, Lopez Rodriguez MJ, Sapina AM, Lopez LA, and Sacristan AR. Probable transmission of brucellosis by breast milk. Journal of Tropical Pediatrics. 2006;52(5): 380-381.

[12] Kato Y, Masuda G, Itoda I, Imamura A, Ajisawa A, and Negishi M. Brucellosis in a returned traveler and his wife: probable person-to-person transmission of *Brucella melitensis* Journal of Travel Medicine. 2007;14(5):343-345.

[13] Mantur BG, Mangalgi SS, and Mulimani M. *Brucella melitensis*—a sexually transmissible agent? Lancet. 1996;347(9017):1763.

[14] Stantic-Pavlinic M, Cec V, and Mehlc J. Brucellosis in spouses and the possibility of interhuman infection. Infection. 1983;11(6):313-314.

[15] Ficht TA, and Adams LG. In: Barrett Alan DT and Stanberry LR, eds. *Vaccines for Biodefense and Emerging and Neglected Diseases*; 2009:807-829.

[16] Pappas G, Akritidis N, Bosilkovski M, and Tsianos E. Brucellosis. New England Journal of Medicine. 2005;352(22):2325-2336.

[17] Pappas G, Papadimitriou P, Akritidis N, Christou L, and Tsianos EV. The new global map of human brucellosis. Lancet Infectious Diseases. 2006;6(2):91-99.

[18] Franco MP, Mulder M, Gilman RH, and Smits HL. Human brucellosis. Lancet Infectious Diseases. 2007;7(12):775-786.

[19] Godfroid J, Cloeckaert A, Liautard JP, Kohler S, Fretin D, Walravens K, Garin-Bastuji B, and Letesson JJ. From the discovery of the Malta fever's agent to the discovery of a marine mammal reservoir, brucellosis has continuously been a re-emerging zoonosis. Veterinary Research. 2005;36(3):313-326.

[20] Perkins SD, Smither SJ, and Atkins HS. Towards a *Brucella* vaccine for humans. FEMS Microbiology Reviews. 2010;34(3):379-394.

[21] Roth F, Zinsstag J, Orkhon D, Chimed-Ochir G, Hutton G, Cosivi O, Carrin G, and Otte J. Human health benefits from livestock vaccination for brucellosis: case study. Bulletin of the World Health Organization. 2003;81(12):867-876.

[22] Zinsstag J, Roth F, Orkhon D, Chimed-Ochir G, Nansalmaa M, Kolar J, and Vounatsou P. A model of animal-human brucellosis transmission in Mongolia. Preventive Veterinary Medicine. 2005;69(1-2):77-95.

[23] Alton GG. In: Duncan JR and Nielsen K, eds. *Animal Brucellosis*. Boston; 1990:383-409.

[24] Blasco JM. Control and eradication strategies for *Brucella melitensis* infection in sheep and goats. Prilozi. 2010;31(1):145-165.

[25] FAO. *Brucella melitensis* in Eurasia and the Middle East. FAO Animal Production and Health Proceedings. 2009;10.

[26] Nicoletti P. Brucellosis: past, present and future. Prilozi. 2010;31(1):21-32.

[27] Maudlin I, and Weber-Mosdorf S. The control of neglected zoonotic diseases. WHO/SDE/FOS/2006.1. 2006.

[28] McDermott J, Grace D, and Zinsstag J. Economics of brucellosis impact and control in low-income countries. Revue Scientifique et Technique (International Office of Epizootics). 2013;32(1):249-261.

[29] Adone R, and Pasquali P. Epidemiosurveillance of brucellosis. Revue Scientifique et Technique (International Office of Epizootics). 2013;32(1):199-205.

[30] Crespo León F. Brucelosis ovina y caprina. World Organisation for Animal Health (OIE), Paris; 1994:1-450.

[31] Kolar J. Some experience from brucellosis control with Rev. 1 vaccine in a heavily infected country- Mongolia. FAO/WHO/OIE Round Table on the Use of Rev. 1 Vaccine in Small Ruminants and Cattle, Alfort, France; 1995:77-81.

[32] EFSA. Porcine brucellosis (*Brucella suis*): scientific opinion of the Panel on Animal Health and Welfare 2009; http://www.efsa.europa.eu/de/scdocs/doc/1144.pdf.

[33] Crespo León F, Saez Llorente JL, Reviriego Gordejo FJ, Rodriguez Ferri EF, and Duran FM. Complementary tools for the control and eradication of caprine and ovine brucellosis in the European Union. Revue Scientifique et Technique (International Office of Epizootics). 2012;31(3):985-996.

[34] Smits HL. Brucellosis in pastoral and confined livestock: prevention and vaccination. Revue Scientifique et Technique (International Office of Epizootics). 2013;32(1): 219-228;

[35] Rodriguez Ferri EF, and Crespo León F. Brucelosis. Veterinaria en Castilla y León. 2000;13:13-43.

[36] Kreizinger Z, Foster JT, Ronai Z, Sulyok KM, Wehmann E, Janosi S, and Gyuranecz M. Genetic relatedness of *Brucella suis* biovar 2 isolates from hares, wild boars and domestic pigs. Veterinary Microbiology. 2014;172(3-4):492-498.

[37] Rhyan JC, Nol P, Quance C, Gertonson A, Belfrage J, Harris L, Straka K, and Robbe-Austerman S. Transmission of brucellosis from elk to cattle and bison, Greater Yellowstone area, U.S.A., 2002-2012. Emerging Infectious Diseases. 2013;19(12): 1992-1995.

[38] Reviriego FJ, Moreno MA, and Dominguez L. Risk factors for brucellosis seroprevalence of sheep and goat flocks in Spain. Preventive Veterinary Medicine. 2000;44(3-4): 167-173.

[39] Robinson A. Guidelines for coordinated human and animal brucellosis surveillance. FAO Animal Production and Health Paper. 2003;156.

[40] Diaz-Aparicio E, and Diaz. Epidemiology of brucellosis in domestic animals caused by *Brucella melitensis, Brucella suis* and *Brucella abortus*. Revue Scientifique et Technique (International Office of Epizootics). 2013;32(1):53-60.

[41] Blasco JM, and Molina-Flores B. Control and eradication of *Brucella melitensis* infection in sheep and goats. Veterinary Clinics of North America: Food Animal Practice. 2011;27(1):95-104.

[42] Alvarez J, Saez JL, Garcia N, Serrat C, Perez-Sancho M, Gonzalez S, Ortega MJ, GouJ, Carbajo L, Garrido F, et al. Management of an outbreak of brucellosis due to *B. melitensis* in dairy cattle in Spain. Research in Veterinary Science. 2010;90(2):208-211

[43] Saez JL, Sanz C, Duran M, Garcia P, Fernandez F, Minguez O, Carbajo L, Mardones F, Perez A, Gonzalez S, et al. Comparison of depopulation and S19-RB51 vaccination strategies for control of bovine brucellosis in high prevalence areas. Veterinary Record. 2014;174(25):634.

[44] Garin-Bastuji B, Blasco JM, Grayon M, and Verger JM. *Brucella melitensis* infection in sheep: present and future. Veterinary Research. 1998;29(3-4):255-274.

[45] Nicoletti P. Further evaluations of serologic test procedures used to diagnose brucellosis. American Journal of Veterinary Research. 1969;30(10):1811-1816.

[46] Kolar J. Diagnosis and control of brucellosis in small ruminants. Preventive Veterinary Medicine. 1984;2(1-4):215-225.

[47] Blasco JM, Garin-Bastuji B, Marin CM, Gerbier G, Fanlo J, Jimenez de Bagues MP, and Cau C. Efficacy of different rose bengal and complement fixation antigens for the diagnosis of *Brucella melitensis* infection in sheep and goats. Veterinary Record. 1994;134(16):415-420.

[48] Jacques I, Olivier-Bernardin V, and Dubray G. Efficacy of ELISA compared to conventional tests (RBPT and CFT) for the diagnosis of *Brucella melitensis* infection in sheep. Veterinary Microbiology. 1998;64(1):61-73.

[49] Diaz-Aparicio E, Aragon V, Marin C, Alonso B, Font M, Moreno E, Perez-Ortiz S, Blasco JM, Diaz R, and Moriyon I. Comparative analysis of *Brucella* serotype A and M and *Yersinia enterocolitica* O:9 polysaccharides for serological diagnosis of brucellosis in cattle, sheep, and goats. Journal of Clinical Microbiology. 1993;31(12):3136-3141.

[50] Nielsen K, Gall D, Smith P, Balsevicius S, Garrido F, Ferrer MD, Biancifiori F, Dajer A, Luna E, Samartino L, et al. Comparison of serological tests for the detection of ovine and caprine antibody to *Brucella melitensis*. Revue Scientifique et Technique (International Office of Epizootics). 2004;23(3):979-987.

[51] Poester FP, Samartino LE, and Santos RL. Pathogenesis and pathobiology of brucellosis in livestock. Revue Scientifique et Technique (International Office of Epizootics). 2013;32(1):105-115.

[52] Godfroid J, Nielsen K, and Saegerman C. Diagnosis of brucellosis in livestock and wildlife. Croatian Medical Journal. 2010;51(4):296-305..

[53] Nielsen K. Diagnosis of brucellosis by serology. Veterinary Microbiology. 2002;90(1-4):447-459.

[54] Nielsen K, Smith P, Yu W, Nicoletti P, Jungersen G, Stack J, and Godfroid J. Serological discrimination by indirect enzyme immunoassay between the antibody response to *Brucella* spp. and *Yersinia enterocolitica* O:9 in cattle and pigs. Veterinary Immunology and Immunopathology. 2006;109(1-2):69-78.

[55] McGiven JA, Nicola A, Commander NJ, Duncombe L, Taylor AV, Villari S, Dainty A, Thirlwall R, Bouzelmat N, Perrett LL, et al. An evaluation of the capability of existing and novel serodiagnostic methods for porcine brucellosis to reduce false positive serological reactions. Veterinary Microbiology. 2012;160(3-4):378-386.

[56] Zaccheus MV, Ali T, Cloeckaert A, Zygmunt MS, Weintraub A, Iriarte M, Moriyon I, and Widmalm G. The epitopic and structural characterization of *Brucella suis* biovar 2 *O*-polysaccharide demonstrates the existence of a new M-negative C-negative smooth *Brucella* serovar. PloS one. 2013;8(1):e53941.

[57] Scientific Committee on Animal Health and Animal Welfare. Brucellosis in Sheep and Goats. 2001 European Commission SANCO/C.2/AII/R23/2001, 1-89.

[58] Ragan V, Vroegindewey G, and Babcock S. International standards for brucellosis prevention and management. Revue Scientifique et Technique (International Office of Epizootics). 2013;32(1):189-198.

[59] Oie. Bovine Brucellosis. Manual of diagnostic tests and vaccines for terrestrial animals. 2009; Chapter 2.4.3.

[60] Morgan WJ, Mackinnon DJ, Lawson JR, and Cullen GA. The rose bengal plate agglutination test in the diagnosis of brucellosis. Veterinary Record. 1969;85(23):636-641.

[61] OIE. Porcine brucellosis. Manual of diagnostic tests and vaccines for terrestrial animals. 2008; Chapter 2.8.5.

[62] OIE. Caprine and Ovine Brucellosis (excluding *Brucella ovis*). Manual of diagnostic tests and vaccines for terrestrial animals. 2009; Chapter 2.7.2.

[63] Abernethy DA, Menzies FD, McCullough SJ, McDowell SW, Burns KE, Watt R, Gordon AW, Greiner M, and Pfeiffer DU. Field trial of six serological tests for bovine brucellosis. Veterinary Journal. 2012;191(3):364-370.

[64] Matope G, Muma JB, Toft N, Gori E, Lund A, Nielsen K, and Skjerve E. Evaluation of sensitivity and specificity of RBT, c-ELISA and fluorescence polarisation assay for diagnosis of brucellosis in cattle using latent class analysis. Veterinary Immunology and Immunopathology. 2011;141(1-2):58-63.

[65] Sanogo M, Thys E, Achi YL, Fretin D, Michel P, Abatih E, Berkvens D, and Saegerman C. Bayesian estimation of the true prevalence, sensitivity and specificity of the rose bengal and indirect ELISA tests in the diagnosis of bovine brucellosis. Veterinary Journal. 2013;195(1):114-120.

[66] Minas A, Stournara A, Minas M, Stack J, Petridou E, Christodoulopoulos G, and Krikelis V. Validation of a fluorescence polarization assay (FPA) performed in microplates and comparison with other tests used for diagnosing *B. melitensis* infection in sheep and goats. Journal of Immunological Methods. 2007;320(1-2):94-103.

[67] Ramirez-Pfeiffer C, Diaz-Aparicio E, Gomez-Flores R, Rodriguez-Padilla C, Morales-Loredo A, and Alvarez-Ojeda G. Use of the *Brucella melitensis* native hapten to diagnose brucellosis in goats by a rapid, simple, and specific fluorescence polarization assay. Clinical and Vaccine Immunology. 2008;15(6):911-915.

[68] Gall D, and Nielsen K. Serological diagnosis of bovine brucellosis: a review of test performance and cost comparison. Revue Scientifique et Technique (International Office of Epizootics). 2004;23(3):989-1002.

[69] Greiner M, Verloo D, and de MF. Meta-analytical equivalence studies on diagnostic tests for bovine brucellosis allowing assessment of a test against a group of comparative tests. Preventive Veterinary Medicine. 2009;92(4):373-381.

[70] Munoz PM, Marin CM, Monreal D, Gonzalez D, Garin-Bastuji B, Diaz R, Mainar-Jaime RC, Moriyon I, and Blasco JM. Efficacy of several serological tests and antigens for diagnosis of bovine brucellosis in the presence of false-positive serological results due to *Yersinia enterocolitica* O:9. Clinical and Diagnostic Laboratory Immunology. 2005;12(1):141-151.

[71] Garcia-Bocanegra I, Allepuz A, Perez JJ, Alba A, Giovannini A, Arenas A, Candeloro L, Pacios A, Saez JL, and Gonzalez MA. Evaluation of different enzyme-linked im-

munosorbent assays for the diagnosis of brucellosis due to *Brucella melitensis* in sheep. Veterinary Journal. 2014;199(3):439-445.

[72] Muktaderul A, Md.Ariful I, Mst.Minara K, and Byeong-Kirl B. Evaluation of four serological tests for the detection of brucellosis in goats and cattle under the field condition of Bangladesh. Asian Journal of Biological Sciences. 2011;4:477-482.

[73] Rahman AK, Saegerman C, Berkvens D, Fretin D, Gani MO, Ershaduzzaman M, Ahmed MU, and Emmanuel A. Bayesian estimation of true prevalence, sensitivity and specificity of indirect ELISA, rose bengal test and slow agglutination test for the diagnosis of brucellosis in sheep and goats in Bangladesh. Preventive Veterinary Medicine. 2013;110(2):242-252.

[74] Munoz PM, Blasco JM, Engel B, de Miguel MJ, Marin CM, Dieste L, and Mainar-Jaime RC. Assessment of performance of selected serological tests for diagnosing brucellosis in pigs. Veterinary Immunology and Immunopathology. 2012;146(2): 150-158.

[75] Praud A, Gimenez O, Zanella G, Dufour B, Pozzi N, Antras V, Meyer L, and Garin-Bastuji B. Estimation of sensitivity and specificity of five serological tests for the diagnosis of porcine brucellosis. Preventive Veterinary Medicine. 2012;104(1-2):94-100.

[76] Dieste-Perez L, Blasco JM, de Miguel MJ, Moriyon I, and Munoz PM. Diagnostic performance of serological tests for swine brucellosis in the presence of false positive serological reactions. Journal of Microbiological Methods. 2015;111C:57-63.

[77] Diaz-Aparicio E, Marin C, Alonso-Urmeneta B, Aragon V, Perez-Ortiz S, Pardo M, Blasco JM, Diaz R, and Moriyon I. Evaluation of serological tests for diagnosis of *Brucella melitensis* infection of goats. Journal Clinical Microbiology. 1994;32(5):1159-1165.

[78] Alton GG, Jones LM, Angus RD, and Verger JM. Techniques for the brucellosis laboratory. Paris, France: Inra Publications; 1988.

[79] Minas A, Stournara A, Minas M, Papaioannou A, Krikelis V, and Tselepidis S. Validation of fluorescence polarization assay (FPA) and comparison with other tests used for diagnosis of *B. melitensis* infection in sheep. Veterinary Microbiology. 2005;111(3-4):211-221.

[80] Chappel RJ, and Hayes J. Comparison of radioimmunoassay with the complement fixation test and the indirect haemolysis test in the field diagnosis of bovine brucellosis. Journal of Hygiene. 1983;90(1):67-70.

[81] Blasco JM, Marin C, Jimenez de BM, Barberan M, Hernandez A, Molina L, Velasco J, Diaz R, and Moriyon I. Evaluation of allergic and serological tests for diagnosing *Brucella melitensis* infection in sheep. Journal Clinical Microbiology. 1994;32(8): 1835-1840.

[82] Garin-Bastuji B, Blasco JM, Marin C, and Albert D. The diagnosis of brucellosis in sheep and goats, old and new tools. Small Ruminant Research. 2006;62:63-70.

[83] Mainar-Jaime RC, Munoz PM, de Miguel MJ, Grillo MJ, Marin CM, Moriyon I, and Blasco JM. Specificity dependence between serological tests for diagnosing bovine brucellosis in *Brucella*-free farms showing false positive serological reactions due to *Yersinia enterocolitica* O:9. Canadian Veterinary Journal. 2005;46(10):913-916.

[84] Robson JM, Harrison MW, Wood RN, Tilse MH, McKay AB, and Brodribb TR. Brucellosis: re-emergence and changing epidemiology in Queensland. Medical Journal of Australia. 1993;159(3):153-158.

[85] Stoffregen WC, Olsen SC, and Bricker BJ. Parenteral vaccination of domestic pigs with *Brucella abortus* strain RB51. American Journal of Veterinary Research. 2006;67(10):1802-1808.

[86] Rogers RJ, Cook DR, Ketterer PJ, Baldock FC, Blackall PJ, and Stewart RW. An evaluation of three serological tests for antibody to *Brucella suis* in pigs. Australian Veterinary Journal. 1989;66(3):77-80.

[87] Dieste-Perez L, Barberan M, Munoz PM, Moriyon I, and Blasco JM. Clinical and histological features of brucellin skin test responses in *Brucella suis* biovar 2 infected pigs. Veterinary Immunology and Immunopathology. 2015;163(1-2):77-85.

[88] Perrett LL, McGiven JA, Brew SD, and Stack JA. Evaluation of competitive ELISA for detection of antibodies to *Brucella* infection in domestic animals. Croatian Medical Journal. 2010;51(4):314-319.

[89] Carlsson HE, Hurvell B, and Lindberg AA. Enzyme-linked immunosorbent assay (ELISA) for titration of antibodies against *Brucella abortus* and *Yersinia enterocolitica*. Acta Pathologica Microbiologica Scandinavica Series C. 1976;84(3):168-176.

[90] Minas A, Stournara A, Christodoulopoulos G, and Katsoulos PD. Validation of a competitive ELISA for diagnosis of *Brucella melitensis* infection in sheep and goats. Veterinary Journal. 2008;177(3):411-417.

[91] Nielsen K, Smith P, Yu WL, Elmgren C, Halbert G, Nicoletti P, Perez B, Conde S, Samartino L, Nicola A, et al. Validation of a second generation competitive enzyme immunoassay (CELISA) for the diagnosis of brucellosis in various species of domestic animals. Veterinary Immunology and Immunopathology. 2008;125(3-4):246-250.

[92] Burriel AR, Christodoulopoulod G, Bisias G, and Fthenakis GC. Comparison of fluorescence polarization assay, indirect ELISA and competitive ELISA methods for diagnosis of *Brucella melitensis* infection in small ruminants. Small Ruminant Research. 2004;54(3):243-247.

[93] Nielsen KH, Kelly L, Gall D, Nicoletti P, and Kelly W. Improved competitive enzyme immunoassay for the diagnosis of bovine brucellosis. Veterinary Immunology and Immunopathology. 1995;46(3-4):285-291.

[94] Paulo PS, Vigliocco AM, Ramondino RF, Marticorena D, Bissi E, Briones G, Gorchs C, Gall D, and Nielsen K. Evaluation of primary binding assays for presumptive sero-

diagnosis of swine brucellosis in Argentina. Clinical and Diagnostic Laboratory Immunology. 2000;7(5):828-831.

[95] Fensterbank R. Brucellosis in cattle, sheep and goats: diagnosis, control and vaccination. In: Office International des Epizooties, ed. Technical Series; 1987:9-35.

[96] Mahajan NK, and Kulshreshtha RC. Comparison of serological tests for *Brucella melitensis* infection in sheep. Tropical Animal Health and Production. 1991;23(1):11-16.

[97] Waghela S, Wandera JG, and Wagner GG. Comparison of four serological tests in the diagnosis of caprine brucellosis. Research in Veterinary Science. 1980;28(2):168-171.

[98] Radwan AI, Bekairi SI, Al-Mukayel AA, and Abu Agla OS. Control of ovine brucellosis in Najdi sheep in Saudi Arabia. Tropical Animal Health and Production. 1984;16(4):213-218.

[99] McGiven JA, Stack JA, Perrett LL, Tucker JD, Brew SD, Stubberfield E, and MacMillan AP. Harmonisation of European tests for serological diagnosis of *Brucella* infection in bovines. Revue Scientifique et Technique (International Office of Epizootics). 2006;25(3):1039-1053.

[100] O'Grady D, Byrne W, Kelleher P, O'Callaghan H, Kenny K, Heneghan T, Power S, Egan J, and Ryan F. A comparative assessment of culture and serology in the diagnosis of brucellosis in dairy cattle. Veterinary Journal. 2014;199(3):370-375.

[101] Ferris RA, Schoenbaum MA, and Crawford RP. Comparison of serologic tests and bacteriologic culture for detection of brucellosis in swine from naturally infected herds. Journal of the American Veterinary Medical Association. 1995;207(10): 1332-1333.

[102] Lord VR, Cherwonogrodzky JW, Marcano MJ, and Melendez G. Serological and bacteriological study of swine brucellosis. Journal Clinical Microbiology. 1997;35(1): 295-297.

[103] Vanzini VR, Aguirre NP, Valentini BS, Torioni de Echaide S, Lugaresi CI, Marchesino MD, and Nielsen K. Comparison of an indirect ELISA with the *Brucella* milk ring test for detection of antibodies to *Brucella abortus* in bulk milk samples. Veterinary Microbiology. 2001;82(1):55-60.

[104] Jones LM, and Marly J. Titration of a *Brucella* protein allergen in sheep sensitized with *Brucella melitensis* Annals of Veterinary Research. 1975;6(2):173-178.

[105] Dieste-Perez L, Blasco JM, de Miguel MJ, Marin CM, Barberan M, Conde-Alvarez R, Moriyon I, and Munoz PM. Performance of skin tests with allergens from *B. melitensis* B115 and rough *B. abortus* mutants for diagnosing swine brucellosis. Veterinary Microbiology. 2014;168(1):161-168.

[106] Pouillot R, Garin-Bastuji B, Gerbier G, Coche Y, Cau C, Dufour B, and Moutou F. The brucellin skin test as a tool to discriminate false positive serological reactions in bovine brucellosis. Veterinary Research. 1997;28(4):365-374.

[107] Riber U, and Jungersen G. Cell-mediated immune responses differentiate infections with *Brucella suis* from *Yersinia enterocolitica* serotype O:9 in pigs. Veterinary Immunology and Immunopathology. 2007;116(1-2):13-25.

[108] Fensterbank R. Allergic diagnosis of brucellosis. In: Nijhoff, ed. *Brucella melitensis*; 1985:167-172. Dordrecht.

[109] Velasco J, Diaz R, Grillo MJ, Barberan M, Marin C, Blasco JM, and Moriyon I. Antibody and delayed-type hypersensitivity responses to *Ochrobactrum anthropi* cytosolic and outer membrane antigens in infections by smooth and rough *Brucella* spp. Clinical and Diagnostic Laboratory Immunology. 1997;4(3):279-284.

[110] Jiang X, and Baldwin CL. Effects of cytokines on intracellular growth of *Brucella abortus*. Infection and Immunity. 1993;61(1):124-134.

[111] Kim S, Lee DS, Watanabe K, Furuoka H, Suzuki H, and Watarai M. Interferon-gamma promotes abortion due to *Brucella* infection in pregnant mice. BMC Microbiology. 2005;5:22.

[112] Vitry MA, Hanot Mambres D, De Trez C, Akira S, Ryffel B, Letesson JJ, and Muraille E. Humoral immunity and CD4+ Th1 cells are both necessary for a fully protective immune response upon secondary infection with *Brucella melitensis*. Journal of Immunology. 2014;192(8):3740-3752.

[113] Weynants V, Godfroid J, Limbourg B, Saegerman C, and Letesson JJ. Specific bovine brucellosis diagnosis based on in vitro antigen-specific gamma interferon production. Journal Clinical Microbiology. 1995;33(3):706-712.

[114] Duran-Ferrer M, Leon L, Nielsen K, Caporale V, Mendoza J, Osuna A, Perales A, Smith P, De-Frutos C, Gomez-Martin B, et al. Antibody response and antigen-specific gamma-interferon profiles of vaccinated and unvaccinated pregnant sheep experimentally infected with *Brucella melitensis*. Veterinary Microbiology. 2004;100(3-4): 219-231.

[115] Perez-Sancho M, Duran-Ferrer M, Garcia-Seco T, Macias P, Garcia N, Martinez I, Ruiz E, Legaz E, Diez-Guerrier A, Gonzalez S, et al. Interferon-gamma responses in sheep exposed to virulent and attenuated *Brucella melitensis* strains. Veterinary Immunology and Immunopathology. 2014;160(1-2):123-128.

[116] Elberg SS, and Meyer KF. Caprine immunization against brucellosis; a summary of experiments on the isolation, properties and behaviour of a vaccine strain. Bulletin of the World Health Organization. 1958;19(4):711-724.

[117] Corbel, MJ. Brucellosis in humans and animals. World Health Organization, Food and Agriculture Organization of the United Nations, and World Organization for

Animal Health. World Health Organization. 2006; http://www.who.int/csr/resources/publications/Brucellosis.pdf.

[118] De Miguel MJ, Marin CM, Munoz PM, Dieste L, Grillo MJ, and Blasco JM. Development of a selective culture medium for primary isolation of the main *Brucella* species. Journal of Clinical Microbiology. 2011;49(4):1458-1463.

[119] Blasco JM. Estado Actual de la Brucelosis en España. Profesion Veterinaria. 2004;15(58):22-34.

[120] McGiven JA. New developments in the immunodiagnosis of brucellosis in livestock and wildlife. Revue Scientifique et Technique (International Office of Epizootics). 2013;32(1):163-176.

[121] Hornitzky M, and Searson J. The relationship between the isolation of *Brucella abortus* and serological status of infected, non-vaccinated cattle. Australian Veterinary Journal. 1986;63(6):172-174.

[122] Ferreira AC, Almendra C, Cardoso R, Pereira MS, Beja-Pereira A, Luikart G, and Correa de Sa MI. Development and evaluation of a selective medium for *Brucella suis*. Research in Veterinary Science. 2012;93(2):565-567.

[123] Her M, Cho DH, Kang SI, Cho YS, Hwang IY, Bae YC, Yoon H, Heo YR, Jung SC, and Yoo H. The development of a selective medium for the *Brucella abortus* strains and its comparison with the currently recommended and used medium. Diagnostic Microbiology and Infectious Disease. 2010;67(1):15-21.

[124] Yu WL, and Nielsen K. Review of Detection of *Brucella* spp. by Polymerase Chain Reaction. Croatian Medical Journal. 2010;51(4):306-313.

[125] Nan W, Tan P, Wang Y, Xu Z, Mao K, Peng D, and Chen Y. Duplex PCR for differentiation of the vaccine strain *Brucella suis* S2 and B. suis biovar 1 from other strains of *Brucella* spp. Veterinary Journal. 2014;201(3):427-428.

[126] Kang SI, Lee SE, Kim JY, Lee K, Kim JW, Lee HK, Sung SR, Heo YR, Jung SC, and Her M. A new *Brucella canis* species-specific PCR assay for the diagnosis of canine brucellosis. Comparative Immunology, Microbiology and Infectious diseases. 2014;37(4):237-241.

[127] Gopaul KK, Sells J, Lee R, Beckstrom-Sternberg SM, Foster JT, and Whatmore AM. Development and assessment of multiplex high resolution melting assay as a tool for rapid single-tube identification of five *Brucella* species. BMC research notes. 2014.

[128] Hinic V, Brodard I, Thomann A, Cvetnic Z, Makaya PV, Frey J, and Abril C. Novel identification and differentiation of *Brucella melitensis*, *B. abortus*, *B. suis*, *B. ovis*, *B. canis*, and *B. neotomae* suitable for both conventional and real-time PCR systems. Journal of Microbiological Methods. 2008;75(2):375-378.

[129] Bounaadja L, Albert D, Chenais B, Henault S, Zygmunt MS, Poliak S, and Garin-Bastuji B. Real-time PCR for identification of *Brucella* spp.: a comparative study of IS *711*, *bcsp31* and *per* target genes. Veterinary Microbiology. 2009;137(1-2):156-164.

[130] Garcia-Yoldi D, Marin CM, de Miguel MJ, Munoz PM, Vizmanos JL, and Lopez-Goni I. Multiplex PCR assay for the identification and differentiation of all *Brucella* species and the vaccine strains *Brucella abortus* S19 and RB51 and *Brucella melitensis* Rev1. Clinical Chemistry. 2006;52(4):779-781.

[131] Huber B, Scholz HC, Lucero N, and Busse HJ. Development of a PCR assay for typing and subtyping of *Brucella* species. International Journal of Medical Microbiology. 2009;299(8):563-573.

[132] Mayer-Scholl A, Draeger A, Gollner C, Scholz HC, and Nockler K. Advancement of a multiplex PCR for the differentiation of all currently described *Brucella* species. Journal of Microbiological Methods. 2010;80(1):112-114.

[133] Mirnejad R, Doust RH, Kachuei R, Mortazavi SM, Khoobdel M, and Ahamadi A. Simultaneous detection and differentiates of *Brucella abortus* and *Brucella melitensis* by combinatorial PCR. Asian Pacific Journal of Tropical Medicine. 2012;5(1):24-28.

[134] Rantakokko-Jalava K, and Jalava J. Optimal DNA isolation method for detection of bacteria in clinical specimens by broad-range PCR. Journal of Clinical Microbiology. 2002;40(11):4211-4217.

[135] Bricker BJ. PCR as a diagnostic tool for brucellosis. Veterinary Microbiology. 2002;90(1-4):435-446.

[136] O'Leary S, Sheahan M, and Sweeney T. *Brucella abortus* detection by PCR assay in blood, milk and lymph tissue of serologically positive cows. Research in Veterinary Science. 2006;81(2):170-176.

[137] Tomaso H, Kattar M, Eickhoff M, Wernery U, Al DS, Straube E, Neubauer H, and Scholz HC. Comparison of commercial DNA preparation kits for the detection of Brucellae in tissue using quantitative real-time PCR. BMC Infectious Diseases. 2010;10:100.

[138] Godfroid J, Scholz HC, Barbier T, Nicolas C, Wattiau P, Fretin D, What more AM, Cloeckaert A, Blasco JM, Moriyon I, et al. Brucellosis at the animal/ecosystem/human interface at the beginning of the 21st century. Preventive Veterinary Medicine. 2011;102(2):118-131.

[139] Olsen SC. Recent developments in livestock and wildlife brucellosis vaccination. Revue Scientifique et Technique (International Office of Epizootics). 2013;32(1):207-217.

[140] Moriyon I, Grillo MJ, Monreal D, Gonzalez D, Marin C, Lopez-Goni I, Mainar-Jaime RC, Moreno E, and Blasco JM. Rough vaccines in animal brucellosis: structural and genetic basis and present status. Veterinary Research. 2004;35(1):1-38.

[141] Elzer PH, Hagius SD, Davis DS, DelVecchio VG, and Enright FM. Characterization of the caprine model for ruminant brucellosis. Veterinary Microbiology. 2002;90(1-4): 425-431.

[142] Bosseray N. *Brucella melitensis* Rev. 1 living attenuated vaccine: stability of markers, residual virulence and immunogenicity in mice. Biologicals: Journal of the International Association of Biological Standardization. 1991;19(4):355-363.

[143] Elberg SS, and Meyer KF. Caprine immunization against brucellosis; a summary of experiments on the isolation, properties and behaviour of a vaccine strain. Bulletin of the World Health Organization. 1958;19(4):711-724.

[144] Zundel E, Verger JM, Grayon M, and Michel R. Conjunctival vaccination of pregnant ewes and goats with *Brucella melitensis* Rev 1 vaccine: safety and serological responses. Annals of Veterinary Research. 1992;23(2):177-188.

[145] Thomas EL, Bracewell CD, and Corbel MJ. Characterisation of *Brucella abortus* strain 19 cultures isolated from vaccinated cattle. Veterinary Record. 1981;108(5):90-93.

[146] Jimenez de Bagues MP, Marin CM, Barberan M, and Blasco JM. Responses of ewes to *B. melitensis* Rev1 vaccine administered by subcutaneous or conjunctival routes at different stages of pregnancy. Annals of Veterinary Research. 1989;20(2):205-213.

[147] Pacheco WA, Genovez ME, Pozzi CR, Silva MP, Azevedo SS, Did CC, Piatti RM, Pinheiro ES, Castro V, Miyashiro S, et al. Excretion of *Brucella abortus* vaccine B19 strain during a reproductive cycle in dairy cows. Brazilian Journal of Microbiology. 2012:594-601.

[148] Jones LM, and Marly J. Serological and bacteriological studies of ewes vaccinated with *Brucella melitensis* strain Rev. 1 during lactation. Annals of Veterinary Research. 1975;6(1):67-71.

[149] Alton GG. Duration of the immunity produced in goats by the Rev. 1 *Brucella melitensis* vaccine. Journal of Comparative Pathology. 1966;76(3):241-253.

[150] Alton GG. Further studies on the duration of the immunity produced in goats by the Rev. 1 *Brucella melitensis* vaccine. Journal of Comparative Pathology. 1968;78(2): 173-178.

[151] Lord VR, Schurig GG, Cherwonogrodzky JW, Marcano MJ, and Melendez GE. Field study of vaccination of cattle with *Brucella abortus* strains RB51 and 19 under high and low disease prevalence. American Journal of Veterinary Research. 1998;59(8): 1016-1020.

[152] Diaz-Aparicio E, Hernandez L, and Suarez-Guemes F. Protection against brucellosis in goats, five years after vaccination with reduced-dose *Brucella melitensis* Rev 1 vaccine. Tropical Animal Health and Production. 2004;36(2):117-121.

[153] Nicoletti P. In: Nielsen K and Duncan JR, eds. *Animal Brucellosis*. Boca Raton: CRC Press; 1990:248-299.

[154] Scharp DW, al Khalaf SA, al Muhanna MW, Cheema RA, and Godana W. Use of mass vaccination with a reduced dose of REV 1 vaccine for *Brucella melitensis* control in a population of small ruminants. Tropical Animal Health and Production. 1999;31(3):135-141.

[155] Beckett FW, and MacDiarmid SC. The effect of reduced-dose *Brucella abortus* strain 19 vaccination in accredited dairy herds. British Veterinary Journal. 1985;141(5):507-514.

[156] Blasco JM. A review of the use of *B. melitensis* Rev 1 vaccine in adult sheep and goats. Preventive Veterinary Medicine. 1997;31(3-4):275-283.

[157] Crowther RW, Orphanides A, and Polydorou K. Vaccination of adult sheep with reduced doses of *Brucella melitensis* strain Rev. 1: safety and serological responses. Tropical Animal Health and Production. 1977;9(2):85-91.

[158] Confer AW, Hall SM, Faulkner CB, Espe BH, Deyoe BL, Morton RJ, and Smith RA. Effects of challenge dose on the clinical and immune responses of cattle vaccinated with reduced doses of *Brucella abortus* strain 19. Veterinary Microbiology. 1985;10(6): 561-575.

[159] Woodard LF, and Jasman RL. Comparative efficacy of an experimental S45/20 bacterin and a reduced dose of strain 19 vaccine against bovine brucellosis. American Journal of Veterinary Research. 1983;44(5):907-910.

[160] al-Khalaf SA, Mohamad BT, and Nicoletti P. Control of brucellosis in Kuwait by vaccination of cattle, sheep and goats with *Brucella abortus* strain 19 or *Brucella melitensis* strain Rev. 1. Tropical Animal Health and Production. 1992;24(1):45-49.

[161] Al-Shamakh IH. A brief review of the national project for the control of brucellosis in the Kingdom of Saudi Arabia. FAO/WHO/OIE Round Table, on the use of Rev.-1 vaccine in small ruminants and cattle. CNVA Alfort, France, September 1995.

[162] Nicoletti P. A preliminary report on the efficacy of adult cattle vaccination using Strain 19 in selected dairy herds in Florida. Proceedings of Annual Meeting of United States of Animal Health Association. 197680):91-106.

[163] Nicoletti P. The effects of adult cattle vaccination with strain 19 on the incidence of brucellosis in dairy herds in Florida and Puerto Rico. Proceedings of the Annual Meeting of the United States Animal Health Association. 1979(83):75-80.

[164] Fensterbank R, and Plommet M. Vaccination against bovine brucellosis with a low dose of strain 19 administered by the conjunctival route. IV. Comparison between two methods of vaccination. Annals of Veterinary Research. 1979;10(1):131-139.

[165] Ali Kojouri G, and Gholami M. Post vaccination follow-up of *Brucella melitensis* in blood stream of sheep by PCR assay. Comparative Clinical Pathology. 2009;18(4): 439-442.

[166] Banai M, Abramson M, Mayer I, Chechick K, Hoida G, Zamir O, Bardenstein S, Cohen A, and Davidson M. Problems associated with the persistence and possible horizontal transfer of *Brucella melitensis* Rev. I vaccine in connection with serological surveillance in Israel. FAO/WHO/OIE Round Table on the use of Rev. 1 vaccine in small ruminants an cattle CNEVA Alfort, France; 1995:69-76.

[167] Sales Henriques HLR, Hueston WD, Hoblet KH, and Shulaw WP. Field trials evaluating the safety and serologic reactions of reduced-dose *Brucella melitensis* Rev 1 vaccination in adult sheep. Preventive Veterinary Medicine. 1992;13(3):205-215.

[168] Stournara A, Minas A, Bourtzi-Chatzopoulou E, Stack J, Koptopoulos G, Petridou E, and Sarris K. Assessment of serological response of young and adult sheep to conjunctival vaccination with Rev-1 vaccine by fluorescence polarization assay (FPA) and other serological tests for *B. melitensis*. Veterinary Microbiology. 2007;119(1): 53-64.

[169] Lantier F and Fensterbank R. Kinetics of Rev1 infection in sheep. In: Verger JM and Plommet M, eds. *Brucella melitensis*. Martinus Nijhoff, Dordrecht; 1985:247-251.

[170] Tolari F, and Salvi G. Segnalazione di un caso di orchite bilaterale in un capretto in sequito a vaccinatzione con Rev. 1. Estrato dagli Anm Faculta Med Vet. 1980:33.

[171] Corbel MJ, Stuart FA, Brewer RA, Jeffrey M, and Bradley R. Arthropathy associated with *Brucella abortus* strain 19 vaccination in cattle. II. Experimental studies. British Veterinary Journal. 1989;145(4):347-355.

[172] Olsen SC, and Stoffregen WS. Essential role of vaccines in brucellosis control and eradication programs for livestock. Expert Review of Vaccines. 2005;4(6):915-928.

[173] Banai M. Control of small ruminant brucellosis by use of *Brucella melitensis* Rev. 1 vaccine: laboratory aspects and field observations. Veterinary Microbiology. 2002;90(1-4):497-519.

[174] Blasco JM, and Diaz R. *Brucella melitensi*s Rev-1 vaccine as a cause of human brucellosis. Lancet. 1993;342(8874):805.

[175] Meyer ME. Characterization of *Brucella abortus* strain 19 isolated from human and bovine tissues and fluids. American Journal of Veterinary Research. 1985;46(4):902-904.

[176] Pivnick H, Worton H, Smith DL, and Barnum D. Infection of veterinarians in Ontario by *Brucella abortus* strain 19. Canadian journal of public healthRevue canadienne de sante publique. 1966;57(5):225-231.

[177] Vincent P, Joubert L, and Prave M. Two occupational cases of brucellar infection after inoculation of B 19 vaccine. Bulletin de l'Academie Veterinaire de France. 1970;43(2): 89-97.

[178] Grillo MJ, Bosseray N, and Blasco JM. In vitro markers and biological activity in mice of seed lot strains and commercial *Brucella melitensis* Rev 1 and *Brucella abortus* B19 vaccines. Biologicals: Journal of the International Association of Biological Standardization. 2000;28(2):119-127.

[179] Alton GG. In: Verger J, and Plommet M eds. *Brucella melitensis* Dordrecht/Boston/ Lancaster: Martinus Nijhoff; 1985:215-227.

[180] Mukherjee F, Jain J, Grillo MJ, Blasco JM, and Nair M. Evaluation of *Brucella abortus* S19 vaccine strains by bacteriological tests, molecular analysis of ery loci and virulence in BALB/c mice. Biologicals: Journal of the International Association of Biological Standardization. 2005;33(3):153-160.

[181] Menzies PI. Vaccination programs for reproductive disorders of small ruminants. Animal Reproduction Science. 2012;130(3-4):162-172.

[182] Garcia-Yoldi D, Le FP, Marin CM, de Miguel MJ, Munoz PM, Vergnaud G, and Lopez-Goni I. Assessment of genetic stability of *Brucella melitensis* Rev 1 vaccine strain by multiple-locus variable-number tandem repeat analysis. Vaccine. 2007;25(15): 2858-2862.

[183] Alton GG. Rev. 1 *Brucella melitensis* vaccine. Serological reactions in Maltese goats. Journal of Comparative Pathology. 1967;77(3):327-329.

[184] Alton GG, Fensterbank R, and Plommet AM. La brucellose de la chevre. In: Yvor P and Perrin G eds. *Les maladies de la chevre*. 1984.

[185] Herr S, Ehret WJ, Ribeiro LM, and Chaparro F. The persistence of serological reactions following heifer vaccination with *Brucella abortus* strain 19 on brucellosis-free farms. Journal of the South African Veterinary Association. 1990;61(1):11-13.

[186] Plommet M, and Plommet AM. Vaccination against bovine brucellosis with a low dose of strain 19 administered by the conjunctival route. Annals of Veterinary Research. 1976;7(1):1-8.

[187] Fensterbank R, Pardon P, and Marly J. Comparison between subcutaneous and conjunctival route of vaccination with Rev. 1 strain against *Brucella melitensis* infection in ewes. Annals of Veterinary Research. 1982;13(4):295-301.

[188] Verger JM, Grayon M, Zundel E, Lechopier P, and Olivier-Bernardin V. Comparison of the efficacy of *Brucella suis* strain 2 and *Brucella melitensis* Rev. 1 live vaccines against a *Brucella melitensis* experimental infection in pregnant ewes. Vaccine. 1995;13(2):191-196.

[189] Delgado S, Fernandez M, and C rmenes P. Influence of age and stage of gestation on serological response to subcutaneous or conjunctival *Brucella melitensis* strain Rev. 1 vaccination in ewes. Small Ruminant Research. 1996;19(1):63-68.

[190] McGiven JA, Tucker JD, Perrett LL, Stack JA, Brew SD, and MacMillan AP. Validation of FPA and cELISA for the detection of antibodies to *Brucella abortus* in cattle sera and comparison to SAT, CFT, and iELISA. Journal of Immunological Methods. 2003;278(1-2):171-178.

[191] Nielsen K. The serological response of cattle immunized with *Yersinia enterocolitica* O: 9 or O:16 to *Yersinia* and *Brucella abortus* antigens in enzyme immunoassays. Veterinary Immunology and Immunopathology. 1990;24(4):373-382.

[192] Debbarh HS, Cloeckaert A, Zygmunt MS, and Dubray G. Identification of sero-reactive *Brucella melitensis* cytosoluble proteins which discriminate between antibodies elicited by infection and Rev. 1 vaccination in sheep. Veterinary Microbiology. 1995;44(1):37-48.

[193] Cloeckaert A, Baucheron S, Vizcaino N, and Zygmunt MS. Use of recombinant BP26 protein in serological diagnosis of *Brucella melitensis* infection in sheep. Clinical and Diagnostic Laboratory Immunology 2001;8(4):772-775.

[194] Salih-Alj DH, Cloeckaert A, Bezard G, Dubray G, and Zygmunt MS. Enzyme-linked immunosorbent assay with partially purified cytosoluble 28-kilodalton protein for serological differentiation between *Brucella melitensis*-infected and *B. melitensis* Rev. 1-vaccinated sheep. Clinical and Diagnostic Laboratory Immunology. 1996;3(3): 305-308.

[195] Debbarh HS, Zygmunt MS, Dubray G, and Cloeckaert A. Competitive enzyme-linked immunosorbent assay using monoclonal antibodies to the *Brucella melitensis* BP26 protein to evaluate antibody responses in infected and *B. melitensis* Rev. 1 vaccinated sheep. Veterinary Microbiology. 1996;53(3-4):325-337.

[196] Xin T, Yang H, Wang N, Wang F, Zhao P, Wang H, Mao K, Zhu H, and Ding J. Limitations of the BP26 protein-based indirect enzyme-linked immunosorbent assay for diagnosis of Brucellosis. Clinical and Vaccine Immunology: CVI. 2013;20(9): 1410-1417.

[197] Ciocchini AE, Serantes DA, Melli LJ, Guidolin LS, Iwashkiw JA, Elena S, Franco C, Nicola AM, Feldman MF, Comerci DJ, et al. A bacterial engineered glycoprotein as a novel antigen for diagnosis of bovine brucellosis. Veterinary Microbiology. 2014;172(3-4):455-465.

[198] Baldi PC, Giambartolomei GH, Goldbaum FA, Abdon LF, Velikovsky CA, Kittelberger R, and Fossati CA. Humoral immune response against lipopolysaccharide and cytoplasmic proteins of *Brucella abortus* in cattle vaccinated with *B. abortus* S19 or experimentally infected with *Yersinia enterocolitica* serotype O:9. Clinical and Diagnostic Laboratory Immunology. 1996;3(4):472-476.

[199] Pajuaba AC, Silva DA, and Mineo JR. Evaluation of indirect enzyme-linked immunosorbent assays and IgG avidity assays using a protein A-peroxidase conjugate for serological distinction between *Brucella abortus* S19-vaccinated and -infected cows. Clinical and Vaccine Immunology: CVI. 2010;17(4):588-595.

[200] Blasco JM, Diaz R, Moriyon I, and Salvo MD. Evaluation of a radial immunodiffusion test for diagnosing brucellosis in sheep and its possible value for differentiating infected from *Brucella melitensis* Rev 1 vaccinated sheep. Developments in Biological Standardization. 1984;56:507-511.

[201] Diaz R, Garatea P, Jones LM, and Moriyon I. Radial immunodiffusion test with a *Brucella* polysaccharide antigen for differentiating infected from vaccinated cattle. Journal of Clinical Microbiology. 1979;10(1):37-41.

[202] Kittelberger R, Reichel MP, Joyce MA, and Staak C. Serological crossreactivity between *Brucella abortus* and *Yersinia enterocolitica* O:9. III. Specificity of the in vitro antigen-specific gamma interferon test for bovine brucellosis diagnosis in experimentally *Yersinia enterocolitica* 0:9-infected cattle. Veterinary Microbiology. 1997;57(4):361-371.

[203] Jimenez de Bagues MP, Marin CM, Blasco JM, Moriyon I, and Gamazo C. An ELISA with *Brucella* lipopolysaccharide antigen for the diagnosis of *B. melitensis* infection in sheep and for the evaluation of serological responses following subcutaneous or conjunctival *B. melitensis* strain Rev 1 vaccination. Veterinary Microbiology. 1992;30(2-3): 233-241.

[204] Jones LM, Berman DT, Moreno E, Deyoe BL, Gilsdorf MJ, Huber JD, and Nicoletti P. Evaluation of a radial immunodiffusion test with polysaccharide B antigen for diagnosis of bovine brucellosis. Journal of Clinical Microbiology. 1980;12(6):753-760.

[205] Cosivi O, and Corbel MJ. WHO consultation on the development of new/improved brucellosis vaccines. 17 December 1997, Geneva, Switzerland. Biologicals: Journal of the International Association of Biological Standardization. 1998;26(4):361-363.

[206] Gonzalez D, Grillo MJ, de Miguel MJ, Ali T, Arce-Gorvel V, Delrue RM, Conde-Alvarez R, Munoz P, Lopez-Goñi I, Iriarte M, et al. Brucellosis vaccines: assessment of *Brucella melitensis* lipopolysaccharide rough mutants defective in core and *O*-polysaccharide synthesis and export. PLoS One. 2008;3(7):e2760.

[207] Cloeckaert A, Jacques I, de WP, Dubray G, and Limet JN. Protection against *Brucella melitensis* or *Brucella abortus* in mice with immunoglobulin G (IgG), IgA, and IgM monoclonal antibodies specific for a common epitope shared by the *Brucella* A and M smooth lipopolysaccharides. Infections and Immunity. 1992;60(1):312-315.

[208] Limet J, Plommet AM, Dubray G, and Plommet M. Immunity conferred upon mice by anti-LPS monoclonal antibodies in murine brucellosis. Annales de l' Institute Pasteur Immunology. 1987;138(3):417-424.

[209] Montaraz JA, Winter AJ, Hunter DM, Sowa BA, Wu AM, and Adams LG. Protection against *Brucella abortus* in mice with *O*-polysaccharide-specific monoclonal antibodies. Infections and Immunity. 1986;51(3):961-963.

[210] Adone R, Francia M, Pistoia C, Petrucci P, Pesciaroli M, and Pasquali P. Protective role of antibodies induced by *Brucella melitensis* B115 against *B. melitensis* and *Brucella abortus* infections in mice. Vaccine. 2012;30(27):3992-3995.

[211] Barrio MB, Grillo MJ, Munoz PM, Jacques I, Gonzalez D, de Miguel MJ, Marin CM, Barberan M, Letesson JJ, Gorvel JP, et al. Rough mutants defective in core and *O*-polysaccharide synthesis and export induce antibodies reacting in an indirect ELISA with smooth lipopolysaccharide and are less effective than Rev 1 vaccine against *Brucella melitensis* infection of sheep. Vaccine. 2009;27(11):1741-1749.

[212] Adone R, Francia M, and Ciuchini F. *Brucella melitensis* B115-based complement fixation test to detect antibodies induced by *Brucella* rough strains. Journal of Applied Microbiology. 2008;105(2):567-574.

[213] Ivanov AV, Salmakov KM, Olsen SC, and Plumb GE. A live vaccine from *Brucella abortus* strain 82 for control of cattle brucellosis in the Russian Federation. Animal Health Research Reviews. 2011;12(1):113-121.

[214] Nicoletti P. Vaccination against *Brucella*. Advances in Biotechnology Processes. 1990;13:147-168.

[215] Schurig GG, Roop RM, Bagchi T, Boyle S, Buhrman D, and Sriranganathan N. Biological properties of RB51; a stable rough strain of *Brucella abortus*. Veterinary Microbiology. 1991;28(2):171-188.

[216] Ugalde JE, Comerci DJ, Leguizamon MS, and Ugalde RA. Evaluation of *Brucella abortus* phosphoglucomutase (*pgm*) mutant as a new live rough-phenotype vaccine. Infection and Immunity. 2003;71(11):6264-6269.

[217] Stevens MG, Hennager SG, Olsen SC, and Cheville NF. Serologic responses in diagnostic tests for brucellosis in cattle vaccinated with *Brucella abortus* 19 or RB51. Journal of Clinical Microbiology. 1994;32(4):1065-1066.

[218] Uza FA, Samartino L, Schurig G, Carrasco A, Nielsen K, Cabrera RF, and Taddeo HR. Effect of vaccination with *Brucella abortus* strain RB51 on heifers and pregnant cattle. Veterinary Research Communications. 2000;24(3):143-151.

[219] Cloeckaert A, Zygmunt MS, and Guilloteau LA. *Brucella abortus* vaccine strain RB51 produces low levels of M-like O-antigen. Vaccine. 2002;20(13-14):1820-1822.

[220] Olsen SC, Evans D, Hennager SG, Cheville NF, and Stevens MG. Serologic responses of *Brucella abortus* strain 19 calfhood-vaccinated cattle following adult vaccination with strain RB51. Journal of Veterinary Diagnostic Investigation. 1996;8(4):451-454.

[221] Palmer MV, Cheville NF, and Jensen AE. Experimental infection of pregnant cattle with the vaccine candidate *Brucella abortus* strain RB51: pathologic, bacteriologic, and serologic findings. Veterinary Pathology. 1996;33(6):682-691.

[222] Palmer MV, Olsen SC, and Cheville NF. Safety and immunogenicity of *Brucella abortus* strain RB51 vaccine in pregnant cattle. American Journal of Veterinary Research. 1997;58(5):472-477.

[223] Van Metre DC, Kennedy GA, Olsen SC, Hansen GR, and Ewalt DR. Brucellosis induced by RB51 vaccine in a pregnant heifer. Journal of American Veterinary Medicine Association. 1999;215(10):1491-1493.

[224] Cheville NF, Olsen SC, Jensen AE, Stevens MG, Palmer MV, and Florance AM. Effects of age at vaccination on efficacy of *Brucella abortus* strain RB51 to protect cattle against brucellosis. American Journal of Veterinary Research. 1996;57(8):1153-1156.

[225] Olsen SC. Immune responses and efficacy after administration of a commercial *Brucella abortus* strain RB51 vaccine to cattle. Veterinary Therapeutics. 2000;1(3):183-191.

[226] Lord VR, Cherwonogrodzky JW, Schurig GG, Lord RD, Marcano MJ, and Melendez GE. Venezuelan field trials of vaccines against brucellosis in swine. American Journal of Veterinary Research. 1998;59(5):546-551.

[227] el Idrissi AH, Benkirane A, el MM, Bouslikhane M, Berrada J, and Zerouali A. Comparison of the efficacy of *Brucella abortus* strain RB51 and *Brucella melitensis* Rev. 1 live vaccines against experimental infection with *Brucella melitensis* in pregnant ewes. Revue Scientifique et Technique (International Office of Epizootics). 2001;20(3):741-747.

[228] Herrera E, Rivera A, Palomares EG, Hernandez-Castro R, and Diaz-Aparicio E. Isolation of *Brucella melitensis* from a RB51-vaccinated seronegative goat. Tropical Animal Health and Production. 2011;43(6):1069-1070.

[229] Martínez DI, Morales JA, Peniche AE, Molina B RMA, Loeza R, Robledo ML, Morales JF, and Flores-Castro R. Use of RB51 vaccine for small ruminants brucellosis prevention in Veracruz, Mexico. International Journal of Diary Sciences. 2010;5(1):10-17.

[230] Adone R, Ciuchini F, Marianelli C, Tarantino M, Pistoia C, Marcon G, Petrucci P, Francia M, Riccardi G, and Pasquali P. Protective properties of rifampin-resistant rough mutants of *Brucella melitensis*. Infection and Immunity. 2005;73(7):4198-4204.

[231] Adone R, Francia M, and Ciuchini F. Evaluation of *Brucella melitensis* B115 as rough-phenotype vaccine against *B. melitensis* and *B. ovis* infections. Vaccine. 2008;26(38): 4913-4917.

[232] Winter AJ, Schurig GG, Boyle SM, Sriranganathan N, Bevins JS, Enright FM, Elzer PH, and Kopec JD. Protection of BALB/c mice against homologous and heterologous species of *Brucella* by rough strain vaccines derived from *Brucella melitensis* and *Brucella suis* biovar 4. American Journal of Veterinary Research. 1996;57(5):677-683.

[233] Stoffregen WC, Johnson CS, and Olsen SC. Immunogenicity and safety of a natural rough mutant of *Brucella suis* as a vaccine for swine. Research in Veterinary Science. 2013;95(2):451-458.

[234] Schumaker B. Risks of *Brucella abortus* spillover in the Greater Yellowstone area. Revue Scientifique et Technique. 2013;32(1):71-77.

[235] European Commission. Health and Consumer Directoriate-General. Task force on monitoring animal disease eradication (2009). Working document on eradication of bovine, sheep and goats brucellosis of the Task force on monitoring animal disease eradication in the EU. SANCO/6095/2009. http://ec.europa.eu/food/animal/diseases/eradication/eradication_bovine_sheep_goats_brucellosis_en.pdf

[236] Manthei CA. In: Association USLSS ed. 63rd Annual Meeting, US Live Stock Sanitary Association.1959:91-97.

[237] Erasmus JA, and Erasmus MC. The use of reduced-dose *Brucella abortus* strain 19 vaccine in the control of bovine brucellosis. Journal of the South African Veterinary Association. 1987;58(2):71-75.

[238] Sanz C, Saez JL, Alvarez J, Cortes M, Pereira G, Reyes A, Rubio F, Martin J, Garcia N, Dominguez L, et al. Mass vaccination as a complementary tool in the control of a severe outbreak of bovine brucellosis due to *Brucella abortus* in Extremadura, Spain. Preventive Veterinary Medicine. 2010;97(2):119-125.

[239] Olsen SC, Bricker B, Palmer MV, Jensen AE, and Cheville NF. Responses of cattle to two dosages of *Brucella abortus* strain RB51: serology, clearance and efficacy. Research in Veterinary Science. 1999;66(2):101-105.

[240] Poester FP, Goncalves VS, Paixao TA, Santos RL, Olsen SC, Schurig GG, and Lage AP. Efficacy of strain RB51 vaccine in heifers against experimental brucellosis. Vaccine. 2006;24(25):5327-5334.

[241] Martins H, Garin-Bastuji B, Lima F, Flor L, Pina FA, and Boinas F. Eradication of bovine brucellosis in the Azores, Portugal—outcome of a 5-year programme (2002-2007) based on test-and-slaughter and RB51 vaccination. Preventive Veterinary Medicine. 2009;90(1-2):80-89.

[242] Blasco JM, and Moriyon I. Eradication of bovine brucellosis in the Azores, Portugal--outcome of a 5-year programme (2002-2007) based on test-and-slaughter and RB51 vaccination. Preventive Veterinary Medicine. 2010;94(1-2):154-157.

[243] Samartino LE, Fort M, Gregoret R, and Schurig GG. Use of *Brucella abortus* vaccine strain RB51 in pregnant cows after calfhood vaccination with strain 19 in Argentina. Preventive Veterinary Medicine. 2000;45(3-4):193-199.

[244] Bercovich Z. Maintenance of *Brucella abortus*-free herds: a review with emphasis on the epidemiology and the problems in diagnosing brucellosis in areas of low prevalence. Veterinary Quarterly. 1998;20(3):81-88.

[245] Benkirane A. Ovine and caprine brucellosis: world distribution and control/eradication strategies in West Asia/North Africa region. Small Ruminant Research. 2006;62:19-25.

[246] Racloz V, Schelling E, Chitnis N, Roth F, and Zinsstag J. Persistence of brucellosis in pastoral systems. Revue Scientifique et Technique (International Office of Epizootics). 2013;32(1):61-70.

[247] European Commission. Health and Consumer Directoriate-General.Task force on monitoring animal disease, e. (2009). Working document on eradication of bovine, sheep and goats brucellosis of the Task force on monitoring animal disease eradication in the EU.SANCO/6095/2009. http://ec.europa.eu/food/animal/diseases/eradication/eradication_bovine_sheep_goats_brucellosis_en.pdf

[248] Adone R, Francia M, Pistoia C, Pesciaroli M, and Pasquali P. *B. melitensis* rough strain B115 is protective against heterologous *Brucella* spp. infections. Vaccine. 2011;29(14): 2523-2529..

[249] Avila-Calderon ED, Lopez-Merino A, Jain N, Peralta H, Lopez-Villegas EO, Sriranganathan N, Boyle SM, Witonsky S, and Contreras-Rodriguez A. Characterization of outer membrane vesicles from *Brucella melitensis* and protection induced in mice. Clinical and Developmental Immunology. 2012:352-493.

[250] Edmonds MD, Cloeckaert A, Hagius SD, Samartino LE, Fulton WT, Walker JV, Enright FM, Booth NJ, and Elzer PH. Pathogenicity and protective activity in pregnant goats of a *Brucella melitensis Deltaomp25* deletion mutant. Research in Veterinary Science. 2002;72(3):235-239.

[251] Magnani DM, Harms JS, Durward MA, and Splitter GA. Nondividing but metabolically active gamma-irradiated *Brucella melitensis* is protective against virulent *B. melitensis* challenge in mice. Infection and Immunity. 2009;77(11):5181-5189.

[252] Sislema-Egas F, Cespedes S, Fernandez P, Retamal-Diaz A, Saez D, and Onate A. Evaluation of protective effect of DNA vaccines encoding the BAB1_0263 and BAB1_0278 open reading frames of *Brucella abortus* in BALB/c mice. Vaccine. 2012;30(50):7286-7291

[253] Tibor A, Jacques I, Guilloteau L, Verger JM, Grayon M, Wansard V, and Letesson JJ. Effect of P39 gene deletion in live *Brucella* vaccine strains on residual virulence and protective activity in mice. Infection and Immunity. 1998;66(11):5561-5564.

[254] Yang X, Hudson M, Walters N, Bargatze RF, and Pascual DW. Selection of protective epitopes for *Brucella melitensis* by DNA vaccination. Infection and Immunity. 2005;73(11):7297-7303.

[255] Perez-Sancho M, Adone R, Garcia-Seco T, Tarantino M, Diez-Guerrier A, Drumo R, Francia M, Dominguez L, Pasquali P, and Alvarez J. Evaluation of the immunogenic-

ity and safety of *Brucella melitensis* B115 vaccination in pregnant sheep. Vaccine. 2014;32(16):1877-1881.

[256] WAHID—OIE World Animal Health Information System; http://www.oie.int/wahis_2/public/wahid.php/Wahidhome/Home.

[257] Deqiu S, Donglou X, and Jiming Y. Epidemiology and control of brucellosis in China. Veterinary Microbiology. 2002;90(1-4):165-182.

[258] Alton G. *Brucella melitensis*. In: Animal Brucellosis, Nielsen KH, and Duncan JR, eds. CRC Press, Boca Raton, Florida, USA; 1990:383-409.

[259] Iowa State University. Porcine and Rangiferine Brucellosis: *Brucella suis*. Enzootic abortion, Contagious Abortion. Undulant Fever. The Centre of Food Security and Public Health. Iowa State University. 2009; http://www.cfsph.iastate.edu/Factsheets/es/brucella-suis.pdf

[260] Animal and Plant Health Inspection Service, United States Department of Agriculture. Swine Brucellosis. Control/Eradication. State-Federal-Industry Uniform Methods and Rules; 1998.

[261] Grupo de Trabajo sobre Prevención, control y Erradicación de la Brucelosis en América Latina y el Caribe. Programa Regional para la Prevención, Control, y Erradicación de la Brucelosis en América Latina y el Caribe. Instituto Panamericano de Protección de Alimentos y Zoonosis Programa de Salud Pública Veterinaria. 1994.

[262] Resolución 63/2013. Créase el "Registro Nacional de Establecimientos Oficialmente Libres de Brucelosis Porcina". Servicio Nacional de Sanidad y Calidad Agroalimentaria (SENASA); http://www.senasa.gov.ar/contenido.php?to=n&in=1592&io=22788.

[263] Eales KM, Norton RE, and Ketheesan N. Brucellosis in northern Australia. American Journal of Tropical Medicine and Hygiene. 2010;83(4):876-878.

[264] Department of Agriculture and Fisheries. *Brucella suis*. https://www.daff.qld.gov.au/animal-industries/animal-health-and-diseases/a-z-list/brucellosis/brucella-suis.

[265] Althouse GC, and Rossow K. The potential risk of infectious disease dissemination via artificial insemination in swine. Reproduction in Domestic Animals. 2011;46 Suppl 2:64-67.

[266] Stoffregen WC, Olsen SC, Jack WC, Bricker BJ, Palmer MV, Jensen AE, Halling SM, and Alt DP. Diagnostic characterization of a feral swine herd enzootically infected with Brucella. Journal of Veterinary Diagnostic and Investigation. 2007;19(3):227-237.

[267] Dieste-Perez L, Fraile L, de Miguel MJ, Barberan M, Blasco JM, and Muñoz PM. Studies on a suitable antibiotic therapy for treating swine brucellosis. Journal of Veterinary Pharmacology and Therapeutics. 2014.